Recent Advances in the Treatment of Hypertension

Recent Advances in the Treatment of Hypertension

Editor

Fabio Angeli

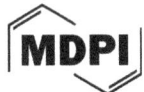

Basel • Beijing • Wuhan • Barcelona • Belgrade • Novi Sad • Cluj • Manchester

Editor
Fabio Angeli
Department of Medicine and
Technological Innovation (DiMIT)
University of Insubria
Varese
Italy

Editorial Office
MDPI
St. Alban-Anlage 66
4052 Basel, Switzerland

This is a reprint of articles from the Special Issue published online in the open access journal *Journal of Cardiovascular Development and Disease* (ISSN 2308-3425) (available at: www.mdpi.com/ journal/jcdd/special_issues/hypertension_treatment).

For citation purposes, cite each article independently as indicated on the article page online and as indicated below:

Lastname, A.A.; Lastname, B.B. Article Title. *Journal Name* **Year**, *Volume Number*, Page Range.

ISBN 978-3-0365-8793-6 (Hbk)
ISBN 978-3-0365-8792-9 (PDF)
doi.org/10.3390/books978-3-0365-8792-9

© 2023 by the authors. Articles in this book are Open Access and distributed under the Creative Commons Attribution (CC BY) license. The book as a whole is distributed by MDPI under the terms and conditions of the Creative Commons Attribution-NonCommercial-NoDerivs (CC BY-NC-ND) license.

Contents

About the Editor vii

Preface ix

Fabio Angeli
New Perspectives and Strategies for the Management of Hypertension
Reprinted from: *J. Cardiovasc. Dev. Dis.* **2023**, *10*, 346, doi:10.3390/jcdd10080346 1

Fabio Angeli, Gianpaolo Reboldi, Monica Trapasso, Gabriella Santilli, Martina Zappa and Paolo Verdecchia
Blood Pressure Increase following COVID-19 Vaccination: A Systematic Overview and Meta-Analysis
Reprinted from: *J. Cardiovasc. Dev. Dis.* **2022**, *9*, 150, doi:10.3390/jcdd9050150 4

Fabio Angeli, Paolo Verdecchia, Antonella Balestrino, Claudio Bruschi, Piero Ceriana and Luca Chiovato et al.
Renin Angiotensin System Blockers and Risk of Mortality in Hypertensive Patients Hospitalized for COVID-19: An Italian Registry
Reprinted from: *J. Cardiovasc. Dev. Dis.* **2022**, *9*, 15, doi:10.3390/jcdd9010015 13

Paolo Verdecchia, Claudio Cavallini and Fabio Angeli
Advances in the Treatment Strategies in Hypertension: Present and Future
Reprinted from: *J. Cardiovasc. Dev. Dis.* **2022**, *9*, 72, doi:10.3390/jcdd9030072 25

Jacopo Marazzato, Federico Blasi, Michele Golino, Paolo Verdecchia, Fabio Angeli and Roberto De Ponti
Hypertension and Arrhythmias: A Clinical Overview of the Pathophysiology-Driven Management of Cardiac Arrhythmias in Hypertensive Patients
Reprinted from: *J. Cardiovasc. Dev. Dis.* **2022**, *9*, 110, doi:10.3390/jcdd9040110 41

Giorgio Gentile, Kathryn Mckinney and Gianpaolo Reboldi
Tight Blood Pressure Control in Chronic Kidney Disease
Reprinted from: *J. Cardiovasc. Dev. Dis.* **2022**, *9*, 139, doi:10.3390/jcdd9050139 58

Yuko Okamoto, Toru Miyoshi, Keishi Ichikawa, Yoichi Takaya, Kazufumi Nakamura and Hiroshi Ito
Cardio-Ankle Vascular Index as an Arterial Stiffness Marker Improves the Prediction of Cardiovascular Events in Patients without Cardiovascular Diseases
Reprinted from: *J. Cardiovasc. Dev. Dis.* **2022**, *9*, 368, doi:10.3390/jcdd9110368 74

Jacomina P. du Plessis, Leandi Lammertyn, Aletta E. Schutte and Cornelie Nienaber-Rousseau
H-Type Hypertension among Black South Africans and the Relationship between Homocysteine, Its Genetic Determinants and Estimates of Vascular Function
Reprinted from: *J. Cardiovasc. Dev. Dis.* **2022**, *9*, 447, doi:10.3390/jcdd9120447 82

Humberto Badillo-Alonso, Marisol Martínez-Alanis, Ramiro Sánchez-Huesca, Abel Lerma and Claudia Lerma
Effectiveness of the Combination of Enalapril and Nifedipine for the Treatment of Hypertension versus Empirical Treatment in Primary Care Patients
Reprinted from: *J. Cardiovasc. Dev. Dis.* **2023**, *10*, 243, doi:10.3390/jcdd10060243 98

Pasquale Ambrosino, Tiziana Bachetti, Silvestro Ennio D'Anna, Brurya Galloway, Andrea Bianco and Vito D'Agnano et al.
Mechanisms and Clinical Implications of Endothelial Dysfunction in Arterial Hypertension
Reprinted from: *J. Cardiovasc. Dev. Dis.* **2022**, *9*, 136, doi:10.3390/jcdd9050136 . . . . **111**

Anil T John, Moniruddin Chowdhury, Md. Rabiul Islam, Imtiyaz Ali Mir, Md Zobaer Hasan and Chao Yi Chong et al.
Effectiveness of High-Intensity Interval Training and Continuous Moderate-Intensity Training on Blood Pressure in Physically Inactive Pre-Hypertensive Young Adults
Reprinted from: *J. Cardiovasc. Dev. Dis.* **2022**, *9*, 246, doi:10.3390/jcdd9080246 . . . . **129**

Valeria Visco, Carmine Izzo, Costantino Mancusi, Antonella Rispoli, Michele Tedeschi and Nicola Virtuoso et al.
Artificial Intelligence in Hypertension Management: An Ace up Your Sleeve
Reprinted from: *J. Cardiovasc. Dev. Dis.* **2023**, *10*, 74, doi:10.3390/jcdd10020074 . . . . **141**

About the Editor

Fabio Angeli

Professor Fabio Angeli, MD, currently works in the Department of Medicine and Technological Innovation (DiMIT) of the University of Insubria, Varese, Italy.

He is the Chief of the Divisions of (i) General Internal Medicine and (ii) Cardiac Rehabilitation at the Maugeri Care and Research Institute (IRCCS) of Tradate, Varese (Italy). He is also the President of Nursery School at the University of Insubria, Varese (Italy). He has focused on clinical cardiovascular research, including Hypertension, Cardiovascular Disease Prevention, Atrial Fibrillation, Heart Failure and Coronary Syndromes.

He has articles published by leading journals in the field of Cardiology and Internal Medicine and he is responsible for planning and management of mono-centre and multi-centre Clinical Studies in connection with other Universities and Hospitals.

His awards include the American Heart Association Best Manuscript Award 2012 (Population Science; Day-Night Dip and Early-Morning Surge in Blood Pressure in Hypertension Prognostic Implications); Expertscape's one of the world's top experts in the field of hypertension research and treatment; high impact paper in Hypertension (Summer Collection award 2019) from American Heart Association (with the article "Sudden Cardiac Death in Hypertensive Patients"); biographical record in Who's Who in Medicine and Healthcare, and Who's Who in Science and Engineer; Top Italian Scientist, VIA-Academy.

Preface

Hypertension is the leading preventable risk factor for cardiovascular disease and all-cause mortality worldwide. Despite its global prevalence remaining very high, the last few years have been characterized by an impressive paucity of innovative studies; moreover, the proportion of treated hypertensive patients with 'controlled hypertension' remains very low (about 23% in women and 18% in men, worldwide).

The Special Issue "Recent Advances in the Treatment of Hypertension" of the *Journal of Cardiovascular Development and Disease* included articles discussing several pertinent issues in this area of research, including pathophysiology, risk stratification, control and management of hypertension. Two research articles also evaluated the role of hypertension in the pandemic era of the severe acute respiratory syndrome Coronavirus 2 infection.

In conclusion, to curb the detrimental impact of hypertension and its rise in prevalence worldwide, we need significant progress from a combination of new strategies, education and technology. This Special Issue highlighted new insights and re-evaluated preexisting evidences and strategies to improve the management, control and risk stratification of hypertension.

Fabio Angeli
Editor

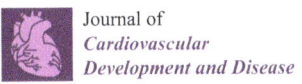

Editorial
New Perspectives and Strategies for the Management of Hypertension

Fabio Angeli [1,2]

1. Department of Medicine and Technological Innovation (DiMIT), University of Insubria, 21100 Varese, Italy; fabio.angeli@uninsubria.it
2. Department of Medicine and Cardiopulmonary Rehabilitation, Istituti Clinici Scientifici Maugeri IRCCS, 21049 Tradate, Italy

Hypertension is the leading preventable risk factor for cardiovascular disease and all-cause mortality worldwide [1]. Moreover, the global prevalence of hypertension remains high [2], and treatment of high blood pressure (BP) is the most common reason for the prescription of chronic drugs and for office visits [3,4].

According to epidemiological information provided by the United States National Health and Nutrition Examination Surveys (NHANES), the prevalence of hypertension in the United States is about 30% [3,4]. However, applying the new definition of hypertension recommended by the American College of Cardiology/American Heart Association (ACC/AHA, BP $\geq$ 140 mmHg systolic or $\geq$ 90 mmHg diastolic, or taking antihypertensive medication) the prevalence of hypertension among adults in the United States was 47% from 1999 to 2000, 41.7% percent from 2013 to 2014, and 45.4% from 2017 to 2018 [4]. The global prevalence of hypertension is similar to that in the United States, although it varies by country [2].

Despite such impressive prevalence, the last few years have been characterized by a notable paucity of innovative studies, and the proportion of treated hypertensive patients with "controlled hypertension" remains very low worldwide. Specifically, it has recently been estimated that such a proportion approaches 23% in women and 18% in men [5].

This Special Issue "Recent Advances in the Treatment of Hypertension" collects articles from the Americas, Africa, Asia, Australia, and Europe discussing several pertinent issues in this area of research, on topics spanning pathophysiology, risk stratification, control and management of hypertension.

Humberto Badillo-Alonso and coworkers report results from a randomized clinical trial comparing the effectiveness of the combination of enalapril and nifedipine for the treatment of hypertension versus empirical treatment [6]. They demonstrated that combined treatment was 31% more efficacious than conventional empirical treatment, which yielded an incremental clinical utility of 18% with high tolerability among patients in primary care [6].

A cross-section investigation analyzing data from the South African arm of the Prospective Urban and Rural Epidemiology (PURE–SA) study reported an H-type hypertension (hypertension associated with homocysteine levels $\geq$ 10 µmol/L) prevalence of 23% among all participants and a 45% prevalence among those with hypertension in a relatively large sample of Black South Africans recruited from both rural and urban communities [7].

A retrospective, single-center cohort study including outpatients with cardiovascular disease risk factors but without known cardiovascular disease evaluated the prognostic impact of cardio-ankle vascular index (CAVI) [8]. Importantly, results showed that CAVI improved the prediction of cardiovascular events (the addition of CAVI to a conventional risk score for coronary heart disease in Japan significantly improved the C statics from 0.642 to 0.713; $p = 0.04$) [8].

Anil T John and co-workers present the results of a 5-week randomized–controlled trial evaluating the effectiveness of high-intensity interval training (HIIT) and continuous moderate-intensity training (CMT) on BP of physically inactive pre-hypertensive young adults [9]. Both HIIT and CMT decreased BP; however, HIIT yielded more beneficial results in terms of reducing all the components of BP (systolic, diastolic, and mean arterial pressure) [9].

Two investigations from Italy analyze the role of hypertension in the era of the severe acute respiratory syndrome coronavirus 2 (SARS-CoV-2) pandemic [10]. An analysis of a pre-designed registry of patients hospitalized for coronavirus disease 2019 (COVID-19) with subsequent prospective collection of data demonstrated that exposure to angiotensin receptor blockers reduced mortality in 566 hypertensive patients hospitalized for COVID-19 [11,12]. After the evidence of a BP increase during the acute phase of SARS-CoV-2 infection [13], a systematic review and meta-analysis (including 357,387 subjects) also evaluated an increase in BP after COVID-19 vaccination as a potential adverse reaction [14,15]. Pooled results showed that the proportion of abnormal/increased BP after vaccination was 3.20% (95% CI: 1.62–6.21), and that proportions of cases of stage III hypertension or hypertensive urgencies and emergencies was 0.6% (95% CI: 0.1% to 5.1%) [15].

Finally, five review articles are included in this Special Issue. They discuss the role of artificial intelligence [16], the prognostic value of a tight BP control in chronic kidney disease [17], implications of endothelial dysfunction as therapeutic target [18] in hypertension and other conditions [19], the link between hypertension and cardiac arrhythmias [20,21], and recent advances in the management of hypertensive patients with a potential clinical role in the years to come (including renal denervation) [22].

In summary, to curb the detrimental impact of hypertension and its increase in prevalence worldwide, we need significant progress from a combination of new strategies, education, and technology [22]. This Special Issue includes reports gathering new insights and re-evaluating pre-existing evidence and strategies to improve the management, control, and risk stratification of hypertension.

Conflicts of Interest: The authors declare no conflict of interest.

References

1. Mills, K.T.; Stefanescu, A.; He, J. The global epidemiology of hypertension. *Nat. Rev. Nephrol.* **2020**, *16*, 223–237. [CrossRef]
2. Kearney, P.M.; Whelton, M.; Reynolds, K.; Muntner, P.; Whelton, P.K.; He, J. Global burden of hypertension: Analysis of worldwide data. *Lancet* **2005**, *365*, 217–223. [CrossRef]
3. Muntner, P.; Carey, R.M.; Gidding, S.; Jones, D.W.; Taler, S.J.; Wright, J.T., Jr.; Whelton, P.K. Potential US Population Impact of the 2017 ACC/AHA High Blood Pressure Guideline. *Circulation* **2018**, *137*, 109–118. [CrossRef]
4. Muntner, P.; Hardy, S.T.; Fine, L.J.; Jaeger, B.C.; Wozniak, G.; Levitan, E.B.; Colantonio, L.D. Trends in Blood Pressure Control among US Adults with Hypertension, 1999–2000 to 2017–2018. *JAMA* **2020**, *324*, 1190–1200. [CrossRef]
5. NCD Risk Factor Collaboration (NCD-RisC). Worldwide trends in hypertension prevalence and progress in treatment and control from 1990 to 2019: A pooled analysis of 1201 population-representative studies with 104 million participants. *Lancet* **2021**, *398*, 957–980. [CrossRef]
6. Badillo-Alonso, H.; Martinez-Alanis, M.; Sanchez-Huesca, R.; Lerma, A.; Lerma, C. Effectiveness of the Combination of Enalapril and Nifedipine for the Treatment of Hypertension versus Empirical Treatment in Primary Care Patients. *J. Cardiovasc. Dev. Dis.* **2023**, *10*, 243. [CrossRef] [PubMed]
7. Du Plessis, J.P.; Lammertyn, L.; Schutte, A.E.; Nienaber-Rousseau, C. H-Type Hypertension among Black South Africans and the Relationship between Homocysteine, Its Genetic Determinants and Estimates of Vascular Function. *J. Cardiovasc. Dev. Dis.* **2022**, *9*, 447. [CrossRef] [PubMed]
8. Okamoto, Y.; Miyoshi, T.; Ichikawa, K.; Takaya, Y.; Nakamura, K.; Ito, H. Cardio-Ankle Vascular Index as an Arterial Stiffness Marker Improves the Prediction of Cardiovascular Events in Patients without Cardiovascular Diseases. *J. Cardiovasc. Dev. Dis.* **2022**, *9*, 368. [CrossRef] [PubMed]
9. John, A.T.; Chowdhury, M.; Islam, M.R.; Mir, I.A.; Hasan, M.Z.; Chong, C.Y.; Humayra, S.; Higashi, Y. Effectiveness of High-Intensity Interval Training and Continuous Moderate-Intensity Training on Blood Pressure in Physically Inactive Pre-Hypertensive Young Adults. *J. Cardiovasc. Dev. Dis.* **2022**, *9*, 246. [CrossRef] [PubMed]
10. Angeli, F.; Zappa, M.; Reboldi, G.; Trapasso, M.; Cavallini, C.; Spanevello, A.; Verdecchia, P. The pivotal link between ACE2 deficiency and SARS-CoV-2 infection: One year later. *Eur. J. Intern. Med.* **2021**, *93*, 28–34. [CrossRef]

11. Angeli, F.; Verdecchia, P.; Balestrino, A.; Bruschi, C.; Ceriana, P.; Chiovato, L.; Dalla Vecchia, L.A.; Fanfulla, F.; La Rovere, M.T.; Perego, F.; et al. Renin Angiotensin System Blockers and Risk of Mortality in Hypertensive Patients Hospitalized for COVID-19: An Italian Registry. *J. Cardiovasc. Dev. Dis.* **2022**, *9*, 15. [CrossRef] [PubMed]
12. Verdecchia, P.; Reboldi, G.; Cavallini, C.; Mazzotta, G.; Angeli, F. ACE-inhibitors, angiotensin receptor blockers and severe acute respiratory syndrome caused by coronavirus. *G. Ital. Cardiol.* **2020**, *21*, 321–327.
13. Angeli, F.; Zappa, M.; Oliva, F.M.; Spanevello, A.; Verdecchia, P. Blood pressure increase during hospitalization for COVID-19. *Eur. J. Intern. Med.* **2022**, *104*, 110–112. [CrossRef]
14. Zappa, M.; Verdecchia, P.; Spanevello, A.; Visca, D.; Angeli, F. Blood pressure increase after Pfizer/BioNTech SARS-CoV-2 vaccine. *Eur. J. Intern. Med.* **2021**, *90*, 111–113. [CrossRef] [PubMed]
15. Angeli, F.; Reboldi, G.; Trapasso, M.; Santilli, G.; Zappa, M.; Verdecchia, P. Blood Pressure Increase following COVID-19 Vaccination: A Systematic Overview and Meta-Analysis. *J. Cardiovasc. Dev. Dis.* **2022**, *9*, 150. [CrossRef] [PubMed]
16. Visco, V.; Izzo, C.; Mancusi, C.; Rispoli, A.; Tedeschi, M.; Virtuoso, N.; Giano, A.; Gioia, R.; Melfi, A.; Serio, B.; et al. Artificial Intelligence in Hypertension Management: An Ace up Your Sleeve. *J. Cardiovasc. Dev. Dis.* **2023**, *10*, 74. [CrossRef]
17. Gentile, G.; McKinney, K.; Reboldi, G. Tight Blood Pressure Control in Chronic Kidney Disease. *J. Cardiovasc. Dev. Dis.* **2022**, *9*, 139. [CrossRef]
18. Ambrosino, P.; Bachetti, T.; D'Anna, S.E.; Galloway, B.; Bianco, A.; D'Agnano, V.; Papa, A.; Motta, A.; Perrotta, F.; Maniscalco, M. Mechanisms and Clinical Implications of Endothelial Dysfunction in Arterial Hypertension. *J. Cardiovasc. Dev. Dis.* **2022**, *9*, 136. [CrossRef]
19. Angeli, F.; Verdecchia, P.; Karthikeyan, G.; Mazzotta, G.; Del Pinto, M.; Repaci, S.; Gatteschi, C.; Gentile, G.; Cavallini, C.; Reboldi, G. New-onset hyperglycemia and acute coronary syndrome: A systematic overview and meta-analysis. *Curr. Diabetes Rev.* **2010**, *6*, 102–110. [CrossRef]
20. Marazzato, J.; Blasi, F.; Golino, M.; Verdecchia, P.; Angeli, F.; De Ponti, R. Hypertension and Arrhythmias: A Clinical Overview of the Pathophysiology-Driven Management of Cardiac Arrhythmias in Hypertensive Patients. *J. Cardiovasc. Dev. Dis.* **2022**, *9*, 110. [CrossRef]
21. Angeli, F.; Reboldi, G.; Verdecchia, P. Hypertension, inflammation and atrial fibrillation. *J. Hypertens* **2014**, *32*, 480–483. [CrossRef] [PubMed]
22. Verdecchia, P.; Cavallini, C.; Angeli, F. Advances in the Treatment Strategies in Hypertension: Present and Future. *J. Cardiovasc. Dev. Dis.* **2022**, *9*, 72. [CrossRef] [PubMed]

Disclaimer/Publisher's Note: The statements, opinions and data contained in all publications are solely those of the individual author(s) and contributor(s) and not of MDPI and/or the editor(s). MDPI and/or the editor(s) disclaim responsibility for any injury to people or property resulting from any ideas, methods, instructions or products referred to in the content.

Systematic Review

Blood Pressure Increase following COVID-19 Vaccination: A Systematic Overview and Meta-Analysis

Fabio Angeli [1,2,*], Gianpaolo Reboldi [3], Monica Trapasso [4], Gabriella Santilli [3], Martina Zappa [1] and Paolo Verdecchia [5]

1. Department of Medicine and Surgery, University of Insubria, 21100 Varese, Italy; marty-italy92@hotmail.it
2. Department of Medicine and Cardiopulmonary Rehabilitation, Istituti Clinici Scientifici Maugeri IRCCS, 21049 Tradate, Italy
3. Department of Medicine, and Centro di Ricerca Clinica e Traslazionale (CERICLET), University of Perugia, 06100 Perugia, Italy; paolo.reboldi@unipg.it (G.R.); santilli.gabriella@gmail.com (G.S.)
4. Dipartimento di Igiene e Prevenzione Sanitaria, PSAL, Sede Territoriale di Varese, ATS Insubria, 21100 Varese, Italy; montrapasso@gmail.com
5. Fondazione Umbra Cuore e Ipertensione-ONLUS and Division of Cardiology, Hospital S. Maria della Misericordia, 06100 Perugia, Italy; verdecchiapaolo@gmail.com
* Correspondence: angeli.internet@gmail.com

Abstract: Coronavirus disease 2019 (COVID-19) vaccines proved a strong clinical efficacy against symptomatic or moderate/severe COVID-19 and are considered the most promising approach for curbing the pandemic. However, some questions regarding the safety of COVID-19 vaccines have been recently raised. Among adverse events to vaccines and despite a lack of signal during phase III clinical trials, an increase in blood pressure (BP) after COVID-19 vaccination has been reported as a potential adverse reaction. We systematically analyze this topic and undertook a meta-analysis of available data to estimate the proportion of patients with abnormal BP or raise in BP after vaccination. Six studies entered the final analysis. Overall, studies accrued 357,387 subjects with 13,444 events of abnormal or increased BP. After exclusion of outlier studies, the pooled estimated proportion of abnormal/increased BP after vaccination was 3.20% (95% CI: 1.62–6.21). Proportions of cases of stage III hypertension or hypertensive urgencies and emergencies was 0.6% (95% CI: 0.1% to 5.1%). In conclusion, abnormal BP is not rare after COVID-19 vaccination, but the basic mechanisms of this phenomenon are still unclear and require further research.

Keywords: COVID-19; vaccine; blood pressure; hypertension; adverse drug reaction; BNT162b2; mRNA-1273; Ad26.COV2.S; CVnCoV; ChAdOx1nCoV-19; NVX-CoV2373; Gam-COVID-Vac

1. Introduction

Different therapeutic strategies are under scrutiny to block the transition from infection to severe forms of coronavirus disease 2019 (COVID-19) [1,2]. They include prevention of the viral RNA synthesis and replication, blockade of SARS-CoV-2 from binding to human cell receptors, the restoration of the host's innate immunity, and the modulation of the host's specific receptors or enzymes [1–6].

However, vaccines to prevent SARS-CoV-2 infection are considered the most promising approach, offering the opportunity to come out of the current phase of the pandemic [2,7].

COVID-19 vaccines have been developed using different advanced technologies and several platforms [7–9], including live attenuated vaccines, inactivated vaccines, recombinant protein vaccines, vector vaccines (replication-incompetent vector vaccines, replication-competent vector vaccines, and inactivated virus vector vaccines), DNA vaccines, and RNA vaccines (Table 1). By 18 March 2022 a total of 10,925,055,390 vaccine doses have been administered globally (5,007,662,851 persons vaccinated with at least one dose, and 4,446,884,806 persons fully vaccinated; (https://covid19.who.int/ accessed on 18 March 2022).

Table 1. Main features of COVID-19 vaccines.

Vaccine	Developer	Platform	Doses
BNT162b2 *	Pfizer/BioNTech	mRNA	2
mRNA-1273 *	Moderna	mRNA	2
Ad26.COV2.S *	Janssen/Johnson & Johnson	DNA Adenovirus vector	1
CVnCoV	CureVAC	mRNA	2
ChAdOx1nCoV-19 *	AstraZeneca/University of Oxford/Serum Institute of India	DNA Adenovirus vector	2
NVX-CoV2373 *	Novavax	Recombinant protein	2
Gam-COVID-Vac (Sputnik V)	Gamaleya Institute	DNA Adenovirus vectors	2

* vaccines authorized for use in the European Union (https://www.ema.europa.eu/en/human-regulatory/overview/public-health-threats/coronavirus-disease-covid-19/treatments-vaccines/covid-19-vaccines accessed on 18 March 2022).

Despite the clinical efficacy against symptomatic or moderate/severe COVID-19 ranged from 67% to 95% in several clinical trial [10–15], some questions regarding the safety of COVID-19 vaccines have been recently raised and mainly based on reports of thromboembolic events [16–22]. An extremely carefully monitoring of safety issues showed other rare adverse events occurring after COVID-19 vaccination, including anaphylaxis, myocarditis/pericarditis, and Guillain-Barré Syndrome (https://www.cdc.gov/coronavirus/2019-ncov/vaccines/safety/adverse-events.html accessed on 18 March 2022) [2].

Just recently and despite a lack of signal during the main phase III clinical trials, an increase in blood pressure (BP) after COVID-19 vaccination has been reported [2,23–25].

The main aim of this review was to systematically analyze data on this topic, offering an overview of the clinical implications and potential mechanisms of this phenomenon. Specifically, we undertook a meta-analysis of available data to estimate the proportion of patients with abnormal or raised BP after vaccination.

2. Materials and Methods

2.1. Study Selection and Outcome Measures

We addressed analyses and clinical studies (both retrospective and prospective) meeting all the following inclusion criteria: (a) data on incidence of abnormal or increased BP regardless of the specific vaccination strategy; (b) publication in a peer-reviewed journal before 28 February 2022; (c) no age or language restriction, in order to avoid discriminating papers not written in English ("tower of Babel bias") [26].

2.2. Data Sources and Searches

Candidate studies were searched through MEDLINE, Scopus, Web of Science, and CINHAL, using research Methodology Filters [27]. The following research terms were used: "SARS-CoV-2", "COVID-19", "2019-ncov", "coronavirus", "blood pressure", "hypertension", and "adverse events". We made a further screening of review articles, published proceedings of conferences, and regulatory agencies files [28] in order to identify other relevant studies.

2.3. Data Synthesis

Table 2 shows the clinical studies identified on the basis of the above criteria. Overall, studies accrued 357,387 subjects. Figure 1 shows the flow diagram with the criteria used for selection of studies. We used the Preferred Reporting Items for Systematic Reviews and Meta-Analyses (PRISMA) statement (Table S1) [29]. Data were independently extracted by two authors (FA and PV). Disagreements were discussed in conference.

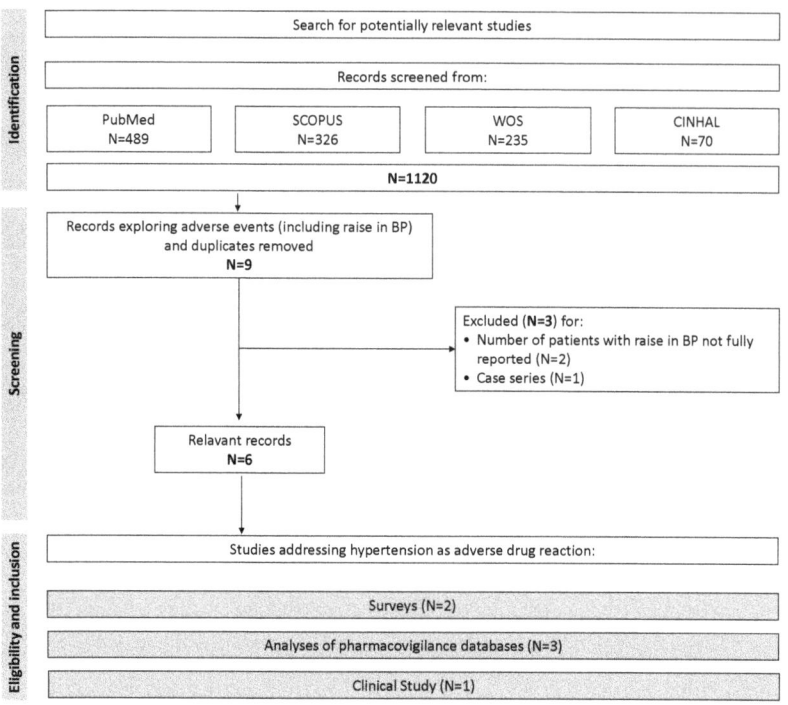

Figure 1. Criteria used for selection of studies.

Three reviewers independently assessed the risk of bias of each of the included studies and discussed their assessments to achieve consensus. The included studies were scored for quality using the Newcastle-Ottawa scale. The scale items assess appropriateness of research design, recruitment strategy, response rate, representativeness of sample, objectivity/reliability of outcome determination, power calculation, and appropriate statistical analyses [30,31]. Score disagreements were resolved by consensus and a final agreed-upon rating was assigned to each study (Table S2) [30,31].

2.4. Data Analysis

Proportions were calculated by dividing the number of patients with the specific endpoint by the total number of patients for each study. We used a generalized linear mixed model (GLMM)—i.e., a random intercept logistic regression model—for the meta-analysis of proportions [32]. We also tested for the presence of statistical outliers using the method described by Harrer et al. [33]. Studies are defined as outliers when their 95% confidence interval lies outside the 95% confidence interval of the pooled effect.

The null hypothesis of homogeneity across individual studies was tested by using the Q test. Pooled estimates were assessed for heterogeneity by using the I^2 statistic [34].

Analyses were performed using R version 4.1.3 (R Foundation for Statistical Computing, Vienna, Austria) and Stata, version 16 (StataCorp LP, College Station, TX, USA).

3. Results

Literature search initially yielded 1120 reports. After removal of duplicates and studies not focused on safety of COVID-19 vaccines, we reviewed nine clinical studies in full text [24,25,35–41].

Table 2. Main features of studies included in the analysis.

Study	Source	Cohort (N)	Year	Vaccine	Outcome Definition	Outcome N	Severe Increase in BP * (N)
Bouhanick et al. [36]	Pharmacovigilance database	91,761	2021	BNT162b2, ChAdOx1nCoV-19, Ad26.COV2.S	Abnormal BP	1776	-
Bouhanick et al. [35]	Patients and healthcare workers	21,909	2022	BNT162b2	Persistent BP ≥ 140/90 (15 min after vaccination)	5197	709
Kaur et al. [38]	Pharmacovigilance database	30,523	2021	BNT162b2, ChAdOx1nCoV-19, mRNA-1273	Abnormal BP	283	36
Lehmann et al. [41]	Pharmacovigilance database	212,053	2021	BNT162b2, ChAdOx1nCoV-19, Ad26.COV2.S, mRNA-1273	Abnormal BP	6130	551
Tran et al. [40]	Cross-sectional online survey	1028	2021	ChAdOx1nCoV-19	Self reported hypertension	52	-
Angeli et al. [25]	Cross-sectional online survey	113	2021	BNT162b2	Raise in home BP > 10 mmHg	6	2

* severe increase in BP included stage III hypertension, hypertensive urgencies, and hypertensive emergencies.

We excluded two studies because of lack of data on the precise number of adverse drug reactions (ADRs) or a clear definition of raise in BP [37,39]. Among the remaining seven studies, we removed one study reporting a case series of vaccinated patients (Figure 1) [24]. Thus, six studies entered the final analysis (Table 2) [25,35,36,38,40,41]. Of these, two were cross-sectional surveys [25,40], three analyzed data from pharmacovigilance databases [36,38,41], and one evaluated BP after 15 min from vaccination among a cohort of patients and healthcare workers [35].

3.1. Excluded Studies

Meylan and co-workers reported a case series of nine patients with stage III hypertension documented within minutes of vaccination, of which eight were symptomatic [24] (Table S3). BP was measured with an oscillometric validated manometer with at least three sets of separate values at 5-min intervals [24]. Median age was 73 years, and eight of nine patients had a history of arterial hypertension with most patients on antihypertensive therapy [24]. All but one patient received the BNT162b2 vaccine. Of note, patients had a previous well controlled hypertension. All patients recovered but required at most several hours of monitoring at tertiary center's emergency department [24].

Sanidas and co-workers [37,39] (Table S3) investigated the effects of vaccination on BP in patients with known hypertension and healthy controls. A total of 100 patients between the age of 50 to 70 years old were included [37,39]. They were randomly assigned to one of the approved and available vaccines (BNT162b2, mRNA-1273, Ad26.COV2.S, and ChAdOx1nCoV-19) [37,39]. All participants had systolic BP < 140 mmHg and diastolic BP < 90 mmHg before vaccination and volunteered for home BP measurements and ambulatory BP measurements between the 5th and the 20th day after fully COVID-19 vaccination [37,39]. Patients with known history of hypertension showed a mean home BP equal to 175/97 mmHg. Similar results were also recorded for 24-h mean BP (177/98 mmHg) [37,39]. Healthy controls showed a BP of 158/96 mmHg and 157/95 mmHg during home and ambulatory monitoring, respectively [37,39]. Five of 50 hypertensive patients received additional medication whereas some of the non-hypertensive patients started life modification changes and systematic BP measurements for a possible diagnosis of hypertension [37,39].

Finally, a recent analysis by Ch'ng and coworkers [37,39] (Table S3) collected data from 4906 healthcare workers. BP was measured three times for each staff member using an automated BP monitor. Pre-vaccination BP was recorded when the staff members arrived at the vaccination site; post-vaccination BP was measured immediately after vaccination and 15–30 min later in a waiting room [37,39]. Mean pre-vaccination systolic and diastolic BP were 130.1 mmHg and 80.2 mmHg, respectively. When compared with baseline, BP was increased in more than half of the subjects immediately and 30 min post vaccination. The mean changes immediately after vaccination were +2.3/2.4 mmHg for systolic/diastolic BP [37,39].

3.2. Included Studies

The retrospective analysis by Bouhanick and co-workers, describing the prevalence of high BP after vaccination, exhibited the largest proportion of this phenomenon [35]. They retrospectively investigated BP profile of vaccinated patients and healthcare workers to describe the course of BP values after the first and the second injection of vaccine and to assess the prevalence of high BP values in this population. Notably, BP was measured 15 min after vaccine injection and measurements were performed with a validated automatic electronic device [35]. A total of 21,909 subjects had complete data on BP (61.7% were women, mean age was 59 years). Among these subjects, 8121 people (37.1%) exhibited systolic and/or diastolic BP above 140 and/or 90 mmHg after the first injection. Among the subjects with high BP after the first injection, 64% were still hypertensive after the second one [35].

Interrogations of pharmacovigilance databases [36,38,41] showed proportions of abnormal or increased BP after vaccination ranging from 0.93% to 2.89%.

Proportions from surveys, specifically designed to evaluate BP changes after vaccination, was about 5% (5.06% in the analysis by Tran and co-workers [40] and 5.31% in the sample from Angeli and co-workers [25]).

More specifically, the Italian prospective survey [25] showed that among 113 health care workers who received the Pfizer vaccine, 6 subjects (5.3%) showed a rise in systolic or diastolic BP at home ≥ 10 mmHg during the first five days after the first dose of the vaccine when compared with the five days before the vaccine (the BP rise required an intensification of BP-lowering treatment in 4 subjects) [25]. Interestingly, the subjects with documented infection by SARS-COV-2 over the previous year showed a higher frequency of systemic reactions to vaccine when compared with those without history of documented infection (38% vs. 10%, $p = 0.004$). History of COVID-19 was associated with a higher incidence of rise in BP when compared with subjects without previous exposure to SARS-CoV-2 (23% vs. 3%, $p = 0.002$). Symptomatic tachycardia was noted in 7 and 3 respondents after the first and second dose of vaccine, respectively, and there were no cardiovascular events or severe or immediate allergic reactions during a follow-up of 103 days [25].

Similarly, Tran and co-workers performed a cross-sectional survey including 1028 subjects (899 had one ChAdOx1nCoV-19 dose and the rest received 2 doses) [40]. Abnormal BP after vaccination was recorded in 52 subjects.

Quality assessment of the included studies is reported in Table S2.

3.3. Pooled Analyzses

Overall, the pooled estimated proportion of abnormal or increased BP after vaccination was 3.91% (95% confidence interval [CI]: 1.25–11.56, $p < 0.01$; Figure 2). Nonetheless, two studies were identified as statistical outliers [35,38]. As depicted in Figure 3, after the exclusion of these 2 studies [35,38], the pooled proportion of abnormal or increased BP after vaccination was 3.20% (95% CI: 1.62–6.21, $p < 0.01$).

We also evaluated the proportion of cases of stage III hypertension or hypertensive urgencies and emergencies. Four studies reported the proportion of patients who developed these outcomes after COVID-19 vaccination (range: 0.1% to 3.2%). The pooled proportion of these events was 0.6% (95% CI: 0.1–5.1%).

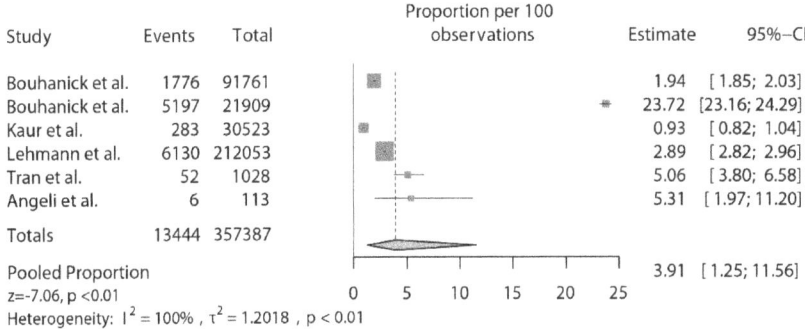

Figure 2. Proportions of increased BP after vaccination [25,35,36,38,40,41].

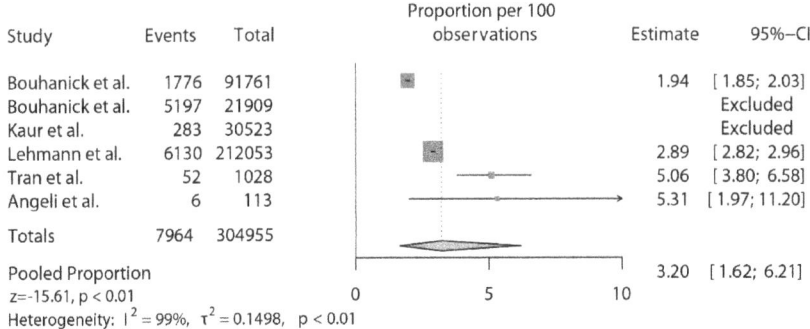

Figure 3. Proportions of increased BP after vaccination, after the exclusion of outlier studies [25,35,36,38,40,41].

4. Discussion

To the best of our knowledge, this is the first systematic review designed to investigate the occurrence of abnormal or increased BP after COVID-19 vaccination. The main novelty of our study is the evidence that a raise in BP after COVID-19 vaccination is not unusual. The proportions of patients with abnormal BP or with a significant increase in BP ranged from 0.93% to 23.72%, with a pooled point estimate of 3.91% (3.20% excluding statistical outliers). Moreover, the estimate of stage III hypertension or hypertensive urgencies and emergencies following COVID-19 vaccination was 0.6% (95% CI: 0.1–5.1%).

As aforementioned, the design of the study largely affected such proportions, with the highest value recorded in a retrospective study carried out in healthcare workers who received the BNT162b2 vaccine in a University Hospital in Toulouse [35]. Specifically, Bouhanick and co-workers [35] reported the course of BP after the injection of vaccine and assessed the incidence of high BP values in this population [35]. BP was measured 15 min after vaccination in all patients who received a first or a second injection. Subjects remained seated for 15 min after injection, and hypertension was defined as BP greater than or equal to 140/90 mmHg (grade III hypertension was declared if BP was greater than or equal to 180/111 mmHg) [35]. As remarked by the authors, the main limitation of this study was the lack of pre-vaccination control of BP and, thus, the proportion of subjects with high BP observed after the injection may reflect an unknown or insufficiently controlled hypertension [35].

Conversely, analyses of pharmacovigilance databases and clinical surveys, showed rates of abnormal BP or significantly increased BP after vaccination ranging from 0.93% to 2.89% (Figure 2).

The precise basic mechanism of this phenomenon is still unclear and further studies are required to investigate the association between COVID-19 vaccination and hypertension [2,23,42]. Stress response, white-coat effect, and the possible role of excipients [24] might contribute to explain the high prevalence of abnormal BP values recorded immediately after vaccination. Nonetheless, the resulting features of COVID-19 vaccination resemble those of active COVID-19 disease [2,23,43,44]. It is well known that the entry of severe acute respiratory syndrome coronavirus 2 (SARS-CoV-2) occurs through the angiotensin-converting enzyme 2 (ACE2) receptors of the host cells [1,3,6,45–48]. Recent observations support the notion that when a vaccinated cell dies or are destroyed by the immune system, the debris may release a large amount of Spike proteins and protein fragments (free-floating Spike proteins) [2,23]. Spike proteins produced upon vaccination have the native-like mimicry of SARS-CoV-2 Spike protein's receptor binding functionality and prefusion structure [49]. The native-like conformation of the Spike protein produced by vaccines has the potential to interact with ACE2, leading to its internalization and degradation [50]. The loss of ACE2 receptor activity from the outer layer of the cell membrane, as mediated by the interaction between ACE2 and SARS-CoV-2 Spike proteins, leads to less angiotensin II inactivation resulting from a reduced generation of antiotensin$_{1-7}$. It is well known that angiotensin$_{1-7}$ binds to the Mas receptor and reduces several effects of angiotensin 2 including inflammation, reabsorption of renal sodium, release of vasopressin and aldosterone, and fibrosis [46,47,51]. Thus, the imbalance between angiotensin II overactivity and of antiotensin$_{1-7}$ deficiency after vaccination may trigger a raise in BP [45–47].

Our systematic review and meta-analysis has several limitations. First, studies included in our analysis did not use a control group to unmask the real effect of COVID-19 vaccination on BP and showed a low accounting comparability (Table S2). Second, and as aforementioned, time of BP recording (from 15 min to several days after vaccination) clearly affects the rates of BP increase after vaccination. Finally, pharmacovigilance databases provided the largest cohorts of subjects exploring this phenomenon. However, they analyzed the rates of BP increase as a self-reported phenomenon.

5. Conclusions

Vaccines to prevent SARS-CoV-2 infection elicit an immune neutralizing response, and they are the most promising approach for curbing the pandemic.

However, some concerns regarding the safety of COVID-19 vaccines have been recently raised, including an increase in BP. Our systematic review and meta-analysis of observational studies specifically investigated this phenomenon.

Overall, included studies accrued 357,387 subjects with 13,444 events of abnormal or increased BP. The pooled proportions of abnormal/increased BP or stage III hypertension recorded following vaccination (3.20% and 0.6%, respectively) showed that this event should not be considered sporadic. However, in view of the small number of included studies and their inherent quality limitations (different times of observation, definition of BP increase, and a lack of a control group), the observed phenomenon requires further investigation in controlled settings.

Supplementary Materials: The following supporting information can be downloaded at: https://www.mdpi.com/article/10.3390/jcdd9050150/s1, Table S1: PRISMA checklist; Table S2: Assessment of the quality of included studies using the Newcastle-Ottawa Scale; Table S3: Main characteristics of excluded studies.

Author Contributions: Conceptualization, F.A., G.R., M.T. and P.V.; methodology, F.A, G.R. and P.V.; formal analysis, investigation, and data curation, F.A., P.V., G.R., G.S. and M.Z.; writing—original draft preparation, F.A., G.R., M.T. and P.V.; writing—review and editing, F.A., G.R., M.T., G.S., M.Z. and P.V. All authors have read and agreed to the published version of the manuscript.

Funding: This research received no external funding.

Data Availability Statement: The data underlying this article is fully reported in tables and figures.

Conflicts of Interest: The authors declare no conflict of interest.

References

1. Angeli, F.; Reboldi, G.; Verdecchia, P. SARS-CoV-2 Infection and ACE2 Inhibition. *J. Hypertens* **2021**, *39*, 1555–1558. [CrossRef] [PubMed]
2. Angeli, F.; Spanevello, A.; Reboldi, G.; Visca, D.; Verdecchia, P. SARS-CoV-2 vaccines: Lights and shadows. *Eur. J. Intern. Med.* **2021**, *88*, 1–8. [CrossRef] [PubMed]
3. Angeli, F.; Reboldi, G.; Verdecchia, P. Ageing, ACE2 deficiency and bad outcome in COVID-19. *Clin. Chem. Lab. Med.* **2021**, *59*, 1607–1609. [CrossRef] [PubMed]
4. Angeli, F.; Verdecchia, P.; Balestrino, A.; Bruschi, C.; Ceriana, P.; Chiovato, L.; Dalla Vecchia, L.A.; Fanfulla, F.; La Rovere, M.T.; Perego, F.; et al. Renin Angiotensin System Blockers and Risk of Mortality in Hypertensive Patients Hospitalized for COVID-19: An Italian Registry. *J. Cardiovasc. Dev. Dis.* **2022**, *9*, 15. [CrossRef]
5. Angeli, F.; Verdecchia, P.; Reboldi, G. RAAS Inhibitors and Risk of Covid-19. *N. Engl. J. Med.* **2020**, *383*, 1990–1991. [CrossRef]
6. Verdecchia, P.; Angeli, F.; Reboldi, G. Angiotensin-converting enzyme inhibitors, angiotensin II receptor blockers and coronavirus. *J. Hypertens* **2020**, *38*, 1190–1191. [CrossRef]
7. Kaur, S.P.; Gupta, V. COVID-19 Vaccine: A comprehensive status report. *Virus Res.* **2020**, *288*, 198114. [CrossRef]
8. Connors, M.; Graham, B.S.; Lane, H.C.; Fauci, A.S. SARS-CoV-2 Vaccines: Much Accomplished, Much to Learn. *Ann. Intern. Med.* **2021**, *174*, 687–690. [CrossRef]
9. Bakhiet, M.; Taurin, S. SARS-CoV-2: Targeted managements and vaccine development. *Cytokine Growth Factor Rev.* **2021**, *58*, 16–29. [CrossRef]
10. ChAdOx1 nCoV-19/AZD1222. Available online: https://www.astrazeneca.com/content/astraz/media-centre/press-releases/2021/azd1222-us-phase-iii-primary-analysis-confirms-safety-and-efficacy.html (accessed on 8 April 2021).
11. FDA Briefing Document. Janssen Ad26.COV2.S Vaccine for the Prevention of COVID-19. Vaccines and Related Biological Products Advisory Committee Meeting. 26 February 2021. Available online: https://www.fda.gov/media/146217/download (accessed on 8 April 2021).
12. Baden, L.R.; El Sahly, H.M.; Essink, B.; Kotloff, K.; Frey, S.; Novak, R.; Diemert, D.; Spector, S.A.; Rouphael, N.; Creech, C.B.; et al. Efficacy and Safety of the mRNA-1273 SARS-CoV-2 Vaccine. *N. Engl. J. Med.* **2021**, *384*, 403–416. [CrossRef]
13. Polack, F.P.; Thomas, S.J.; Kitchin, N.; Absalon, J.; Gurtman, A.; Lockhart, S.; Perez, J.L.; Perez Marc, G.; Moreira, E.D.; Zerbini, C.; et al. Safety and Efficacy of the BNT162b2 mRNA Covid-19 Vaccine. *N. Engl. J. Med.* **2020**, *383*, 2603–2615. [CrossRef]
14. Sadoff, J.; Le Gars, M.; Shukarev, G.; Heerwegh, D.; Truyers, C.; de Groot, A.M.; Stoop, J.; Tete, S.; Van Damme, W.; Leroux-Roels, I.; et al. Interim Results of a Phase 1-2a Trial of Ad26.COV2.S Covid-19 Vaccine. *N. Engl. J. Med.* **2021**, *384*, 1824–1835. [CrossRef]
15. Voysey, M.; Clemens, S.A.C.; Madhi, S.A.; Weckx, L.Y.; Folegatti, P.M.; Aley, P.K.; Angus, B.; Baillie, V.L.; Barnabas, S.L.; Bhorat, Q.E.; et al. Safety and efficacy of the ChAdOx1 nCoV-19 vaccine (AZD1222) against SARS-CoV-2: An interim analysis of four randomised controlled trials in Brazil, South Africa, and the UK. *Lancet* **2021**, *397*, 99–111. [CrossRef]
16. Wise, J. Covid-19: European countries suspend use of Oxford-AstraZeneca vaccine after reports of blood clots. *BMJ* **2021**, *372*, n699. [CrossRef]
17. Joint CDC and FDA Statement on Johnson & Johnson COVID-19 Vaccine. Available online: https://www.fda.gov/news-events/press-announcements/joint-cdc-and-fda-statement-johnson-johnson-covid-19-vaccine (accessed on 14 April 2021).
18. Greinacher, A.; Thiele, T.; Warkentin, T.E.; Weisser, K.; Kyrle, P.A.; Eichinger, S. Thrombotic Thrombocytopenia after ChAdOx1 nCov-19 Vaccination. *N. Engl. J. Med.* **2021**, *384*, 2092–2101. [CrossRef]
19. Schultz, N.H.; Sorvoll, I.H.; Michelsen, A.E.; Munthe, L.A.; Lund-Johansen, F.; Ahlen, M.T.; Wiedmann, M.; Aamodt, A.H.; Skattor, T.H.; Tjonnfjord, G.E.; et al. Thrombosis and Thrombocytopenia after ChAdOx1 nCoV-19 Vaccination. *N. Engl. J. Med.* **2021**, *384*, 2124–2130. [CrossRef]
20. Shiravi, A.A.; Ardekani, A.; Sheikhbahaei, E.; Heshmat-Ghahdarijani, K. Cardiovascular Complications of SARS-CoV-2 Vaccines: An Overview. *Cardiol. Ther.* **2022**, *11*, 13–21. [CrossRef]
21. Jackson, L.A.; Anderson, E.J.; Rouphael, N.G.; Roberts, P.C.; Makhene, M.; Coler, R.N.; McCullough, M.P.; Chappell, J.D.; Denison, M.R.; Stevens, L.J.; et al. An mRNA Vaccine against SARS-CoV-2—Preliminary Report. *N. Engl. J. Med.* **2020**, *383*, 1920–1931. [CrossRef]
22. Ostergaard, S.D.; Schmidt, M.; Horvath-Puho, E.; Thomsen, R.W.; Sorensen, H.T. Thromboembolism and the Oxford-AstraZeneca COVID-19 vaccine: Side-effect or coincidence? *Lancet* **2021**, *397*, 1441–1443. [CrossRef]
23. Angeli, F.; Reboldi, G.; Trapasso, M.; Verdecchia, P. Hypertension after COVID-19 vaccination. *G. Ital. Cardiol.* **2022**, *23*, 10–14. [CrossRef]
24. Meylan, S.; Livio, F.; Foerster, M.; Genoud, P.J.; Marguet, F.; Wuerzner, G.; Center, C.C.V. Stage III Hypertension in Patients After mRNA-Based SARS-CoV-2 Vaccination. *Hypertension* **2021**, *77*, e56–e57. [CrossRef]
25. Zappa, M.; Verdecchia, P.; Spanevello, A.; Visca, D.; Angeli, F. Blood pressure increase after Pfizer/BioNTech SARS-CoV-2 vaccine. *Eur. J. Intern. Med.* **2021**, *90*, 111–113. [CrossRef]
26. Gregoire, G.; Derderian, F.; Le Lorier, J. Selecting the language of the publications included in a meta-analysis: Is there a Tower of Babel bias? *J. Clin. Epidemiol.* **1995**, *48*, 159–163. [CrossRef]
27. Haynes, R.B.; Wilczynski, N.; McKibbon, K.A.; Walker, C.J.; Sinclair, J.C. Developing optimal search strategies for detecting clinically sound studies in MEDLINE. *J. Am. Med. Inform. Assoc.* **1994**, *1*, 447–458. [CrossRef]

28. McAuley, L.; Pham, B.; Tugwell, P.; Moher, D. Does the inclusion of grey literature influence estimates of intervention effectiveness reported in meta-analyses? *Lancet* **2000**, *356*, 1228–1231. [CrossRef]
29. Moher, D.; Liberati, A.; Tetzlaff, J.; Altman, D.G.; Group, P. Preferred reporting items for systematic reviews and meta-analyses: The PRISMA statement. *BMJ* **2009**, *339*, b2535. [CrossRef]
30. McPheeters, M.L.; Kripalini, S.; Peterson, N.B.; Idowu, R.T. Quality Improvement Interventions To Address Health Disparities. Evidence Report/ technology Assessment. Rockville (MD): Agency for Healthcare Research and Quality (US). 2012. Available online: http://www.ncbi.nlm.nih.gov/pubmedhealth/PMH0049222/pdf/TOC.pdf (accessed on 18 March 2022).
31. Wells, G.A.; Shea, B.; O'Connell, D.; Peterson, J.; Welch, V. The Newcastle-Ottawa Scale (NOS) for Assessing the Quality of Nonrandomized Studies in Meta-Analysis. 2011. Available online: http://www.ohri.ca/programs/clinical_epidemiology/oxford.asp (accessed on 28 February 2022).
32. Stijnen, T.; Hamza, T.H.; Ozdemir, P. Random effects meta-analysis of event outcome in the framework of the generalized linear mixed model with applications in sparse data. *Stat. Med.* **2010**, *29*, 3046–3067. [CrossRef]
33. Harrer, M.; Cuijpers, P.; Furukawa, T.A.; Erbert, D.D. *Doing Meta-Analysis with R: A Hands-On Guide*, 1st ed.; Chapman and Hall/CRC: New York, NY, USA, 2021. [CrossRef]
34. Higgins, J.P.; Thompson, S.G.; Deeks, J.J.; Altman, D.G. Measuring inconsistency in meta-analyses. *BMJ* **2003**, *327*, 557–560. [CrossRef] [PubMed]
35. Bouhanick, B.; Brusq, C.; Bongard, V.; Tessier, S.; Montastruc, J.L.; Senard, J.M.; Montastruc, F.; Herin, F. Blood pressure measurements after mRNA-SARS-CoV-2 tozinameran vaccination: A retrospective analysis in a university hospital in France. *J. Hum. Hypertens* **2022**, 1–2. [CrossRef] [PubMed]
36. Bouhanick, B.; Montastruc, F.; Tessier, S.; Brusq, C.; Bongard, V.; Senard, J.M.; Montastruc, J.L.; Herin, F. Hypertension and Covid-19 vaccines: Are there any differences between the different vaccines? A safety signal. *Eur. J. Clin. Pharmacol.* **2021**, *77*, 1937–1938. [CrossRef] [PubMed]
37. Ch'ng, C.C.; Ong, L.M.; Wong, K.M. Changes in Blood Pressure After Pfizer/Biontech Sars-Cov-2 Vaccination. *Res. Sq.* **2022**. [CrossRef]
38. Kaur, R.J.; Dutta, S.; Charan, J.; Bhardwaj, P.; RTandon, A.; Yadav, D.; Islam, S.; Haque, M. Cardiovascular Adverse Events Reported from COVID-19 Vaccines: A Study Based on WHO Database. *Int. J. Gen. Med.* **2021**, *14*, 3909–3927. [CrossRef]
39. Sanidas, E.; Anastasiou, T.; Papadopoulos, D.; Velliou, M.; Mantzourani, M. Short term blood pressure alterations in recently COVID-19 vaccinated patients. *Eur. J. Intern. Med.* **2022**, *96*, 115–116. [CrossRef]
40. Tran, V.N.; Nguyen, H.A.; Le, T.T.A.; Truong, T.T.; Nguyen, P.T.; Nguyen, T.T.H. Factors influencing adverse events following immunization with AZD1222 in Vietnamese adults during first half of 2021. *Vaccine* **2021**, *39*, 6485–6491. [CrossRef]
41. Lehmann, K. Suspected Cardiovascular Side Effects of two Covid-19 Vaccines. *J. Biol. Today's World* **2021**, *10*, 1–6. [CrossRef]
42. Angeli, F.; Masnaghetti, S.; Visca, D.; Rossoni, A.; Taddeo, S.; Biagini, F.; Verdecchia, P. Severity of COVID-19: The importance of being hypertensive. *Monaldi Arch. Chest Dis.* **2020**, *90*. [CrossRef]
43. Kyriakidis, N.C.; Lopez-Cortes, A.; Gonzalez, E.V.; Grimaldos, A.B.; Prado, E.O. SARS-CoV-2 vaccines strategies: A comprehensive review of phase 3 candidates. *NPJ Vaccines* **2021**, *6*, 28. [CrossRef]
44. Angeli, F.; Verdecchia, P.; Reboldi, G. Pharmacotherapy for hypertensive urgency and emergency in COVID-19 patients. *Expert Opin. Pharm.* **2022**, *23*, 235–242. [CrossRef]
45. Angeli, F.; Zappa, M.; Reboldi, G.; Trapasso, M.; Cavallini, C.; Spanevello, A.; Verdecchia, P. The pivotal link between ACE2 deficiency and SARS-CoV-2 infection: One year later. *Eur. J. Intern. Med.* **2021**, *93*, 28–34. [CrossRef]
46. Verdecchia, P.; Cavallini, C.; Spanevello, A.; Angeli, F. COVID-19: ACE2centric Infective Disease? *Hypertension* **2020**, *76*, 294–299. [CrossRef]
47. Verdecchia, P.; Cavallini, C.; Spanevello, A.; Angeli, F. The pivotal link between ACE2 deficiency and SARS-CoV-2 infection. *Eur. J. Intern. Med.* **2020**, *76*, 14–20. [CrossRef] [PubMed]
48. Verdecchia, P.; Reboldi, G.; Cavallini, C.; Mazzotta, G.; Angeli, F. ACE-inhibitors, angiotensin receptor blockers and severe acute respiratory syndrome caused by coronavirus. *G. Ital. Cardiol.* **2020**, *21*, 321–327. [CrossRef]
49. Watanabe, Y.; Mendonca, L.; Allen, E.R.; Howe, A.; Lee, M.; Allen, J.D.; Chawla, H.; Pulido, D.; Donnellan, F.; Davies, H.; et al. Native-like SARS-CoV-2 spike glycoprotein expressed by ChAdOx1 nCoV-19/AZD1222 vaccine. *ACS Cent. Sci.* **2021**, *7*, 594–602. [CrossRef] [PubMed]
50. Deshotels, M.R.; Xia, H.; Sriramula, S.; Lazartigues, E.; Filipeanu, C.M. Angiotensin II mediates angiotensin converting enzyme type 2 internalization and degradation through an angiotensin II type I receptor-dependent mechanism. *Hypertension* **2014**, *64*, 1368–1375. [CrossRef]
51. Simoes e Silva, A.C.; Silveira, K.D.; Ferreira, A.J.; Teixeira, M.M. ACE2, angiotensin-(1–7) and Mas receptor axis in inflammation and fibrosis. *Br. J. Pharm.* **2013**, *169*, 477–492. [CrossRef]

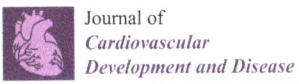

Article

Renin Angiotensin System Blockers and Risk of Mortality in Hypertensive Patients Hospitalized for COVID-19: An Italian Registry

Fabio Angeli [1,2,*], Paolo Verdecchia [3], Antonella Balestrino [4], Claudio Bruschi [5], Piero Ceriana [4], Luca Chiovato [6,7], Laura Adelaide Dalla Vecchia [8], Francesco Fanfulla [4], Maria Teresa La Rovere [9], Francesca Perego [10], Simonetta Scalvini [11], Antonio Spanevello [1,2], Egidio Traversi [9], Dina Visca [1,2], Michele Vitacca [12] and Tiziana Bachetti [13]

1. Department of Medicine and Surgery, University of Insubria, 21100 Varese, Italy; Antonio.spanevello@icsmaugeri.it (A.S.); dina.visca@icsmaugeri.it (D.V.)
2. Department of Medicine and Cardiopulmonary Rehabilitation, Istituti Clinici Scientifici Maugeri IRCCS, 21049 Tradate, Italy
3. Fondazione Umbra Cuore e Ipertensione-ONLUS and Division of Cardiology, Hospital S. Maria Della Misericordia, 06100 Perugia, Italy; verdecchiapaolo@gmail.com
4. Department of Pulmonary Rehabilitation, Istituti Clinici Scientifici Maugeri IRCCS, 27100 Pavia, Italy; antonella.balestrino@icsmaugeri.it (A.B.); piero.ceriana@icsmaugeri.it (P.C.); francesco.fanfulla@icsmaugeri.it (F.F.)
5. Department of Pulmonary Rehabilitation, Istituti Clinici Scientifici Maugeri IRCCS, 27040 Montescano, Italy; claudio.bruschi@icsmaugeri.it
6. Unit of Internal Medicine and Endocrinology, Laboratory for Endocrine Disruptors, Istituti Clinici Scientifici Maugeri IRCCS, 27100 Pavia, Italy; luca.chiovato@icsmaugeri.it
7. Department of Internal Medicine and Therapeutics, University of Pavia, 27100 Pavia, Italy
8. Department of Cardiac Rehabilitation, Istituti Clinici Scientifici Maugeri IRCCS, 20019 Milano, Italy; laura.dallavecchia@icsmaugeri.it
9. Department of Cardiac Rehabilitation, Istituti Clinici Scientifici Maugeri IRCCS, 27040 Montescano, Italy; mariateresa.larovere@icsmaugeri.it (M.T.L.R.); egidio.traversi@icsmaugeri.it (E.T.)
10. Department of Subacute Therapy, Istituti Clinici Scientifici Maugeri IRCCS, 20019 Milano, Italy; francesca.perego@icsmaugeri.it
11. Department of Cardiac Rehabilitation, Istituti Clinici Scientifici Maugeri IRCCS, 25065 Lumezzane, Italy; simonetta.scalvini@icsmaugeri.it
12. Department of Pulmonary Rehabilitation, Istituti Clinici Scientifici Maugeri IRCCS, 25065 Lumezzane, Italy; michele.vitacca@icsmaugeri.it
13. Scientific Direction, Istituti Clinici Scientifici Maugeri IRCCS, 27100 Pavia, Italy; tiziana.bachetti@icsmaugeri.it
* Correspondence: angeli.internet@gmail.com

Abstract: Background: It is uncertain whether exposure to renin–angiotensin system (RAS) modifiers affects the severity of the new coronavirus disease 2019 (COVID-19) because most of the available studies are retrospective. Methods: We tested the prognostic value of exposure to RAS modifiers (either angiotensin-converting enzyme inhibitors [ACE-Is] or angiotensin receptor blockers [ARBs]) in a prospective study of hypertensive patients with COVID-19. We analyzed data from 566 patients (mean age 75 years, 54% males, 162 ACE-Is users, and 147 ARBs users) hospitalized in five Italian hospitals. The study used systematic prospective data collection according to a pre-specified protocol. All-cause mortality during hospitalization was the primary outcome. Results: Sixty-six patients died during hospitalization. Exposure to RAS modifiers was associated with a significant reduction in the risk of in-hospital mortality when compared to other BP-lowering strategies (odds ratio [OR]: 0.54, 95% confidence interval [CI]: 0.32 to 0.90, $p = 0.019$). Exposure to ACE-Is was not significantly associated with a reduced risk of in-hospital mortality when compared with patients not treated with RAS modifiers (OR: 0.66, 95% CI: 0.36 to 1.20, $p = 0.172$). Conversely, ARBs users showed a 59% lower risk of death (OR: 0.41, 95% CI: 0.20 to 0.84, $p = 0.016$) even after allowance for several prognostic markers, including age, oxygen saturation, occurrence of severe hypotension during hospitalization, and lymphocyte count (adjusted OR: 0.37, 95% CI: 0.17 to 0.80, $p = 0.012$). The discontinuation of RAS modifiers during hospitalization did not exert a significant effect ($p = 0.515$). Conclusions:

This prospective study indicates that exposure to ARBs reduces mortality in hospitalized patients with COVID-19.

Keywords: SARS-CoV-2; COVID-19; renin–angiotensin system; ACE2; ACE inhibitors; angiotensin receptor blockers; angiotensin-converting enzyme inhibitors

1. Introduction

At the beginning of the severe acute respiratory syndrome coronavirus 2 (SARS-CoV-2) pandemic, the evidence that angiotensin-converting enzyme 2 (ACE2) acts as the functional receptor for the spike glycoprotein of the virus generated some concerns regarding the potential deleterious effect of renin–angiotensin system (RAS) modifiers, which had been shown to increase ACE2 expression in some experimental models [1].

With advancing knowledge on the role of RAS in the pathogenesis of the new coronavirus disease 2019 (COVID-19), academic literature recognized that, while it has been coopted as the entry point for the SARS-CoV-2 virus on host cells, the ACE2 enzyme also modulates the balance between vasoconstrictors and vasodilators within the heart and kidney, and it plays a significant role in regulating cardiovascular and renal functions [2–4].

Several observational studies conducted to clarify this controversial issue generated mixed results [4]. The majority of the available studies did not show any sign of harm associated with ACE inhibitors (ACE-Is) or angiotensin receptor blockers (ARBs) in patients with COVID-19 (no significant association between the chronic use of RAS modifiers and either the risk to contract an infection or the risk of developing a severe or lethal form of the disease) [4,5]. Conversely, some retrospective clinical studies demonstrated a lower risk of in-hospital death among patients taking ACE-Is or ARBs than among patients not receiving these drugs [6,7].

We designed a prospective study in a cohort of hypertensive patients hospitalized for COVID-19 in order to specifically evaluate the prognostic impact of antihypertensive medications, including RAS modifiers.

2. Materials and Methods

We analyzed data from patients in 5 hospitals of the Lombardy region and belonging to the Maugeri Care and Research Institutes Network. The protocol was approved by the Ethical Committee of our institution, and patients gave their written informed consent to participate.

Details of the protocol have been published [8,9]. Briefly, our study was a pre-designed registry of patients hospitalized for COVID-19 with subsequent prospective collection of data; the primary study outcome was all-cause mortality during hospitalization. Secondary outcomes included death and new hospitalization after 2 years from COVID-19 recovery (follow-up is still ongoing).

Diagnosis of viral infection was confirmed in all patients by using RNA reverse transcription–polymerase chain reaction (RT-PCR) assays from nasopharyngeal swab specimens [10]. Demographic, laboratory, and clinical management data were collected at admission and throughout the entire in-hospital stay. Laboratory parameters were assessed using standard techniques. PaO_2/FIO_2 ratio was used to estimate the severity of respiratory dysfunction, and high-sensitivity cardiac troponin was used as a marker of myocardial injury (as documented by troponin elevation > 5 pg/mL, according to the reference values of our laboratory).

The presence of comorbidities was defined according to documented medical history, as collected by investigators at study site level, including examination of electronic health record data of the Lombardy region. All clinical evaluations were performed by attending physicians during the clinical interview and through examination of medical records. Comorbidities (including type II diabetes, chronic kidney disease, dyslipidemia, hypertension, previous cardiac events) were defined according to current guidelines [11–14]. Previous cardiac events included history of heart failure (symptomatic syndrome, as graded according to the New York Heart Association functional classification or prior hospitalization for acute heart failure requiring intravenous therapy) and coronary artery disease (as defined by at least one of the following criteria: (1) presence of any epicardial coronary vessels with >75% stenosis tested on coronary angiography; (2) history of acute coronary syndrome; (3) coronary revascularization, either percutaneous transluminal coronary angioplasty or coronary artery bypass grafting).

The main exposure of interest was the use of ACE-Is and ARBs (including combinations with other antihypertensive drugs). Specifically, medication exposure was defined as having had active prescriptions of blood pressure (BP)-lowering medications (ACE-Is, ARBs, and other BP-lowering drugs) from at least 30 days before the date of admission. Other BP-lowering drugs included diuretics, beta-blockers, calcium channel blockers, and other antihypertensives, alone or in combination. Sacubitril/valsartan was categorized as an ARB. Even if the medications of interest were being withheld during hospitalization for any acute issues (i.e., hypotension, sepsis, acute kidney injury, and inability to take oral medications), these patients were still included based on their medication exposure. Investigators followed internal guidelines for the treatment of COVID-19 based on the clinical experience of the group. Our internal guidelines included the recommendation to modify the antihypertensive treatment (on clinical judgment) to achieve a systolic blood pressure <140 mmHg and a diastolic blood pressure <90 mmHg during the entire phase of hospitalization.

Statistical analysis. Analyses were performed using Stata, version 16 (StataCorp LP, College Station, TX, USA) and R version 2.9.2 (R Foundation for Statistical Computing, Vienna, Austria). We expressed continuous variables as mean ± standard deviation (SD) and the categorical variables as proportions.

We analyzed differences in proportions between groups using the χ^2 test. Mean values of variables were compared using independent sample *t*-test or analysis of variance, when appropriate.

We evaluated the effect of prognostic factors on mortality using univariable and multivariable logistic regression analyses.

The odds ratios (ORs) from the univariable and multivariable analyses and their corresponding two-sided 95% confidence intervals (CIs) were derived from the regression coefficients in the logistic models. Survival curves were estimated using Kaplan–Meier product limit method and compared with the Mantel (log-rank) test.

We tested the prognostic impact of several variables, which proved a significant influence on mortality in this setting, and we modeled a multivariable model using the covariates that yielded statistical significance in the univariable analysis.

More specifically, we tested the prognostic impact of age (years) [15,16], history of diabetes (yes/no) [16], history of dyslipidemia (yes/no) [17], history of cardiac events (yes/no) [18], history of chronic obstructive pulmonary disease (yes/no) [19], renal function [16], hemoglobin levels (1 g/dL) [20], high-sensitivity C-reactive protein (CRP), troponin elevation, PaO_2/FIO_2 ratio, white blood cell and absolute lymphocyte count (1000/mcl) [17,18], oxygen saturation (%) at admission, history of neoplasm [19], and severe hypotension (yes/no) occurring during hospitalization and requiring inotropic support [17]. For continuous covariates, Youden index analysis was also used to identify the optimal cutoff value for the identification of patients at increased risk of death.

We used Akaike's information criterion (AIC) and the Bayesian information criterion (BIC) to compare performance of different multivariable models. Analyses were performed using a significance level of $\alpha = 0.05$ (2 sided).

3. Results

Overall, 566 hypertensive patients were included in the analysis (mean age 75 years; 54% males; 309 patients treated with RAS modifiers, including ACE-Is and ARBs). None of the patients were receiving a combination of ACE-Is and ARBs. Among patients treated with other BP-lowering drugs (see Materials and Methods), 50 were treated with monotherapy and 207 with combination therapy.

Baseline co-morbidities, specific in-hospital medications, and characteristics commonly used to define severe COVID-19 (age, severe hypotension, lymphocyte count, estimated glomerular filtration rate [eGFR], CRP, and PaO_2/FIO_2 ratio) were well balanced among different BP-lowering drug users (Table 1).

Table 1. Main characteristics of patients included in the analysis.

Variable	Overall (n = 566)	ACE-Is (n = 162)	ARBs (n = 147)	Other BP-Lowering Drugs (n = 257)	p
Age (years)	75 ± 11	74 ± 12	76 ± 10	76 ± 11	0.060
Sex (male, %)	54	62	50	50	0.047
BMI (Kg/m^2)	27.3 ± 5.7	27.6 ± 6.5	26.6 ± 4.2	27.5 ± 5.9	0.334
History					
COPD (%)	16	12	15	20	0.112
Type 2 diabetes (%)	31	30	31	31	0.936
Dyslipidemia (%)	32	28	36	33	0.330
Previous cardiac event (%)	29	30	22	32	0.144
Neoplasm (%)	11	11	15	9	0.139
Hospitalization					
Hydroxychloroquine (%)	58	58	60	56	0.715
Antiretroviral (%)	27	28	25	28	0.834
Macrolides (%)	32	28	38	30	0.298
Aspirin (%)	31	32	30	31	0.919
NSAIDs or glucocorticoids (%)	40	43	45	36	0.149
Oxygen level (%)	95 ± 3	95 ± 3	95 ± 3	95 ± 3	0.715
Severe hypotension	7	6	7	9	0.648
Haemoglobin (g/dL)	11.5 ± 1.8	11.7 ± 1.8	11.2 ± 1.7	11.5 ± 1.8	0.022
Lymphocyte count (× 10^3)	1.51 ± 1.01	1.51 ± 0.66	1.63 ± 1.53	1.44 ± 0.76	0.238
eGFR (mL/min/1.73 m^2)	72 ± 23	73 ± 24	72 ± 21	72 ± 25	0.818
K+ (ng/mL)	4.4 ± 0.6	4.4 ± 0.6	4.3 ± 0.5	4.3 ± 0.6	0.291
Troponin elevation (%)	17	17	16	19	0.649
PaO_2/FIO_2 ratio (mm)	315 ± 129	316 ± 110	309 ± 128	318 ± 141	0.852
High-sensitivity CRP (mg/dL)	11.5 ± 26.4	7.7 ± 18.1	15.5 ± 41.3	11.7 ± 26.4	0.068

Legend: BMI = body mass index; COPD = chronic obstructive pulmonary disease; CRP = C-reactive protein; eGFR = estimated glomerular filtration rate using the Chronic Kidney Disease Epidemiology Collaboration (CKD-EPI) equation; NSAIDs = non-steroidal anti-inflammatory drugs.

During hospitalization, 66 patients died. Among the RAS modifier users, 27 patients (9%) died in hospital, whereas among other BP-lowering drug users, 39 (15%) died. Thus, exposure to RAS modifiers was associated with a significant 46% reduction in the risk of in-hospital mortality when compared with other BP-lowering strategies (OR: 0.54, 95% CI: 0.32 to 0.90, p = 0.019).

We also evaluated the outcomes of hospitalized COVID-19 patients based on their exposure to ACE-Is, ARBs, and other BP-lowering drugs: 162 (29%) were ACE-Is users, 147 (26%) were ARBs users, and 257 (45%) used other antihypertensive medications. The rates of in-hospital mortality were 15%, 10%, and 7% for exposure to other BP-lowering drugs, ACE-Is, and RAS modifiers, respectively. Figure 1 depicts the crude rates of in-hospital death according to the subgroups of antihypertensive therapy. Estimating the risk of death according to logistic regression analysis, the group of ACE-Is users was not significantly associated with a reduced risk of in-hospital mortality when compared with patients treated with other BP-lowering strategies (OR: 0.66, 95% CI: 0.36 to 1.20, p = 0.172). Conversely, ARBs users showed a 59% lower risk of death (OR: 0.41, 95% CI: 0.20 to 0.84, p = 0.016, Figure 1—upper panel). Similar results were obtained using the Kaplan–Meier product limit method (Figure 1—lower panel).

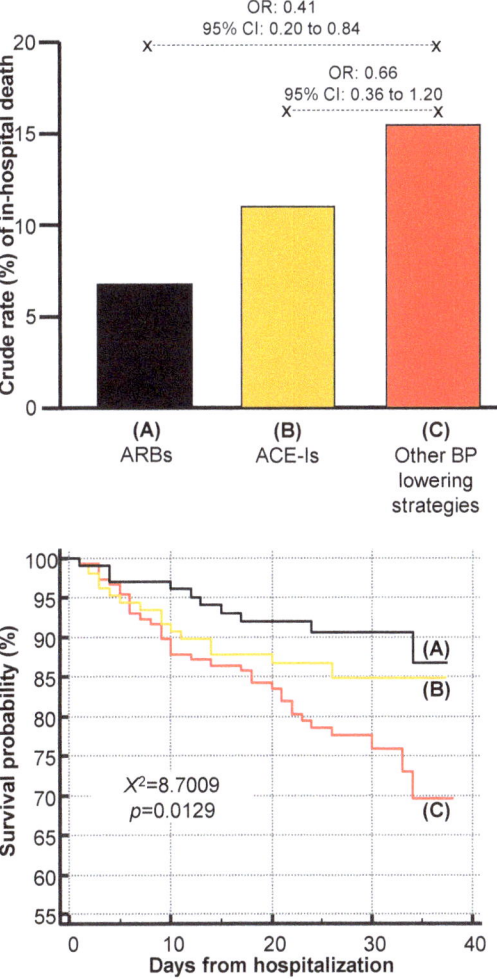

Figure 1. Risk of in-hospital death among hypertensive patients hospitalized for COVID-19 according to subgroups of antihypertensive therapy (upper panel). Survival curves (lower panel) were estimated using Kaplan–Meier product limit method and compared with the Mantel (log-rank) test. Legend: ACE-Is = ACE inhibitors; ARBs = angiotensin receptor blockers; BP = blood pressure; CI = confidence interval; OR = odds ratio.

Among other covariates tested as predictors of in-hospital death (Figure 2), age, chronic obstructive pulmonary disease (COPD), previous cardiac events, a decreased oxygen saturation level recorded at admission, baseline high white blood cell count, severe hypotension occurring during hospitalization, lymphocytopenia at baseline, reduced eGFR at admission, reduced PaO_2/FIO_2 ratio, and increased high-sensitivity CRP were associated with an increased risk of death (all $p < 0.05$, Figure 2).

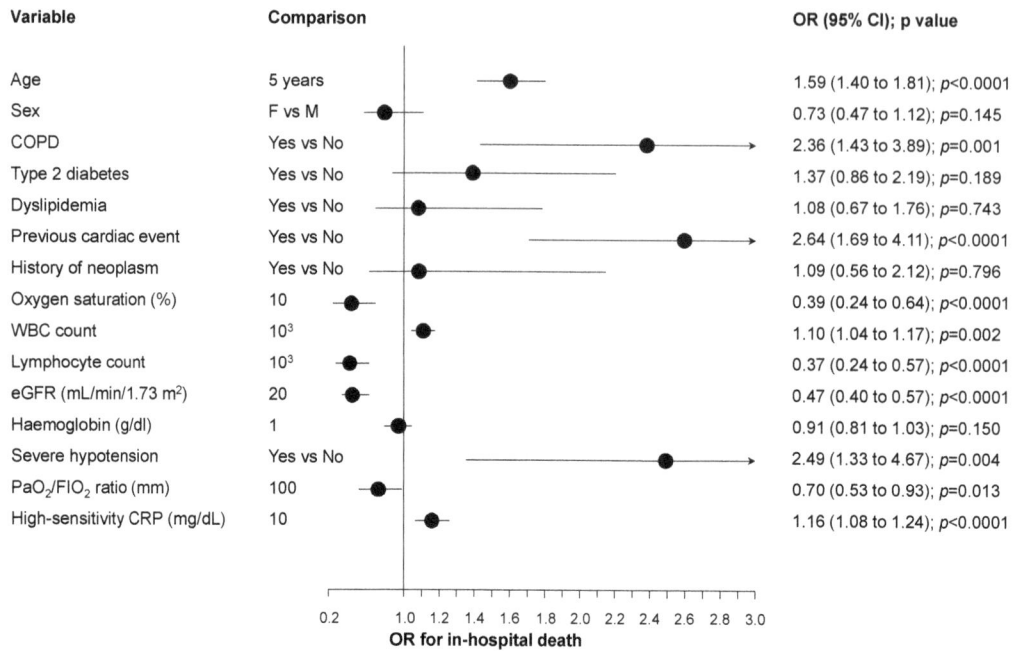

Figure 2. Results of univariable analyses exploring predictors of in-hospital death. Legend: COPD = chronic obstructive pulmonary disease; CRP = C-reactive protein; eGFR = estimated glomerular filtration rate using the Chronic Kidney Disease Epidemiology Collaboration (CKD-EPI) equation; WBC = white blood cell.

Using the categorization of continuous variables according to the optimal cutoff value as identified by the Youden index analysis (see Materials and Methods), the best informative multivariable model (baseline multivariable model, AIC = 358, BIC = 379, Table 2, upper panel) included age, severe hypotension, oxygen saturation, and lymphocyte count.

When we added the exposure to ACE-Is or ARBs (other BP-lowering drugs used as reference) to the baseline model (Table 2, lower panel), ARBs were associated with a significant 63% lower risk of death (OR: 0.37, 95% CI: 0.17 to 0.80, p = 0.012), whereas ACE-Is were associated with a non-significant 27% lower risk of death (OR: 0.73, 95% CI: 0.38 to 1.40, p = 0.339) when compared with other BP-lowering strategies.

Similar results were also obtained after the adjustment of other risk markers that proved statistical significance in the univariable analyses. To further characterize the effect of the severity of COVID-19 at admission as a prognostic modifier, we also evaluated the presence of myocardial injury and pulmonary involvement (see Materials and Methods).

Overall, 99 patients (17%) showed cardiac involvement (high-sensitivity cardiac troponin elevation); the prevalence of troponin elevation was 19%, 17%, and 16% among patients treated with other BP-lowering drugs, ACE-Is, and ARBs, respectively (p = 0.649). The PaO_2/FIO_2 ratio was 318 mm, 316 mm, and 309 mm among patients treated with other BP-lowering drugs, ACE-Is (p = 0.990 vs. other BP-lowering drugs), and ARBs (p = 0.924 vs. other BP-lowering drugs and p = 0.973 vs. ACE-Is), respectively. When compared with the users of other BP-lowering strategies, patients exposed to ARBs showed a significant lower risk of in-hospital death even after adjustment for the significant effect of troponin elevation (p = 0.024) and the PaO_2/FIO_2 ratio (p = 0.012). More specifically, ARBs were associated with a significant 61% lower risk of death (OR: 0.39, 95% CI: 0.19 to 0.82, p = 0.012), whereas ACE-Is were associated with a non-significant 36% lower risk of death (OR: 0.64, 95% CI: 0.35 to 1.18, p = 0.151) when compared with other BP-lowering strategies and after adjustment for troponin elevation. Similar results were obtained after adjustment for the PaO$_2$/FIO$_2$ ratio (OR: 0.40, 95% CI: 0.17 to 0.95, p = 0.037 for ARBs vs. other BP-lowering drugs; OR: 0.76, 95% CI: 0.37 to 1.56, p = 0.456 for ACE-Is vs. other BP-lowering drugs).

The effects of the different BP-lowering drugs on the probability (%) of in-hospital death according to different baseline risk strata (as identified by the presence of risk factors included in the multivariable model) are depicted in Figure 3.

Table 2. Multivariable model exploring the impact of ACE inhibitors and angiotensin receptor blockers on the risk of in-hospital death (lower panel) when added to a baseline multivariable model identified according to information criteria (upper panel).

Variable	Comparison	OR	95% CI	p
Baseline multivariable model				
Age > 80 years	Yes vs. No	2.95	1.68 to 5.19	<0.0001
Severe hypotension	Yes vs. No	3.77	1.68 to 8.45	0.001
Oxygen saturation ≤ 95%	Yes vs. No	2.10	1.18 to 3.71	0.011
Lymphocyte count ≤ 1.23×10^3	Yes vs. No	3.66	2.07 to 6.46	<0.0001
Baseline multivariable model and antihypertensive drug subgroups				
Age > 80 years	Yes vs. No	2.96	1.67 to 5.26	<0.0001
Severe hypotension	Yes vs. No	4.07	1.80 to 9.17	0.001
Oxygen saturation ≤ 95%	Yes vs. No	2.15	1.21 to 3.82	0.009
Lymphocyte count ≤ 1.23×10^3	Yes vs. No	3.65	2.06 to 6.47	<0.0001
BP-lowering drugs				
ACE-Is	Other BP-lowering drugs	0.73	0.38 to 1.40	0.339
ARBs	Other BP-lowering drugs	0.37	0.17 to 0.80	0.012

Legend: BP = blood pressure; ACE-Is = ACE inhibitors; ARBs = angiotensin receptor blockers.

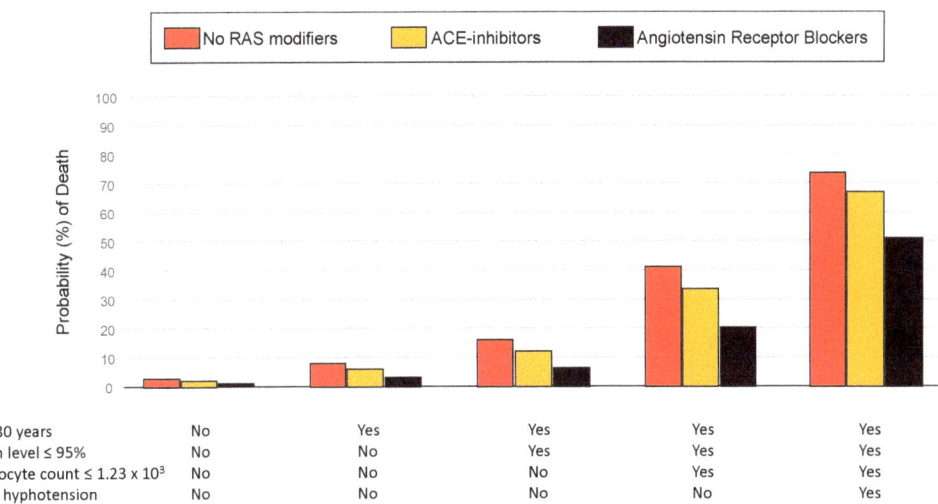

Figure 3. Effects of different blood pressure-lowering drugs on the probability (%) of in-hospital death according to different baseline risk strata (as identified by the presence of independent risk markers of prognosis).

During hospitalization, the discontinuation of ACE-Is, ARBs, and other BP-lowering drugs was 17%, 18%, and 10%, respectively. Of note, the discontinuation of RAS modifiers during hospitalization did not exert a significant confounding impact (p = 0.515).

4. Discussion

The results of our study support the hypothesis that exposure to RAS modifiers reduces the risk of death during hospitalization for COVID-19. When splitting the users of RAS modifiers into ACE-Is and ARBs users, we found that exposure to ACE-Is was not significantly associated with a reduced risk of in-hospital mortality when compared with patients not treated with RAS modifiers. Conversely, ARBs users showed a decreased risk of death even after adjusting for a wide range of prognostic markers.

Some methodological aspects of our study deserve to be highlighted when compared to previous clinical studies. Available clinical studies often did not allow separate analyses of ACE-Is and ARBs, although it may be expected that these two different classes of antihypertensive drugs differently impact the prognosis of COVID-19 [4]. In our cohort, we had the opportunity to evaluate the different impacts of ACE-Is and ARBs on the management of COVID-19 hypertensive patients when compared with other BP-lowering drugs.

The large amount of evidence on the topic is mainly driven by retrospective studies [4,21–29]. Remarkably, our study was not a retrospective collection of clinical data in patients hospitalized for COVID-19 but rather a pre-designed protocol with subsequent prospective collection of data (see Materials and Methods).

Furthermore, exposure to different BP-lowering drugs was measured during a 30-day window before admission as an intention-to-treat analysis, and discontinuation was also evaluated during the entire hospital phase and evaluated as a possible confounding factor.

In other words, even if the medications of interest were being withheld during hospitalization for any acute issues, these patients were still included based on their medication exposure. Such an approach has the potential to avoid the bias related to the evidence that RAS modifiers tend to be continued in healthier patients and discontinued in patients with severe forms of the disease (including hypotension, low eGFR, and new kidney injury) [30].

Finally, we accounted for potential confounders by using a multivariable model adjusted for well-established prognostic factors, including age, severe hypotension, oxygen saturation, and lymphocyte count [9,15–20,31,32]. We also evaluated the effects of different BP-lowering drugs on the risk of in-hospital mortality among different baseline risk strata (as identified by the presence of different risk markers). As expected, the prognostic benefit of ARBs is magnified among patients with advanced age and with other laboratory features of increased risk (Figure 3).

In conclusion, the use of antihypertensive drugs and their potential impact on outcome in COVID-19 patients remain key points. Despite conflicting views in the literature, our results support the preferential use of ARBs.

Although the mechanisms explaining the potential benefits of RAS modifiers are still undetermined, some hypotheses have recently been proposed. There is growing evidence that the blunted ACE2 activity resulting from the reduced expression, downregulation, and dysfunction of these receptors after viral invasion and the resulting imbalance between angiotensin II and angiotensin$_{1-7}$ may play an important role in conditioning inflammatory, thromboembolic, and hemodynamic processes in patients with COVID-19 [3–5,33,34].

Following this line of evidence, by enhancing ACE2 expression [35–38] and limiting the effects of unopposed angiotensin II on the heart, lungs, kidney, and vasculature, RAS-modifiers (and especially ARBs acting distally in the RAS to block the angiotensin II type 1 receptor selectively, Figure 4) have the potential to exert a better protective role in patients with COVID-19 when compared with other BP-lowering drugs [2–4,39–45]. Moreover, we can expect that ARBs exert these effects by both AT1 receptor blockade and angiotensin II type 2 (AT2) receptor stimulation [46,47]. Indeed, it has been reported that AT2 receptor stimulation antagonizes the effects of AT1 receptor stimulation in most tissues, promoting cardiovascular protection by the reduction of inflammation, oxidative stress, fibrosis, vascular remodeling, and vascular smooth muscle cell proliferation [46–49].

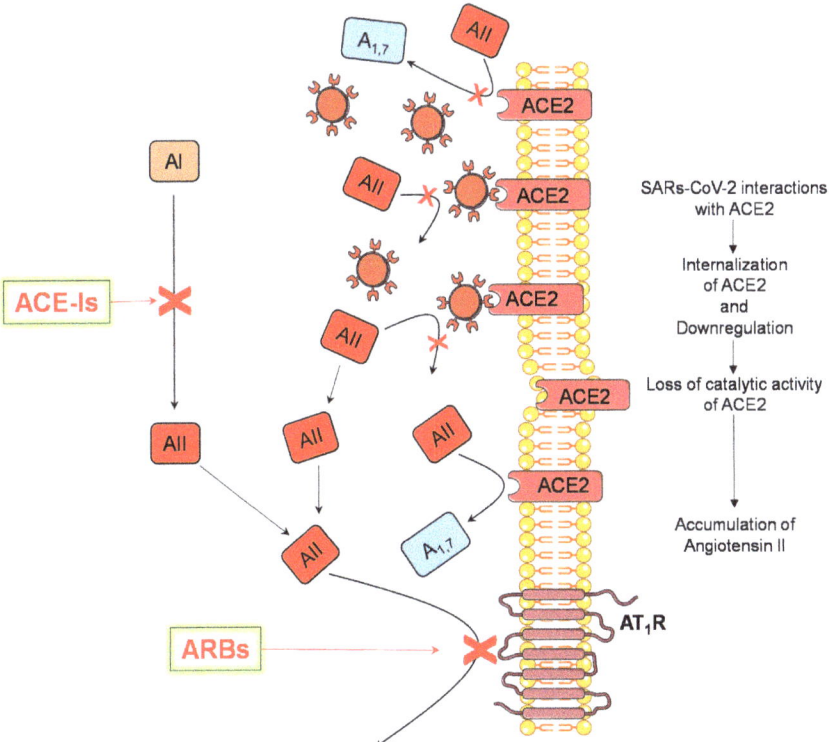

Figure 4. Potential mechanisms of pharmacological modulation of the renin–angiotensin system to reduce the deleterious effects of angiotensin II accumulation. AI = angiotensin I; AII = angiotensin II; $A_{1,7}$ = angiotensin$_{1-7}$; ACE2 = angiotensin-converting enzyme 2; ACE-Is = ACE inhibitors; ARBs = angiotensin receptor blockers; ATR1 = angiotensin II type 1 receptor.

Study limitations. The present study should be interpreted within the context of its potential limitations. First, because the majority of enrolled patients were white, it may be difficult to extrapolate the results to different ethnic groups. Second, during data collection, some evidence was accrued on the prognostic significance of uncontrolled hypertension during hospitalization for COVID-19 [5,50]. In-hospital BP data were not routinely collected, but internal clinical guidelines were followed recommending that systolic BP be kept below 140 mmHg and diastolic BP below 90 mmHg. Third, the type, dosage, and duration of BP-lowering drugs and other cardiovascular concurrent medications, other than reported relevant laboratory results, electrocardiographic and echocardiographic findings, and specific causes of death were not collected. Finally, our study was not designed to evaluate the mechanisms of COVID-19 and the influence of BP-lowering drugs on the pathophysiology of the disease. Although the serum levels of angiotensin II and angiotensin$_{1-7}$ were not measured in our study population, our results may indirectly support the hypothesis of an effect of RAS modifiers on angiotensin II accumulation observed during the acute phase of COVID-19.

Author Contributions: Conceptualization, F.A. and T.B.; methodology, F.A., T.B. and P.V.; formal analysis, investigation, and data curation, F.A., T.B., A.B., C.B., P.C., L.C., L.A.D.V., F.F., M.T.L.R., F.P., S.S., A.S., E.T., D.V. and M.V.; writing—original draft preparation, F.A., T.B. and P.V.; writing—review and editing, F.A., P.V., T.B., A.B., C.B., P.C., L.C., L.A.D.V., F.F., M.T.L.R., F.P., S.S., A.S., E.T., D.V. and M.V. All authors have read and agreed to the published version of the manuscript.

Funding: "Ricerca Corrente" funding scheme of the Ministry of Health, Italy.

Institutional Review Board Statement: The study was conducted according to the guidelines of the Declaration of Helsinki and approved by the Institutional Review Board and Ethics Committee of Istituti Clinici Scientifici Maugeri, Pavia—Italy (protocol number 2415, 23 April 2020).

Informed Consent Statement: Informed consent was obtained from all subjects involved in the study.

Data Availability Statement: The data underlying this article cannot be shared publicly due to the privacy of the individuals that participated in the study. The data will be shared on reasonable request to the corresponding author.

Acknowledgments: We thank Adriana Olivares, Marta Lovagnini, and Riccardo Sideri for their work as data managers.

Conflicts of Interest: The authors declare no conflict of interest.

References

1. Gressens, S.B.; Leftheriotis, G.; Dussaule, J.C.; Flamant, M.; Levy, B.I.; Vidal-Petiot, E. Controversial Roles of the Renin Angiotensin System and Its Modulators during the COVID-19 Pandemic. *Front. Physiol.* **2021**, *12*, 624052. [CrossRef]
2. Angeli, F.; Zappa, M.; Reboldi, G.; Trapasso, M.; Cavallini, C.; Spanevello, A.; Verdecchia, P. The pivotal link between ACE2 deficiency and SARS-CoV-2 infection: One year later. *Eur. J. Intern. Med.* **2021**, *93*, 28–34. [CrossRef]
3. Verdecchia, P.; Cavallini, C.; Spanevello, A.; Angeli, F. The pivotal link between ACE2 deficiency and SARS-CoV-2 infection. *Eur. J. Intern. Med.* **2020**, *76*, 14–20. [CrossRef] [PubMed]
4. Verdecchia, P.; Cavallini, C.; Spanevello, A.; Angeli, F. COVID-19: ACE2centric Infective Disease? *Hypertension* **2020**, *76*, 294–299. [CrossRef] [PubMed]
5. Angeli, F.; Verdecchia, P.; Reboldi, G. Pharmacotherapy for hypertensive urgency and emergency in COVID-19 patients. *Expert Opin. Pharmacother.* **2021**, 1–8. [CrossRef] [PubMed]
6. Mehra, M.R.; Desai, S.S.; Kuy, S.; Henry, T.D.; Patel, A.N. Cardiovascular Disease, Drug Therapy, and Mortality in COVID-19. *N. Engl. J. Med.* **2020**, *382*, e102. [CrossRef] [PubMed]
7. Zhang, P.; Zhu, L.; Cai, J.; Lei, F.; Qin, J.J.; Xie, J.; Liu, Y.M.; Zhao, Y.C.; Huang, X.; Lin, L.; et al. Association of Inpatient Use of Angiotensin-Converting Enzyme Inhibitors and Angiotensin II Receptor Blockers With Mortality Among Patients With Hypertension Hospitalized With COVID-19. *Circ. Res.* **2020**, *126*, 1671–1681. [CrossRef] [PubMed]
8. Angeli, F.; Bachetti, T.; Maugeri Study Group. Temporal changes in co-morbidities and mortality in patients hospitalized for COVID-19 in Italy. *Eur. J. Intern. Med.* **2020**, *82*, 123–125. [CrossRef]
9. Angeli, F.; Marazzato, J.; Verdecchia, P.; Balestrino, A.; Bruschi, C.; Ceriana, P.; Chiovato, L.; Dalla Vecchia, L.A.; De Ponti, R.; Fanfulla, F.; et al. Joint effect of heart failure and coronary artery disease on the risk of death during hospitalization for COVID-19. *Eur. J. Intern. Med.* **2021**, *89*, 81–86. [CrossRef]
10. Li, T. Diagnosis and clinical management of severe acute respiratory syndrome Coronavirus 2 (SARS-CoV-2) infection: An operational recommendation of Peking Union Medical College Hospital (V2.0). *Emerg. Microbes Infect.* **2020**, *9*, 582–585. [CrossRef]
11. Cosentino, F.; Grant, P.J.; Aboyans, V.; Bailey, C.J.; Ceriello, A.; Delgado, V.; Federici, M.; Filippatos, G.; Grobbee, D.E.; Hansen, T.B.; et al. 2019 ESC Guidelines on diabetes, pre-diabetes, and cardiovascular diseases developed in collaboration with the EASD. *Eur. Heart J.* **2020**, *41*, 255–323. [CrossRef]
12. Knuuti, J.; Wijns, W.; Saraste, A.; Capodanno, D.; Barbato, E.; Funck-Brentano, C.; Prescott, E.; Storey, R.F.; Deaton, C.; Cuisset, T.; et al. 2019 ESC Guidelines for the diagnosis and management of chronic coronary syndromes. *Eur. Heart J.* **2020**, *41*, 407–477. [CrossRef]
13. Piepoli, M.F.; Hoes, A.W.; Agewall, S.; Albus, C.; Brotons, C.; Catapano, A.L.; Cooney, M.T.; Corra, U.; Cosyns, B.; Deaton, C.; et al. 2016 European Guidelines on cardiovascular disease prevention in clinical practice: The Sixth Joint Task Force of the European Society of Cardiology and Other Societies on Cardiovascular Disease Prevention in Clinical Practice (constituted by representatives of 10 societies and by invited experts)Developed with the special contribution of the European Association for Cardiovascular Prevention & Rehabilitation (EACPR). *Eur. Heart J.* **2016**, *37*, 2315–2381.
14. Verdecchia, P.; Reboldi, G.; Angeli, F. The 2020 International Society of Hypertension global hypertension practice guidelines-key messages and clinical considerations. *Eur. J. Intern. Med.* **2020**, *82*, 1–6. [CrossRef]
15. Zhou, F.; Yu, T.; Du, R.; Fan, G.; Liu, Y.; Liu, Z.; Xiang, J.; Wang, Y.; Song, B.; Gu, X.; et al. Clinical course and risk factors for mortality of adult inpatients with COVID-19 in Wuhan, China: A retrospective cohort study. *Lancet* **2020**, *395*, 1054–1062. [CrossRef]

16. Iaccarino, G.; Grassi, G.; Borghi, C.; Ferri, C.; Salvetti, M.; Volpe, M. Investigators, Age and Multimorbidity Predict Death among COVID-19 Patients: Results of the SARS-RAS Study of the Italian Society of Hypertension. *Hypertension* **2020**, *76*, 366–372. [CrossRef] [PubMed]
17. Izcovich, A.; Ragusa, M.A.; Tortosa, F.; Lavena Marzio, M.A.; Agnoletti, C.; Bengolea, A.; Ceirano, A.; Espinosa, F.; Saavedra, E.; Sanguine, V.; et al. Prognostic factors for severity and mortality in patients infected with COVID-19: A systematic review. *PLoS ONE* **2020**, *15*, e0241955. [CrossRef]
18. Peng, Y.; Meng, K.; He, M.; Zhu, R.; Guan, H.; Ke, Z.; Leng, L.; Wang, X.; Liu, B.; Hu, C.; et al. Clinical Characteristics and Prognosis of 244 Cardiovascular Patients Suffering From Coronavirus Disease in Wuhan, China. *J. Am. Heart Assoc.* **2020**, *9*, e016796. [CrossRef] [PubMed]
19. Centers for Disease Control and Prevention. Science Brief: Evidence Used to Update the List of Underlying Medical Conditions that Increase a Person's Risk of Severe Illness from COVID-19. Available online: https://www.cdc.gov/coronavirus/2019-ncov/science/science-briefs/underlying-evidence-table.html (accessed on 15 May 2021).
20. Taneri, P.E.; Gómez-Ochoa, S.A.; Llanaj, E.; Raguindin, P.F.; Rojas, L.Z.; Roa-Díaz, Z.M.; Salvador, D.; Groothof, D.; Minder, B.; Kopp-Heim, D.; et al. Anemia and iron metabolism in COVID-19: A systematic review and meta-analysis. *Eur. J. Epidemiol.* **2020**, *35*, 763–773. [CrossRef] [PubMed]
21. Baral, R.; Tsampasian, V.; Debski, M.; Moran, B.; Garg, P.; Clark, A.; Vassiliou, V.S. Association Between Renin-Angiotensin-Aldosterone System Inhibitors and Clinical Outcomes in Patients With COVID-19: A Systematic Review and Meta-analysis. *JAMA Netw. Open* **2021**, *4*, e213594. [CrossRef] [PubMed]
22. Bavishi, C.; Maddox, T.M.; Messerli, F.H. Coronavirus Disease 2019 (COVID-19) Infection and Renin Angiotensin System Blockers. *JAMA Cardiol.* **2020**, *5*, 745–747. [CrossRef] [PubMed]
23. Conversano, A.; Melillo, F.; Napolano, A.; Fominskiy, E.; Spessot, M.; Ciceri, F.; Agricola, E. Renin-Angiotensin-Aldosterone System inhibitors and outcome in patients with SARS-CoV-2 pneumonia. A case series study. *Hypertension* **2020**, *76*, e10–e12. [CrossRef] [PubMed]
24. Danser, A.H.J.; Epstein, M.; Batlle, D. Renin-Angiotensin System Blockers and the COVID-19 Pandemic: At Present There Is No Evidence to Abandon Renin-Angiotensin System Blockers. *Hypertension* **2020**, *75*, 1382–1385. [CrossRef]
25. Esler, M.; Esler, D. Can angiotensin receptor-blocking drugs perhaps be harmful in the COVID-19 pandemic? *J. Hypertens.* **2020**, *38*, 1–2. [CrossRef]
26. Kjeldsen, S.E.; Narkiewicz, K.; Burnier, M.; Oparil, S. Potential protective effects of antihypertensive treatments during the COVID-19 pandemic: From inhibitors of the renin-angiotensin system to beta-adrenergic receptor blockers. *Blood Press* **2021**, *30*, 1–3. [CrossRef] [PubMed]
27. Mehta, N.; Kalra, A.; Nowacki, A.S.; Anjewierden, S.; Han, Z.; Bhat, P.; Carmona-Rubio, A.E.; Jacob, M.; Procop, G.W.; Harrington, S.; et al. Association of Use of Angiotensin-Converting Enzyme Inhibitors and Angiotensin II Receptor Blockers With Testing Positive for Coronavirus Disease 2019 (COVID-19). *JAMA Cardiol.* **2020**, *5*, 1020–1026. [CrossRef] [PubMed]
28. Reynolds, H.R.; Adhikari, S.; Pulgarin, C.; Troxel, A.B.; Iturrate, E.; Johnson, S.B.; Hausvater, A.; Newman, J.D.; Berger, J.S.; Bangalore, S.; et al. Renin-Angiotensin-Aldosterone System Inhibitors and Risk of COVID-19. *N. Engl. J. Med.* **2020**, *382*, 2441–2448. [CrossRef]
29. Richardson, S.; Hirsch, J.S.; Narasimhan, M.; Crawford, J.M.; McGinn, T.; Davidson, K.W.; Barnaby, D.P.; Becker, L.B.; Chelico, J.D.; Cohen, S.L.; et al. Presenting Characteristics, Comorbidities, and Outcomes Among 5700 Patients Hospitalized With COVID-19 in the New York City Area. *JAMA* **2020**, *323*, 2052–2059. [CrossRef] [PubMed]
30. Lahens, A.; Mullaert, J.; Gressens, S.; Gault, N.; Flamant, M.; Deconinck, L.; Joly, V.; Yazdanpanah, Y.; Lescure, F.X.; Vidal-Petiot, E. Association between renin-angiotensin-aldosterone system blockers and outcome in coronavirus disease 2019: Analysing in-hospital exposure generates a biased seemingly protective effect of treatment. *J. Hypertens.* **2021**, *39*, 367–375. [CrossRef]
31. Angeli, F.; Reboldi, G.; Spanevello, A.; De Ponti, R.; Visca, D.; Marazzato, J.; Zappa, M.; Trapasso, M.; Masnaghetti, S.; Fabbri, L.M.; et al. Electrocardiographic features of patients with COVID-19: One year of unexpected manifestations. *Eur. J. Intern. Med.* **2022**, *95*, 7–12. [CrossRef]
32. Angeli, F.; Spanevello, A.; De Ponti, R.; Visca, D.; Marazzato, J.; Palmiotto, G.; Feci, D.; Reboldi, G.; Fabbri, L.M.; Verdecchia, P. Electrocardiographic features of patients with COVID-19 pneumonia. *Eur. J. Intern. Med.* **2020**, *78*, 101–106. [CrossRef]
33. Verdecchia, P.; Angeli, F.; Reboldi, G. Angiotensin-converting enzyme inhibitors, angiotensin II receptor blockers and coronavirus. *J. Hypertens.* **2020**, *38*, 1190–1191. [CrossRef]
34. Mongelli, A.; Barbi, V.; Gottardi Zamperla, M.; Atlante, S.; Forleo, L.; Nesta, M.; Massetti, M.; Pontecorvi, A.; Nanni, S.; Farsetti, A.; et al. Evidence for Biological Age Acceleration and Telomere Shortening in COVID-19 Survivors. *Int. J. Mol. Sci.* **2021**, *22*, 6151. [CrossRef]
35. Ferrario, C.M.; Jessup, J.; Chappell, M.C.; Averill, D.B.; Brosnihan, K.B.; Tallant, E.A.; Diz, D.I.; Gallagher, P.E. Effect of angiotensin-converting enzyme inhibition and angiotensin II receptor blockers on cardiac angiotensin-converting enzyme 2. *Circulation* **2005**, *111*, 2605–2610. [CrossRef] [PubMed]
36. Ishiyama, Y.; Gallagher, P.E.; Averill, D.B.; Tallant, E.A.; Brosnihan, K.B.; Ferrario, C.M. Upregulation of angiotensin-converting enzyme 2 after myocardial infarction by blockade of angiotensin II receptors. *Hypertension* **2004**, *43*, 970–976. [CrossRef]

37. Karram, T.; Abbasi, A.; Keidar, S.; Golomb, E.; Hochberg, I.; Winaver, J.; Hoffman, A.; Abassi, Z. Effects of spironolactone and eprosartan on cardiac remodeling and angiotensin-converting enzyme isoforms in rats with experimental heart failure. *Am. J. Physiol. Heart Circ. Physiol.* **2005**, *289*, H1351–H1358. [CrossRef]
38. Ocaranza, M.P.; Godoy, I.; Jalil, J.E.; Varas, M.; Collantes, P.; Pinto, M.; Roman, M.; Ramirez, C.; Copaja, M.; Diaz-Araya, G.; et al. Enalapril attenuates downregulation of Angiotensin-converting enzyme 2 in the late phase of ventricular dysfunction in myocardial infarcted rat. *Hypertension* **2006**, *48*, 572–578. [CrossRef] [PubMed]
39. Kreutz, R.; Algharably, E.A.E.H.; Azizi, M.; Dobrowolski, P.; Guzik, T.; Januszewicz, A.; Persu, A.; Prejbisz, A.; Riemer, T.G.; Wang, J.G.; et al. Hypertension, the renin-angiotensin system, and the risk of lower respiratory tract infections and lung injury: Implications for COVID-19. *Cardiovasc. Res.* **2020**, *116*, 1688–1699. [CrossRef] [PubMed]
40. Sharma, R.K.; Stevens, B.R.; Obukhov, A.G.; Grant, M.B.; Oudit, G.Y.; Li, Q.; Richards, E.M.; Pepine, C.J.; Raizada, M.K. ACE2 (Angiotensin-Converting Enzyme 2) in Cardiopulmonary Diseases: Ramifications for the Control of SARS-CoV-2. *Hypertension* **2020**, *76*, 651–661. [CrossRef]
41. Angeli, F.; Reboldi, G.; Verdecchia, P. Ageing, ACE2 deficiency and bad outcome in COVID-19. *Clin. Chem. Lab. Med.* **2021**, *59*, 1607–1609. [CrossRef]
42. Angeli, F.; Reboldi, G.; Verdecchia, P. SARS-CoV-2 infection and ACE2 inhibition. *J. Hypertens.* **2021**, *39*, 1555–1558. [CrossRef]
43. Angeli, F.; Reboldi, G.; Trapasso, M.; Verdecchia, P. Hypertension after COVID-19 vaccination. *G. Ital. Cardiol.* **2022**, *23*, 10–14.
44. Verdecchia, P.; Reboldi, G.; Cavallini, C.; Mazzotta, G.; Angeli, F. ACE-inhibitors, angiotensin receptor blockers and severe acute respiratory syndrome caused by coronavirus. *G. Ital. Cardiol.* **2020**, *21*, 321–327.
45. Angeli, F.; Verdecchia, P.; Reboldi, G. RAAS Inhibitors and Risk of COVID-19. *N. Engl. J. Med.* **2020**, *383*, 1990–1991.
46. Wu, L.; Iwai, M.; Nakagami, H.; Chen, R.; Suzuki, J.; Akishita, M.; de Gasparo, M.; Horiuchi, M. Effect of angiotensin II type 1 receptor blockade on cardiac remodeling in angiotensin II type 2 receptor null mice. *Arterioscler. Thromb. Vasc. Biol.* **2002**, *22*, 49–54. [CrossRef]
47. Wu, L.; Iwai, M.; Nakagami, H.; Li, Z.; Chen, R.; Suzuki, J.; Akishita, M.; de Gasparo, M.; Horiuchi, M. Roles of angiotensin II type 2 receptor stimulation associated with selective angiotensin II type 1 receptor blockade with valsartan in the improvement of inflammation-induced vascular injury. *Circulation* **2001**, *104*, 2716–2721. [CrossRef] [PubMed]
48. De Gasparo, M.; Catt, K.J.; Inagami, T.; Wright, J.W.; Unger, T. International union of pharmacology. XXIII. The angiotensin II receptors. *Pharmacol. Rev.* **2000**, *52*, 415–472.
49. Horiuchi, M.; Akishita, M.; Dzau, V.J. Recent progress in angiotensin II type 2 receptor research in the cardiovascular system. *Hypertension* **1999**, *33*, 613–621. [CrossRef]
50. Ran, J.; Song, Y.; Zhuang, Z.; Han, L.; Zhao, S.; Cao, P.; Geng, Y.; Xu, L.; Qin, J.; He, D.; et al. Blood pressure control and adverse outcomes of COVID-19 infection in patients with concomitant hypertension in Wuhan, China. *Hypertens. Res.* **2020**, *43*, 1267–1276. [CrossRef]

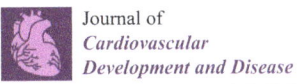

Review

Advances in the Treatment Strategies in Hypertension: Present and Future

Paolo Verdecchia [1,2,*], Claudio Cavallini [2] and Fabio Angeli [3,4]

1. Fondazione Umbra Cuore e Ipertensione-ONLUS, 06100 Perugia, Italy
2. Division of Cardiology, Hospital S. Maria della Misericordia, 06100 Perugia, Italy; claudio.cavallini@ospedale.perugia.it
3. Department of Medicine and Surgery, University of Insubria, 21100 Varese, Italy; fabio.angeli@uninsubria.it
4. Department of Medicine and Cardiopulmonary Rehabilitation, Istituti Clinici Scientifici Maugeri—IRCCS of Tradate, 21049 Tradate, Italy
* Correspondence: verdecchiapaolo@gmail.com

Abstract: Hypertension is the most frequent chronic and non-communicable disease all over the world, with about 1.5 billion affected individuals worldwide. Its impact is currently growing, particularly in low-income countries. Even in high-income countries, hypertension remains largely underdiagnosed and undertreated, with consequent low rates of blood pressure (BP) control. Notwithstanding the large number of clinical observational studies and randomized trials over the past four decades, it is sad to note that in the last few years there has been an impressive paucity of innovative studies. Research focused on BP mechanisms and novel antihypertensive drugs is slowing dramatically. The present review discusses some advances in the management of hypertensive patients, and could play a clinical role in the years to come. First, digital/health technology is expected to be increasingly used, although some crucial points remain (development of non-intrusive and clinically validated devices for ambulatory BP measurement, robust storing systems enabling rapid analysis of accrued data, physician-patient interactions, etc.). Second, several areas should be better outlined with regard to BP diagnosis and treatment targets. Third, from a therapeutic standpoint, existing antihypertensive drugs, which are generally effective and well tolerated, should be better used by exploiting available and novel free and fixed combinations. In particular, spironolactone and other mineral-corticoid receptor antagonists should be used more frequently to improve BP control. In particular, some drugs initially developed for conditions different from hypertension including heart failure and diabetes have demonstrated to lower BP significantly and should therefore be considered. Finally, renal artery denervation is another procedure that has proven effective in the management of hypertension.

Keywords: hypertension; antihypertensive therapy; renal denervation; diabetes; heart failure; chronic disease

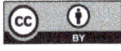

1. Introduction

Because of its high prevalence and important clinical impact, hypertension remains a leading contributor to the risk of cardiovascular disease and death [1–4]. In 2015, about 1.5 billion adults worldwide had a measured office blood pressure (BP) higher than 140 mmHg systolic or 90 mmHg diastolic [5]. According to a recent study, the number of subjects aged 30–79 years with a prior diagnosis of hypertension doubled from 331 million women and 317 million men in 1990 to 626 million women and 652 million men in 2019, despite a stable age-standardized prevalence worldwide [6]. It has been estimated that a systolic BP $\geq$ 140 mmHg explains about 70% of the burden of morbidity and mortality worldwide [7–9].

Despite such impressive growth, the proportion of treated hypertensive subjects with normal BP ('controlled hypertension') remains very low worldwide. It has been estimated that such a proportion approaches 23% in women and 18% in men [6]. Notably, despite an improvement in diagnosis, treatment, and control of hypertension in most developed and high-income countries, important disparities around the world remain. About two-thirds of patients with hypertension actually live in low-income countries [1,10]. Over the past 20 years, there have been no improvements in hypertension awareness, treatment, and control in several countries in sub-Saharan Africa and Oceania [6,11–13].

Thus, a first basic consideration is that, although the prevalence and clinical impact of arterial hypertension is consistently growing worldwide, its control remains disappointing, particularly in low-income countries.

A second consideration is that, despite the huge number of observational studies and randomized controlled trials completed over the past four decades, the last few years have been characterized by an impressive paucity of innovative studies. In a comprehensive review, Dzau noted that research on new antihypertensive drugs and therapeutic targets is slowing dramatically [14]. In addition, there has been no recent attempt to develop clinical applications based on the several genomic polymorphisms associated with hypertension [14]. It should be considered that the time lag between initial discovery and the marketing of a new antihypertensive drug may exceed 10 years, with a consequent final cost greater than two billion US dollars [15,16]. Within this framework, industry is directing most efforts to maximize the utilization of old and effective antihypertensive drugs (e.g., development of new combinations, new dosages, etc.) and to redirect these toward hypertension through the use of BP-lowering drugs, initially developed for different diseases (e.g., gliflozines, drugs for heart failure, etc.) [16].

The current review aims to discuss the main trends and perspectives related to the clinical diagnosis and treatment of hypertension over a foreseeable future. More specifically, our review describes the use of new blood-pressure lowering drugs and device-based approaches to achieve better blood pressure control rates and improve cardiovascular outcomes in patients with hypertension are also reviewed. In other words, we offer clinicians some answers to the following question: "what will the management of hypertensive patients be like in 2030?"

2. Digital/Health Technology for Diagnosis and Monitoring

Owing to the refinement of digital/health technology, the marketing of electronic devices for remote BP measurement and transmission is growing. Theoretically, these devices have the potential to improve the diagnosis of hypertension and the achievement of an adequate BP control at the population level. Just to create a parallel with diabetes, Dzau noted in his review that the number of apps for diabetes management was about 1800 in 2016, with an impressive increase in digital diabetes marketing [14]. There is no reason why this growth should not apply to the hypertension field in the near future, although the growth of devices and apps for hypertension seems to be much less explosive than that of the management of diabetes [14].

Unfortunately, not all BP measurement devices on the market have been appropriately validated according to existing guidelines [17,18] and some of those show some limitations and shortcomings [14]. Particular attention is being devoted to cuff-less continuous BP monitoring systems as alternative to current cuff-based systems, although their validity and reliability are still under research [14,19–21]. We believe that some steps are critical to make a new system reliable:

1. The system should be easily wearable, cheap, and non-intrusive. Systems included in normal smartwatches would be ideal;
2. The system should be validated for accuracy at independent academic or hospital centers. It should allow continuous or almost-continuous BP detection over prolonged periods of time of months or even years;
3. The system should be connectable to an easy-to-use protected digital repository, with software allowing easy BP retrieval over variable periods of time for calculation of appropriate statistical measures (BP averages, variability, etc.) and attached graphics;

4. The system should be easily accessible to doctors, thereby enabling rapid check and response for patients and the suggestion of changes in drug treatment or other measures;
5. Clinical research should urgently identify BP measures retrievable from the system which are more appropriate for the prediction of organ damage and, hopefully, prognosis. In other words, research should identify which BP measurements obtained by the system are more important for clinical decisions.

It is hoped that the application of artificial intelligence to these databases, which are expected to include many different types of biological data for each patient, may help doctors and patients in identifying better strategies for hypertension control, possibly in combination with strategies promoting a healthier diet, better physical activity, and a more intelligent use of drugs. The growing use of 'tele-medicine' during the current COVID pandemic should be extended to the management of hypertension. However, there still a long way to go.

3. Definition of Hypertension and Establishment of Treatment Targets

Whereas the European Society of Cardiology and the European Society of Hypertension (ESC/ESH) define hypertension by office BP levels ≥140 mmHg systolic or 90 mmHg diastolic, [22] the American Heart Association (AHA), the American College of Cardiology (ACC) and other scientific societies have endorsed a more 'aggressive' definition based on office BP values ≥130 mmHg systolic or 80 mmHg diastolic [23]. In addition, the International Society of Hypertension (ISH) adopted the 140/90 mmHg definition [24].

Of note, the more aggressive diagnostic targets endorsed by the US guidelines [23] do no imply that all subjects with office BP in the range of 130–139/80–89 mmHg require drug treatment. Instead, the AHA/ACC guidelines suggest to apply more appropriate life-style measures (weight control, smoking cessation, low-sodium diet, etc.) for these subjects, and to reserve drug treatment for cases of inefficacy of non-pharmacologic measures.

Notably, all guidelines share the recommendation that drug treatment should be started immediately for:
(a) Patients with office BP ≥ 160/100 mmHg regardless of other considerations [22–24];
(b) Patients with BP ≥ 140/90 mmHg in the presence of ischemic heart disease, cerebrovascular disease, or heart failure [22–24].

All guidelines suggest that drug treatment should be initiated, regardless of other considerations, in patients with BP persistently ≥ 140/90 mmHg in case of inefficacy of life-style measures [22–24].

In the case of a BP between 130/80 and 140/90 mmHg, the AHA/AHA guidelines recommend drug treatment in patients with overt cardiovascular disease (i.e., secondary prevention), as well as in patients without overt cardiovascular disease (i.e., primary prevention) if their 10-year risk of cardiovascular disease is ≥10% according to the ASCVD calculator [23].

Available guidelines provide different recommendations in terms of BP targets and definitions of BP control. The ISH and the ESC/ESH guidelines recommend a uniform BP target (<140/90 mmHg), and individualized targets based on age, tolerability, and comorbidities. Conversely, the AHA/ACC guidelines recommend an identical BP target (<130/80 mmHg) in all patients, regardless of age and comorbidities. The potential advantages and disadvantages of these different approaches have been discussed in detail [25–27].

Interestingly, the recent 2021 ESC Guidelines on Cardiovascular Prevention [28] introduce the concept that BP targets lower that 130/80 mmHg are always acceptable when a treatment is well tolerated. Such a statement contrasts with prior ESC/ESH guidelines which state that, for safety reasons, systolic BP should not be targeted below 120 mmHg in people younger than 65 years, or below 130 mmHg in older subjects [22].

In summary, hypertension guidelines seem to be oriented towards individualized BP targets according to the general principle that the lowest well-tolerated BP target should be a reasonable target, with the main goal to prevent the most closely BP-related adverse complication of hypertension, which include stroke and heart failure [29].

4. Life-Style Measures

Although frequently not utilized by many patients, life-style measures play a pivotal role in BP control. These measures include weight reduction for overweight or obese subjects, a low sodium diet, smoking cessation, alcohol and caffeine limitations, and regular physical activity [22,23]. We should not neglect of dismiss the importance of these measures in the future management of hypertensive patients.

5. Chronotherapy

Many studies conducted at independent centers have demonstrated beyond any reasonable doubt the overwhelming prognostic impact of nighttime BP [30–32]. On this basis, it has been thought that using antihypertensive drugs in the evening at bedtime, instead of in the morning, could be preferable to control BP, prevent or regress organ damage, and reduce cardiovascular risk. Indeed, some data from a Spanish research group suggested that evening administration could reduce the incidence of major cardiovascular events associated with hypertension [33,34]. However, these data have been harshly criticized for supposed implausibility [35,36]. Other studies have failed to demonstrate a difference between morning and evening administration of antihypertensive drugs in terms of BP control [37,38]. A large randomized study, the TIME study, is underway to provide a final answer to this question [39].

For the time being, it seems reasonable to advise combining morning and evening administration of antihypertensive drugs in selected patients with severe or resistant hypertension, as well as in those with particularly high nighttime BP. Preference should be given to antihypertensive drugs with a long duration of action, capable of covering the entire 24-h period. For example, when choosing among different diuretics, chlorthalidone appears to be the agent of first choice in patients without severe renal failure [40,41]. In a recent study, patients with renal failure (glomerular filtration rate between 15 and 29 mL/min/1.73 m^2 of body surface area) and uncontrolled hypertension were randomized to chlorthalidone or placebo, with the randomization stratified by prior use of loop diuretics. After 12 weeks of treatment, average 24-h systolic BP was 10.5 mmHg lower in the chlorthalidone group than in the placebo group ($p < 0.001$) [42].

6. More Frequent Use of Mineral-Corticoid Receptor Antagonists

In a double-blind, placebo-controlled, within-patient trial (PATHWAY-2) [43], 335 patients with home systolic BP > 130 mmHg, despite maximal therapy, were randomly assigned to receive, for 12 weeks, spironolactone (25–50 mg), bisoprolol (5–10 mg), doxazosin modified release (4–8 mg), and placebo in addition to their baseline BP drugs [43]. Spironolactone reduced home systolic BP more than placebo (−8.7 mm Hg), doxazosin (−4.03 mmHg), and bisoprolol (−4.48 mmHg) [43]. Thus, spironolactone was the most effective antihypertensive agent, regardless of the distribution of baseline plasma renin, although its BP-lowering effect was predicted by plasma renin activity and the aldosterone-renin ratio [44]. Spironolactone reduced thoracic fluid content, differently from the comparative drugs [44].

In a run-out sub-study of PATWAY-2, amiloride, a distal tubular diuretic that inhibits the epithelial sodium channel sensitive to spironolactone, exerted an antihypertensive effect similar to that of spironolactone and was superior to placebo, doxazosin, and bisoprolol [44]. Notably, amiloride lacks the antiandrogen effect of spironolactone, thereby avoiding gynecomastia.

Eplerenone seems to possess a better safety profile than spironolactone and, thus, it might be an alternative to the latter [45,46]. However, hyperkalemia is an adverse effect of mineral-corticoid receptor antagonists that should be carefully considered in patients treated with these drugs.

Anti-aldosterone drugs are currently recommended in patients with resistant hypertension [22,23,47]. It is reasonable to imagine that these drugs will be used more frequently in the future.

7. Endothelin Receptor Antagonists

Endothelin regulates vascular tone and BP, producing a powerful vasoconstrictor effect and contributing to the pathogenesis of hypertension [48,49]. It causes neurohormonal and sympathetic activation, hypertensive end-organ damage, fibrosis, endothelial dysfunction, and increased aldosterone synthesis and secretion [48,49].

Furthermore, endothelin-1 (ET-1, the biologically predominant member of the endothelin peptide family) is an endothelial cell-derived peptide with a wide variety of developmental and physiological functions, which include embryogenesis and nociception [50,51]. More specifically, the endothelin system plays a role in regulating the development of the specific neural crest cell population and its derivatives [51].

Interestingly, aging affects the shift in balance of release and/or activity of endothelium-derived substances, including increased expression, release, and activity of ET-1 [50,52]. The finding that excessive production of ET-1 is present in patients and experimental models of aging [50,52] supports the therapeutic benefits of targeting the endothelin system in elderly hypertensive patients [49]. Finally, the possibility that endothelin receptor antagonists may have a role in the treatment of pre-eclampsia (due to the large increase of endothelin in this condition [53]) is still undetermined.

Based on evidence that endothelin is a very potent endogenous vasoconstrictor [54], some trials have evaluated the antihypertensive efficacy and tolerability of drugs capable to block the endothelin-A and endothelin-B receptors. However, results are quite disappointing and the tolerability of endothelin receptor antagonists remains a concern. Indeed, these drugs may cause some unwanted effects, including fluid retention, flushing, and headache [16], which may limit their use in clinical practice.

Development of darusentan, and endothelin-A blocker, was stopped for safety concerns.

A trial with atrasentan in patients with diabetic nephropathy, was stopped for reasons related to low recruitment, and apparently different from safety.

Aprocinentan, a blocker of both endothelin-A and endothelin-B receptors with a very long pharmacological half-life (about 44 h), proved more effective than placebo and lisinopril [55]. Interestingly, this antihypertensive agent seems to exert additional mechanisms beyond the expected beneficial effects of sustained BP-lowering action (including a decrease in renal vascular resistance and left ventricular hypertrophy) supporting the hypothesis that this new agent could expand our antihypertensive arsenal in resistant hypertension [49,56]. Indeed, aprocitentan in patients with resistant hypertension is currently under investigation in the PRECISION phase III trial (ClinicalTrials identifier: NCT03541174).

8. Neprilysin Combined with Renin-Angiotensin System Inhibition

The heart produces different natriuretic peptides which include the atrial natriuretic peptide, the B-type natriuretic peptide and the C-type natriuretic peptide [57]. These peptides induce potent natriuresis and vasodilation by acting on different cellular receptors, ultimately leading to enhanced intracellular production of cyclic guanil-cyclase [58].

Neprilysin, a zinc endopeptidase, inactivates, not only the cardiac natriuretic peptides, but also bradykinin [59], thereby inducing vasodilatation and natriuresis resulting from a more prolonged action by these agents [59]. Neprilysin was not developed as monotherapy for clinical use, but combined with drugs that inhibit the renin-angiotensin-aldosterone system.

Omepatrilat was the first-in-class combination of naprilysin with an angiotensin-converting-enzyme inhibitor, but its development was abandoned because of occurrence of severe angioedema [60]. In contrast, LCZ696, a more recently developed combination of neprilysin with the angiotensin II receptor blocker valsartan in the same molecule, proved effective and well tolerated in heart failure [61,62] and hypertension [63].

It is reasonable to foresee that LCZ696 will be increasingly used in the future not only in heart failure, but also for improving BP control, particularly in patients with resistant hypertension. Various reasons are currently favoring a preferential development of this drug in patients with heart failure, but the stage is set for a growing role of this drug in the treatment of hypertension [58,64].

9. Angiotensin II Receptor Agonists

Angiotensin II induces vasoconstriction by stimulating the angiotensin 1 receptors, and vasodilatation by stimulating the angiotensin 2 receptors. In experimental and clinical settings, stimulation of angiotensin 2 receptors inhibits fibrosis [65] and induces vasodilatation, natriuresis, and blood pressure reduction [66,67]. Consequently, angiotensin II receptor agonists display an interesting antihypertensive potential and are currently investigated for efficacy and safety [68,69].

10. Sodium-Glucose Cotrasporter-2 Inhibitors

About 97% of glucose secreted at glomerular level is reabsorbed in the proximal renal tubule through the sodium-glucose cotrasporter-2 receptors (SGLT2) [70]. The remaining 3% is reabsorbed by the SGLT1 receptors, also located in the proximal tubule [70]. Inhibition of SGLT2 and SGLT1 receptors results in an increased excretion of glucose with urines with consequent reduction of hemoglobin A1C [70,71].

In pivotal phase III clinical trials, selective SGLT2 receptor inhibitors empagliflozin, canagliflozin, dapagliflozin and ertugliflozin modestly reduced systolic and diastolic BP through various mechanisms which may include natriuresis, osmotic diuresis and reduction of the sympathetic tone [72]. These drugs induced a marked reduction in the risk of heart failure [72]. In patients with heart failure and reduced ejection fraction (HFrEF), both with and without diabetes, empagliflozin and dapagliflozin reduced cardiovascular mortality and the need of re-hospitalizations for heart failure [73,74]. In patients with heart failure with preserved ejection fraction (HFpEF), empagliflozin significantly reduced the risk of cardiovascular death or hospitalization for heart failure by 21% [75].

In the EMPA-REG BP trial, empagliflozin 10 mg and 25 mg reduced 24-h ambulatory BP by 3.44/4.16 mmHg more than placebo and the degree of antihypertensive effect was comparable in the presence of none, one or more than one antihypertensive drug [76].

According to available meta-analyses (Figure 1), the degree of BP reduction induced by SGLT2 receptor antagonists appears to be numerically modest [77–79]. However, these drugs have the advantage of reducing glomerular hyperfiltration through vasoconstriction of the afferent arterioles, thereby reducing proteinuria and progression of kidney disease, with measurable nefroprotective effects in terms of major renal events [80].

Although these drugs are generally well tolerated, concerns have been raised about volume depletion, acute kidney injury, and genital infections as potential adverse effects. The SGLT2 receptor inhibitors have been recently suggested by guidelines as first-line antidiabetic drugs in patients with diabetes at high or very high cardiovascular risk due to organ damage or concomitant risk factors [72]. In the future, the use of these drugs is expected to be more recommended for hypertensive patients with diabetes or heart failure, although their place in subjects with uncomplicated hypertension is still under evaluation.

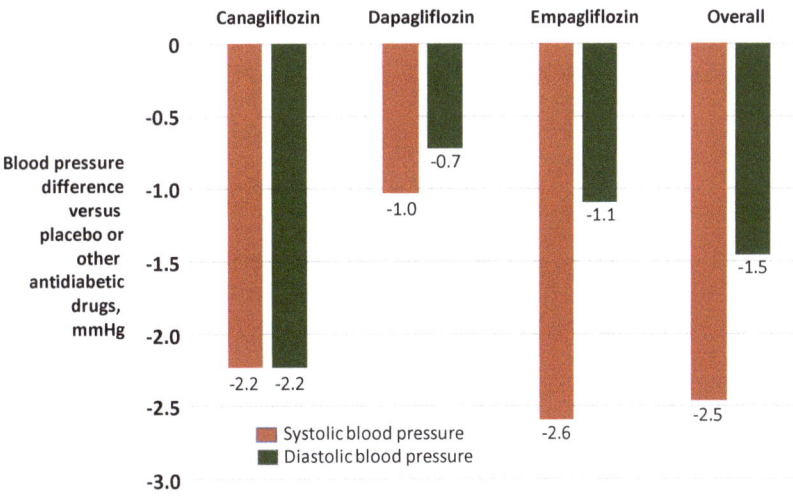

Figure 1. Blood pressure lowering effects of sodium-glucose cotransport-2 inhibitors on blood pressure in patients with diabetes mellitus. Adapted from Mazidi and coworkers [78].

11. Renal Denervation

Renal sympathetic overactivity contributes to the development and progression of hypertension [81–83]. Renal denervation in experimental models of hypertension has been shown to reduce BP and improve renal function, which laid the foundation for its introduction to clinical practice [83,84].

Some clinical trials published over the past 15 years generated many expectations on the clinical utility of renal denervation [85]. Unfortunately, the SIMPLICITY HTN-3 trials failed to demonstrate the superiority of renal denervation over sham control in terms of BP lowering effect [86]. However, the SIMPLICITY HTN-3 trials had several methodological shortcomings. Just to mention some of these limitations, the study erroneously included patients with secondary hypertension (hyperaldosteronism, etc.), 34% of operators had executed only one denervation procedure in the past, drug treatment was much more intense in the 'sham' control group than in the denervation group, denervation was not 'complete' (not all quadrants of renal artery were ablated) in 75% of cases. Thus, the entire issue was reconsidered, with planning and execution of newer better-designed clinical trials, which provided positive results [87–89].

Renal artery denervation has a strong pathophysiological rationale to justify a significant BP lowering effect (Figure 2).

It is well known that sympathetic firing originating from the ganglia located in the central nervous system induces a variety of effects at cardiac, renal, vascular, and muscular levels that ultimately trigger BP elevation. Several mechanistic studies have demonstrated that ablation of efferent and afferent renal nerves is followed by a reduction of the neural 'bursts' of sympathetic activity, detectable by neurography, with parallel reduction in BP [90]. Furthermore, industry produced newer and more effective denervation catheters over the past few years.

In the DENERHTN trial (Figure 3), 106 patients with resistant hypertension were randomized to continue drug treatment with or without renal denervation using radiofrequency. The 'no renal denervation' group did not include a sham procedure. Average 24-h systolic BP at 6 months after the procedure fell by 15.8 mmHg in the denervation group and 9.9 mmHg in the no denervation group ($p = 0.03$) [91].

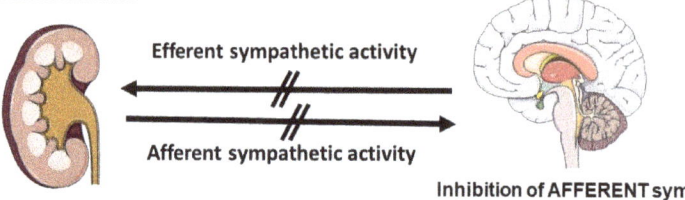

Inhibition of EFFERENT sympathetic activity:
- ✓ ↓ Renal vasoconstriction
- ✓ ↓ Production of renin
- ✓ ↓ Sodium retention

Inhibition of AFFERENT sympathetic activity:
- ✓ ↓ Central sympathetic tone

Figure 2. The main effects of inhibition of afferent and efferent sympathetic activity induced by renal denervation.

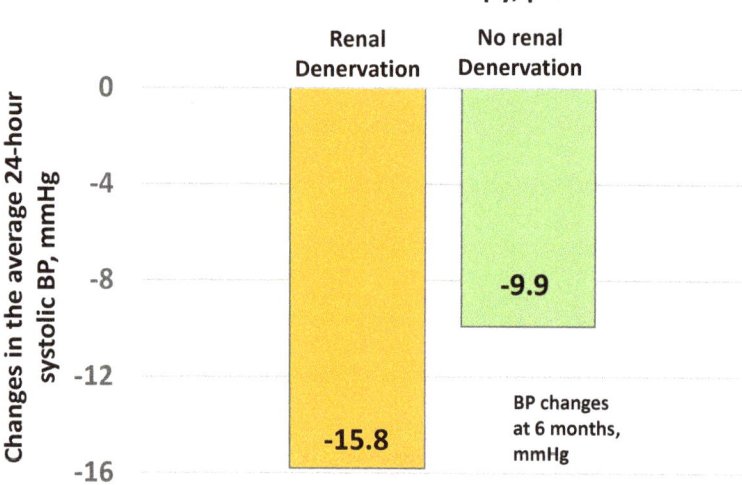

Figure 3. Changes in 24-h systolic BP at 6 months in patients with renal denervation and in a control group not receiving renal denervation. Adapted from Azizi and coworkers [91].

In the SPYRAL HTN-ON MED trial (Figure 4), 80 patients with resistant hypertension were randomized to continue drug treatment with or without (sham procedure) renal denervation using radiofrequency. Average 24-h systolic BP at 6 months after the procedure fell by 9.0 mmHg with renal denervation and only 1.6 mmHg with the sham procedure ($p < 0.05$) [87]. In the SPYRAL HTN-OFF MED Pivotal trial (Figure 4), 331 untreated patients were randomized to a sham procedure or renal denervation using radiofrequency. Average 24-h systolic BP at 3 months after the procedure fell by 4.7 mmHg after renal denervation and by 0.6 mmHg after the sham procedure ($p < 0.05$) [88]. Finally, in the RADIANCE-HTN SOLO (Figure 4), 331 untreated patients were randomized to a Sham procedure or renal denervation using high frequency ultrasounds. Average 24-h systolic BP at 3 months after the procedure fell by 8.5 mmHg after renal denervation and by 2.2 mmHg after the sham procedure ($p < 0.05$) [89]. Overall, these new trials convincingly demonstrated the superiority of renal denervation over the sham procedure in terms of BP reduction at 3 to 6 months.

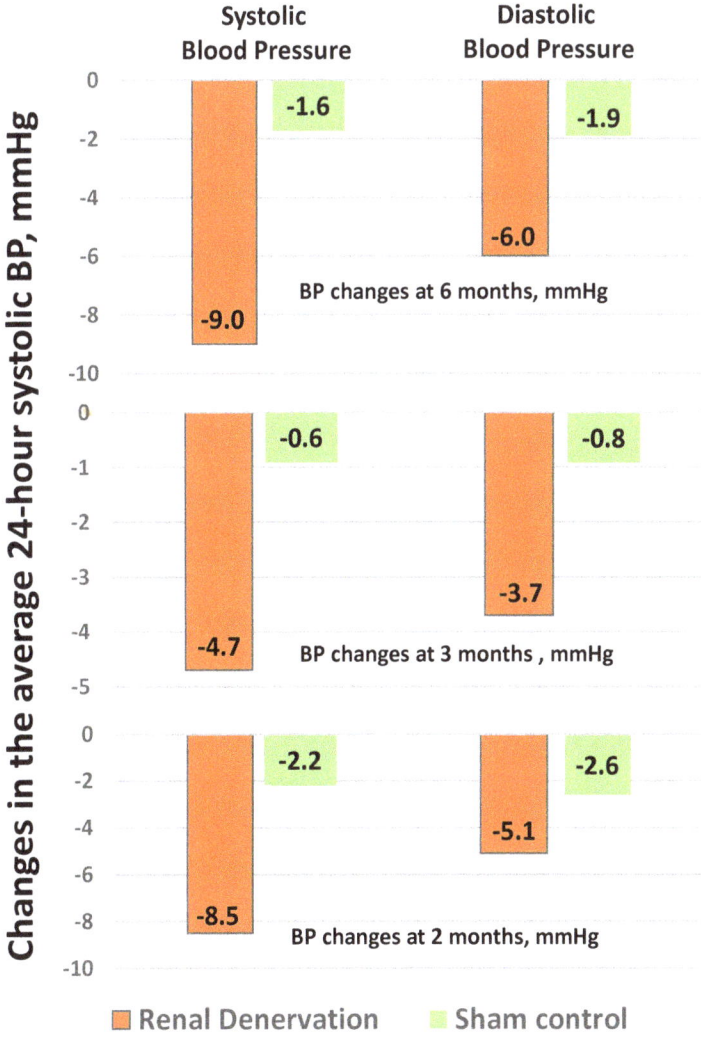

Figure 4. Changes in 24-h systolic BP at different time intervals in patients treated with renal denervation or sham control. Adapted from Azizi and coworkers [87], Bohm and coworkers [88] and Kandzari and coworkers [89].

Concerns remain about the persistence of the antihypertensive effect over the long term. However, encouraging results came from the open and not comparative Global SIMPLICITY Registry (Figure 5), which found no attenuation, or even a slight potentiation, in the antihypertensive effect of renal denervation in the long term (up to three years after the procedure) as compared with pre-procedural levels [92].

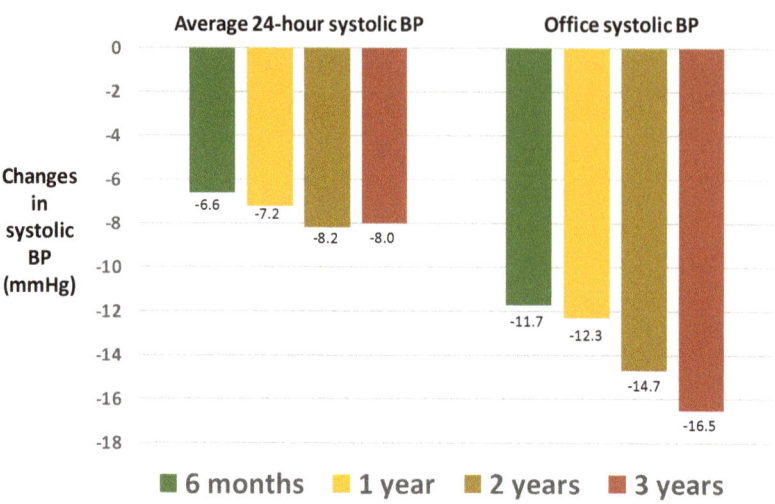

Figure 5. Long-term reduction in systolic BP in the open, non-comparative Global SIMPLICITY Registry. Adapted from Mahfoud and coworkers [89,92].

A clinical trial compared different techniques of denervation and concluded that the ultrasound technique targeted on both main renal artery and its bifurcations was superior to the radiofrequency technique targeted on the main renal artery alone [93].

In conclusion, renal artery denervation has the potential to be further adopted in clinical practice over the next few years. The main contraindication remains renal artery stenosis, which is rare in unselected patients, but relatively higher, up to 30%, in those with more severe or resistant hypertension [94]. Procedural complications of renal denervation (renal artery dissection, post-procedural stenosis) are extremely rare [95].

Ongoing studies should lead to identification of patients more likely to benefit from renal denervation in terms of BP lowering effect. According to a position paper of the Italian Society of Hypertension [95], some clinical conditions (Table 1) should dictate a preferential indication to renal denervation.

Of note, patients with moderate to severe chronic kidney disease were excluded from large international trials, and smaller studies suggest limited utility in this population [96].

Despite the evidence that renal denervation is associated with a low incidence, of mostly, minor complications [94,95,97], an aspect to consider is the question of renal artery stenosis after this procedure. Some anecdotal reports of renal artery stenosis after renal denervation were published, occurring 5–6 months after a successful procedure and leading to a re-elevation of previously depressed BP [98–103].

Thus, when considering renal nerve ablation, arteries with visible stenosis, with calcification or atheromatous plaques, represent relative contraindications [77,78,80].

Finally, available data argue in favor of an incomplete and insufficient ablation of renal sympathetic nerves as a major cause of inadequate BP responses to catheter-based interventions. Indeed, it is not entirely clear whether catheter design and energy delivery may influence the variability of the response to renal nerve ablation and the risk of the development of renal artery stenosis [94,104].

Table 1. Clinical features of patients who may be candidates to renal denervation. Adapted from a position paper of the Italian Society of Hypertension [95].

(A)	Hypertension not controlled by combinations of renin-angiotensin-aldosterone system blockers, diuretics and calcium channel blockers at maximal tolerated dose • Adverse reactions with spironolattone • Low adherence to treatment • Systo-diastolic hypertension • Vascular damage not diffused • High or very high cardiovascular risk • Patient preference
(B)	Essential hypertension stage 1 or 2, either untreated or not controlled with 1–2 drugs • Adverse reaction to several antihypertensive drugs • Low adherence to treatment • High or very high cardiovascular risk • Atrial fibrillation with planned ablation • Patient preference

12. Conclusions

BP is a very potent risk factor. Unfortunately, at variance with other risk factors, such as serum cholesterol, glucose or creatinine, or even body weight or cigarette smoking, BP is extremely variable over time and this may leave uncertainty or even frustration on the real value of what we are measuring. BP recording remains generally intrusive and the precise rules for a correct BP measurement in the clinical practice are scarcely known. Many patients still do not realize that is perfectly normal to find out BP values of 125/70 and 145/85 mmHg at distance of few minutes. Clearly, such imprecision in diagnosis does not help to achieve BP control when needed.

It is hoped that the future will lead to development of accurate and non-intrusive devices for BP measurement in the long-term. From a therapeutic standpoint, we currently dispose of many effective and well tolerated antihypertensive drugs, but a long way is still to do for an optimal use of these drugs, alone or in combination. Unfortunately, research on new antihypertensive drugs dramatically slowed over the past few years. We agree with Bhudia that the future in the management of hypertensive patients remains uncertain [105]. However, significant progress is likely to come over the next few years from a combination of education and technology worldwide.

Author Contributions: Conceptualization, methodology, resources, data curation, writing—original draft preparation, writing—review and editing, visualization, and supervision, P.V., F.A. and C.C. All authors have read and agreed to the published version of the manuscript.

Funding: Study funded in part by the no-profit foundation Fondazione Umbria Cuore e Ipertensione-ONLUS, Perugia, Italy.

Institutional Review Board Statement: Not applicable.

Informed Consent Statement: Not applicable.

Conflicts of Interest: The authors declare no conflict of interest.

References

1. Mills, K.T.; Bundy, J.D.; Kelly, T.N.; Reed, J.E.; Kearney, P.M.; Reynolds, K.; Chen, J.; He, J. Global Disparities of Hypertension Prevalence and Control: A Systematic Analysis of Population-Based Studies From 90 Countries. *Circulation* **2016**, *134*, 441–450. [CrossRef] [PubMed]
2. Verdecchia, P.; Reboldi, G.; Angeli, F.; Trimarco, B.; Mancia, G.; Pogue, J.; Gao, P.; Sleight, P.; Teo, K.; Yusuf, S. Systolic and diastolic blood pressure changes in relation with myocardial infarction and stroke in patients with coronary artery disease. *Hypertension* **2015**, *65*, 108–114. [CrossRef] [PubMed]
3. Reboldi, G.; Angeli, F.; de Simone, G.; Staessen, J.A.; Verdecchia, P.; Cardio-Sis, I. Tight versus standard blood pressure control in patients with hypertension with and without cardiovascular disease. *Hypertension* **2014**, *63*, 475–482. [CrossRef] [PubMed]

4. Angeli, F.; Reboldi, G.; Verdecchia, P. Hypertension, inflammation and atrial fibrillation. *J. Hypertens.* **2014**, *32*, 480–483. [CrossRef] [PubMed]
5. NCD Risk Factor Collaboration (NCD-RisC). Worldwide trends in blood pressure from 1975 to 2015: A pooled analysis of 1479 population-based measurement studies with 19.1 million participants. *Lancet* **2017**, *389*, 37–55. [CrossRef]
6. NCD Risk Factor Collaboration (NCD-RisC). Worldwide trends in hypertension prevalence and progress in treatment and control from 1990 to 2019: A pooled analysis of 1201 population-representative studies with 104 million participants. *Lancet* **2021**, *398*, 957–980. [CrossRef]
7. Forouzanfar, M.H.; Liu, P.; Roth, G.A.; Ng, M.; Biryukov, S.; Marczak, L.; Alexander, L.; Estep, K.; Abate, K.H.; Akinyemiju, T.F.; et al. Global Burden of Hypertension and Systolic Blood Pressure of at Least 110 to 115 mm Hg, 1990–2015. *JAMA* **2017**, *317*, 165–182. [CrossRef]
8. Verdecchia, P.; Angeli, F.; Mazzotta, G.; Garofoli, M.; Reboldi, G. Aggressive blood pressure lowering is dangerous: The J-curve: Con side of the arguement. *Hypertension* **2014**, *63*, 37–40. [CrossRef]
9. de Goma, E.M.; Knowles, J.W.; Angeli, F.; Budoff, M.J.; Rader, D.J. The evolution and refinement of traditional risk factors for cardiovascular disease. *Cardiol. Rev.* **2012**, *20*, 118–129. [CrossRef]
10. Mills, K.T.; Stefanescu, A.; He, J. The global epidemiology of hypertension. *Nat. Rev. Nephrol.* **2020**, *16*, 223–237. [CrossRef]
11. Angeli, F.; Reboldi, G.; Verdecchia, P. "From apennines to andes": Does body mass index affect the relationship between age and blood pressure? *Hypertension* **2012**, *60*, 6–7. [CrossRef] [PubMed]
12. Angeli, F.; Reboldi, G.; Verdecchia, P. Hypertension around the world: New insights from developing countries. *J. Hypertens.* **2013**, *31*, 1358–1361. [CrossRef] [PubMed]
13. Angeli, F.; Reboldi, G.; Verdecchia, P. Modernization and hypertension: Is the link changing? *Hypertens. Res.* **2013**, *36*, 676–678. [CrossRef] [PubMed]
14. Dzau, V.J.; Balatbat, C.A. Future of Hypertension. *Hypertension* **2019**, *74*, 450–457. [CrossRef] [PubMed]
15. DiMasi, J.A.; Grabowski, H.G.; Hansen, R.W. Innovation in the pharmaceutical industry: New estimates of R&D costs. *J. Health Econ.* **2016**, *47*, 20–33. [PubMed]
16. Hunter, P.G.; FChapman, A.; Dhaun, N. Hypertension: Current trends and future perspectives. *Br. J. Clin. Pharmacol.* **2021**, *87*, 3721–3736. [CrossRef] [PubMed]
17. Parati, G.; Stergiou, G.; O'Brien, E.; Asmar, R.; Beilin, L.; Bilo, G.; Clement, D.; de la Sierra, A.; de Leeuw, P.; Dolan, E.; et al. European Society of Hypertension practice guidelines for ambulatory blood pressure monitoring. *J. Hypertens.* **2014**, *32*, 1359–1366. [CrossRef] [PubMed]
18. Stergiou, G.S.; Palatini, P.; Parati, G.; O'Brien, E.; Januszewicz, A.; Lurbe, E.; Persu, A.; Mancia, G.; Kreutz, R.C.; European Society of Hypertension Council and the European Society of Hypertension Working Group on Blood Pressure Monitoring and Cardiovascular Variability. 2021 European Society of Hypertension practice guidelines for office and out-of-office blood pressure measurement. *J. Hypertens.* **2021**, *39*, 1293–1302. [CrossRef] [PubMed]
19. Koren, G.; Nordon, G.; Radinsky, K.; Shalev, V. Machine learning of big data in gaining insight into successful treatment of hypertension. *Pharmacol. Res. Perspect.* **2018**, *6*, e00396. [CrossRef] [PubMed]
20. Madhurantakam, S.; Babu, K.J.; Rayappan, J.B.B.; Krishnan, U.M. Nanotechnology-based electrochemical detection strategies for hypertension markers. *Biosens. Bioelectron.* **2018**, *116*, 67–80. [CrossRef]
21. Park, S.H.; Zhang, Y.; Rogers, J.A.; Gallon, L. Recent advances of biosensors for hypertension and nephrology. *Curr. Opin. Nephrol. Hypertens.* **2019**, *28*, 390–396. [CrossRef] [PubMed]
22. Williams, B.; Mancia, G.; Spiering, W.; Rosei, E.A.; Azizi, M.; Burnier, M.; Clement, D.L.; Coca, A.; de Simone, G.; Dominiczak, A.; et al. Authors/Task Force, 2018 ESC/ESH Guidelines for the management of arterial hypertension: The Task Force for the management of arterial hypertension of the European Society of Cardiology and the European Society of Hypertension: The Task Force for the management of arterial hypertension of the European Society of Cardiology and the European Society of Hypertension. *J. Hypertens.* **2018**, *36*, 1953–2041. [PubMed]
23. Whelton, P.K.; Carey, R.M.; Aronow, W.S.; Casey, D.E., Jr.; Collins, K.J.; Himmelfarb, C.D.; de Palma, S.M.; Gidding, S.; Jamerson, K.A.; Jones, D.W.; et al. 2017 ACC/AHA/AAPA/ABC/ACPM/AGS/APhA/ASH/ASPC/NMA/PCNA Guideline for the Prevention, Detection, Evaluation, and Management of High Blood Pressure in Adults: A Report of the American College of Cardiology/American Heart Association Task Force on Clinical Practice Guidelines. *J. Am. Coll. Cardiol.* **2018**, *71*, e127–e248. [PubMed]
24. Unger, T.; Borghi, C.; Charchar, F.; Khan, N.A.; Poulter, N.R.; Prabhakaran, D.; Ramirez, A.; Schlaich, M.; Stergiou, G.S.; Tomaszewski, M.; et al. 2020 International Society of Hypertension Global Hypertension Practice Guidelines. *Hypertension* **2020**, *75*, 1334–1357. [CrossRef]
25. Angeli, F.; Reboldi, G.; Trapasso, M.; Gentile, G.; Pinzagli, M.G.; Aita, A.; Verdecchia, P. European and US guidelines for arterial hypertension: Similarities and differences. *Eur. J. Intern. Med.* **2019**, *63*, 3–8. [CrossRef]
26. Verdecchia, P.; Angeli, F.; Cavallini, C.; Reboldi, G. Keep Blood Pressure Low, but Not Too Much. *Circ. Res.* **2018**, *123*, 1205–1207. [CrossRef]
27. Verdecchia, P.; Angeli, F. The Seventh Report of the Joint National Committee on the Prevention, Detection, Evaluation and Treatment of High Blood Pressure: The weapons are ready. *Rev. Esp. Cardiol.* **2003**, *56*, 843–847. [CrossRef]

28. Visseren, F.L.J.; Mach, F.; Smulders, Y.M.; Carballo, D.; Koskinas, K.C.; Back, M.; Benetos, A.; Biffi, A.; Boavida, J.M.; Capodanno, D.; et al. 2021 ESC Guidelines on cardiovascular disease prevention in clinical practice. *Eur. Heart J.* **2021**, *42*, 3227–3337. [CrossRef]
29. Verdecchia, P.; Reboldi, G.; Angeli, F. The 2020 International Society of Hypertension global hypertension practice guidelines-key messages and clinical considerations. *Eur. J. Intern. Med.* **2020**, *82*, 1–6. [CrossRef]
30. Tsioufis, C.; Andrikou, I.; Thomopoulos, C.; Syrseloudis, D.; Stergiou, G.; Stefanadis, C. Increased nighttime blood pressure or nondipping profile for prediction of cardiovascular outcomes. *J. Hum. Hypertens.* **2011**, *25*, 281–293. [CrossRef]
31. Verdecchia, P.; Porcellati, C.; Schillaci, G.; Borgioni, C.; Ciucci, A.; Battistelli, M.; Guerrieri, M.; Gatteschi, C.; Zampi, I.; Santucci, A.; et al. Ambulatory blood pressure. An independent predictor of prognosis in essential hypertension. *Hypertension* **1994**, *24*, 793–801. [CrossRef] [PubMed]
32. Yang, W.Y.; Melgarejo, J.D.; Thijs, L.; Zhang, Z.Y.; Boggia, J.; Wei, F.F.; Hansen, T.W.; Asayama, K.; Ohkubo, T.; Jeppesen, J.; et al. Association of Office and Ambulatory Blood Pressure With Mortality and Cardiovascular Outcomes. *JAMA* **2019**, *322*, 409–420. [CrossRef] [PubMed]
33. Hermida, R.C.; Ayala, D.E.; Calvo, C.; Lopez, J.E.; Mojon, A.; Fontao, M.J.; Soler, R.; Fernandez, J.R. Effects of time of day of treatment on ambulatory blood pressure pattern of patients with resistant hypertension. *Hypertension* **2005**, *46*, 1053–1059. [CrossRef] [PubMed]
34. Hermida, R.C.; Ayala, D.E.; Fontao, M.J.; Mojon, A.; Alonso, I.; Fernandez, J.R. Administration-time-dependent effects of spirapril on ambulatory blood pressure in uncomplicated essential hypertension. *Chronobiol. Int.* **2010**, *27*, 560–574. [CrossRef] [PubMed]
35. Guthrie, G.; Poulter, N.; Macdonald, T.; Ford, I.; Mackenzie, I.; Findlay, E.; Williams, B.; Brown, M.; Lang, C.; Webb, D. Chronotherapy in hypertension: The devil is in the details. *Eur. Heart J.* **2020**, *41*, 1606–1607. [CrossRef] [PubMed]
36. Kreutz, R.; Kjeldsen, S.E.; Burnier, M.; Narkiewicz, K.; Oparil, S.; Mancia, G. Blood pressure medication should not be routinely dosed at bedtime. We must disregard the data from the HYGIA project. *Blood Press.* **2020**, *29*, 135–136. [CrossRef] [PubMed]
37. Morgan, T.; Anderson, A.; Jones, E. The effect on 24 h blood pressure control of an angiotensin converting enzyme inhibitor (perindopril) administered in the morning or at night. *J. Hypertens.* **1997**, *15*, 205–211. [CrossRef] [PubMed]
38. Rahman, M.; Greene, T.; Phillips, R.A.; Agodoa, L.Y.; Bakris, G.L.; Charleston, J.; Contreras, G.; Gabbai, F.; Hiremath, L.; Jamerson, K.; et al. A trial of 2 strategies to reduce nocturnal blood pressure in blacks with chronic kidney disease. *Hypertension* **2013**, *61*, 82–88. [CrossRef]
39. Rorie, D.A.; Rogers, A.; Mackenzie, I.S.; Ford, I.; Webb, D.J.; Willams, B.; Brown, M.; Poulter, N.; Findlay, E.; Saywood, W.; et al. Methods of a large prospective, randomised, open-label, blinded end-point study comparing morning versus evening dosing in hypertensive patients: The Treatment In Morning versus Evening (TIME) study. *BMJ Open* **2016**, *6*, e010313. [CrossRef]
40. Kaplan, N.M. Chlorthalidone versus hydrochlorothiazide: A tale of tortoises and a hare. *Hypertension* **2011**, *58*, 994–995. [CrossRef]
41. Kurtz, T.W. Chlorthalidone: Don't call it "thiazide-like" anymore. *Hypertension* **2010**, *56*, 335–337. [CrossRef]
42. Agarwal, R.; ASinha, D.; Cramer, A.E.; Balmes-Fenwick, M.; Dickinson, J.H.; Ouyang, F.; Tu, W. Chlorthalidone for Hypertension in Advanced Chronic Kidney Disease. *N. Engl. J. Med.* **2021**, *385*, 2507–2519. [CrossRef]
43. Williams, B.; MacDonald, T.M.; Morant, S.; Webb, D.J.; Sever, P.; McInnes, G.; Ford, I.; Cruickshank, J.K.; Caulfield, M.J.; Salsbury, J.; et al. Spironolactone versus placebo, bisoprolol, and doxazosin to determine the optimal treatment for drug-resistant hypertension (PATHWAY-2): A randomised, double-blind, crossover trial. *Lancet* **2015**, *386*, 2059–2068. [CrossRef]
44. Williams, B.; MacDonald, T.M.; Morant, S.V.; Webb, D.J.; Sever, P.; McInnes, G.T.; Ford, I.; Cruickshank, J.K.; Caulfield, M.J.; Padmanabhan, S.; et al. Endocrine and haemodynamic changes in resistant hypertension, and blood pressure responses to spironolactone or amiloride: The PATHWAY-2 mechanisms substudies. *Lancet Diabetes Endocrinol.* **2018**, *6*, 464–475. [CrossRef]
45. Struthers, A.; Krum, H.; Williams, G.H. A comparison of the aldosterone-blocking agents eplerenone and spironolactone. *Clin. Cardiol.* **2008**, *31*, 153–158. [CrossRef] [PubMed]
46. Tam, T.S.; Wu, M.H.; Masson, S.C.; Tsang, M.P.; Stabler, S.N.; Kinkade, A.; Tung, A.; Tejani, A.M. Eplerenone for hypertension. *Cochrane Database Syst. Rev.* **2017**, *2*, CD008996. [CrossRef] [PubMed]
47. Carey, R.M.; Calhoun, D.A.; Bakris, G.L.; Brook, R.D.; Daugherty, S.L.; Dennison-Himmelfarb, C.R.; Egan, B.M.; Flack, J.M.; Gidding, S.S.; Judd, E.; et al. Resistant Hypertension: Detection, Evaluation, and Management: A Scientific Statement From the American Heart Association. *Hypertension* **2018**, *72*, e53–e90. [CrossRef]
48. Schiffrin, E.L. Vascular endothelin in hypertension. *Vascul. Pharmacol.* **2005**, *43*, 19–29. [CrossRef]
49. Angeli, F.; Verdecchia, P.; Reboldi, G. Aprocitentan, A Dual Endothelin Receptor Antagonist Under Development for the Treatment of Resistant Hypertension. *Cardiol. Ther.* **2021**, *10*, 397–406. [CrossRef]
50. Barton, M. Aging and endothelin: Determinants of disease. *Life Sci.* **2014**, *118*, 97–109. [CrossRef]
51. Bondurand, N.; Dufour, S.; Pingault, V. News from the endothelin-3/EDNRB signaling pathway: Role during enteric nervous system development and involvement in neural crest-associated disorders. *Dev. Biol.* **2018**, *444* (Suppl. 1), S156–S169. [CrossRef] [PubMed]
52. Goettsch, W.; Lattmann, T.; Amann, K.; Szibor, M.; Morawietz, H.; Munter, K.; Muller, S.P.; Shaw, S.; Barton, M. Increased expression of endothelin-1 and inducible nitric oxide synthase isoform II in aging arteries in vivo: Implications for atherosclerosis. *Biochem. Biophys. Res. Commun.* **2001**, *280*, 908–913. [CrossRef] [PubMed]

53. Verdonk, K.; Saleh, L.; Lankhorst, S.; Smilde, J.E.; van Ingen, M.M.; Garrelds, I.M.; Friesema, E.C.; Russcher, H.; van den Meiracker, A.H.; Visser, W.; et al. Association studies suggest a key role for endothelin-1 in the pathogenesis of preeclampsia and the accompanying renin-angiotensin-aldosterone system suppression. *Hypertension* **2015**, *65*, 1316–1323. [CrossRef] [PubMed]
54. Yanagisawa, M.; Kurihara, H.; Kimura, S.; Tomobe, Y.; Kobayashi, M.; Mitsui, Y.; Yazaki, Y.; Goto, K.; Masaki, T. A novel potent vasoconstrictor peptide produced by vascular endothelial cells. *Nature* **1988**, *332*, 411–415. [CrossRef] [PubMed]
55. Verweij, P.; Danaietash, P.; Flamion, B.; Menard, J.; Bellet, M. Randomized Dose-Response Study of the New Dual Endothelin Receptor Antagonist Aprocitentan in Hypertension. *Hypertension* **2020**, *75*, 956–965. [CrossRef]
56. Trensz, F.; Bortolamiol, C.; Kramberg, M.; Wanner, D.; Hadana, H.; Rey, M.; Strasser, D.S.; Delahaye, S.; Hess, P.; Vezzali, E.; et al. Pharmacological Characterization of Aprocitentan, a Dual Endothelin Receptor Antagonist, Alone and in Combination with Blockers of the Renin Angiotensin System, in Two Models of Experimental Hypertension. *J. Pharmacol. Exp. Ther.* **2019**, *368*, 462–473. [CrossRef]
57. Nakagawa, Y.; Nishikimi, T.; Kuwahara, K. Atrial and brain natriuretic peptides: Hormones secreted from the heart. *Peptides* **2019**, *111*, 18–25. [CrossRef]
58. Malek, V.; Gaikwad, A.B. Neprilysin inhibitors: A new hope to halt the diabetic cardiovascular and renal complications? *Biomed. Pharmacother.* **2017**, *90*, 752–759. [CrossRef] [PubMed]
59. Mills, J.; Vardeny, O. The Role of Neprilysin Inhibitors in Cardiovascular Disease. *Curr. Heart Fail. Rep.* **2015**, *12*, 389–394. [CrossRef] [PubMed]
60. Zanchi, A.; Maillard, M.; Burnier, M. Recent clinical trials with omapatrilat: New developments. *Curr. Hypertens. Rep.* **2003**, *5*, 346–352. [CrossRef]
61. McMurray, J.J.; Packer, M.; Desai, A.S.; Gong, J.; Lefkowitz, M.P.; Rizkala, A.R.; Rouleau, J.L.; Shi, V.C.; Solomon, S.D.; Swedberg, K.; et al. Angiotensin-neprilysin inhibition versus enalapril in heart failure. *N. Engl. J. Med.* **2014**, *371*, 993–1004. [CrossRef] [PubMed]
62. Solomon, S.D.; McMurray, J.J.V.; Anand, I.S.; Ge, J.; Lam, C.S.P.; Maggioni, A.P.; Martinez, F.; Packer, M.; Pfeffer, M.A.; Pieske, B.; et al. Angiotensin-Neprilysin Inhibition in Heart Failure with Preserved Ejection Fraction. *N. Engl. J. Med.* **2019**, *381*, 1609–1620. [CrossRef] [PubMed]
63. Ruilope, L.M.; Dukat, A.; Bohm, M.; Lacourciere, Y.; Gong, J.; Lefkowitz, M.P. Blood-pressure reduction with LCZ696, a novel dual-acting inhibitor of the angiotensin II receptor and neprilysin: A randomised, double-blind, placebo-controlled, active comparator study. *Lancet* **2010**, *375*, 1255–1266. [CrossRef]
64. Reboldi, G.; Gentile, G.; Angeli, F.; Verdecchia, P. Choice of ACE inhibitor combinations in hypertensive patients with type 2 diabetes: Update after recent clinical trials. *Vasc. Health Risk Manag.* **2009**, *5*, 411–427. [CrossRef] [PubMed]
65. Sumners, C.; Peluso, A.A.; Haugaard, A.H.; Bertelsen, J.B.; Steckelings, U.M. Anti-fibrotic mechanisms of angiotensin AT2-receptor stimulation. *Acta Physiol.* **2019**, *227*, e13280. [CrossRef] [PubMed]
66. Kemp, B.A.; Howell, N.L.; Gildea, J.J.; Keller, S.R.; Padia, S.H.; Carey, R.M. AT(2) receptor activation induces natriuresis and lowers blood pressure. *Circ. Res.* **2014**, *115*, 388–399. [CrossRef] [PubMed]
67. Savoia, C.; Ebrahimian, T.; He, Y.; Gratton, J.P.; Schiffrin, E.L.; Touyz, R.M. Angiotensin II/AT2 receptor-induced vasodilation in stroke-prone spontaneously hypertensive rats involves nitric oxide and cGMP-dependent protein kinase. *J. Hypertens.* **2006**, *24*, 2417–2422. [CrossRef] [PubMed]
68. Ghatage, T.; Goyal, S.G.; Dhar, A.; Bhat, A. Novel therapeutics for the treatment of hypertension and its associated complications: Peptide- and nonpeptide-based strategies. *Hypertens. Res.* **2021**, *44*, 740–755. [CrossRef] [PubMed]
69. Verdecchia, P.; Gentile, G.; Angeli, F.; Reboldi, G. Beyond blood pressure: Evidence for cardiovascular, cerebrovascular, and renal protective effects of renin-angiotensin system blockers. *Ther. Adv. Cardiovasc. Dis.* **2012**, *6*, 81–91. [CrossRef] [PubMed]
70. Gallo, L.A.; Wright, E.M.; Vallon, V. Probing SGLT2 as a therapeutic target for diabetes: Basic physiology and consequences. *Diab. Vasc. Dis. Res.* **2015**, *12*, 78–89. [CrossRef]
71. Tahrani, A.A.; Bailey, C.J.; del Prato, S.; Barnett, A.H. Management of type 2 diabetes: New and future developments in treatment. *Lancet* **2011**, *378*, 182–197. [CrossRef]
72. Grant, P.J.; Cosentino, F. The 2019 ESC Guidelines on diabetes, pre-diabetes, and cardiovascular diseases developed in collaboration with the EASD: New features and the 'Ten Commandments' of the 2019 Guidelines are discussed by Professor Peter J. Grant and Professor Francesco Cosentino, the Task Force chairmen. *Eur. Heart J.* **2019**, *40*, 3215–3217. [PubMed]
73. McMurray, J.J.V.; Solomon, S.D.; Inzucchi, S.E.; Kober, L.; Kosiborod, M.N.; Martinez, F.A.; Ponikowski, P.; Sabatine, M.S.; Anand, I.S.; Belohlavek, J.; et al. Dapagliflozin in Patients with Heart Failure and Reduced Ejection Fraction. *N. Engl. J. Med.* **2019**, *381*, 1995–2008. [CrossRef] [PubMed]
74. Packer, M.; Anker, S.D.; Butler, J.; Filippatos, G.; Pocock, S.J.; Carson, P.; Januzzi, J.; Verma, S.; Tsutsui, H.; Brueckmann, M.; et al. Cardiovascular and Renal Outcomes with Empagliflozin in Heart Failure. *N. Engl. J. Med.* **2020**, *383*, 1413–1424. [CrossRef] [PubMed]
75. Anker, S.D.; Butler, J.; Filippatos, G.; Ferreira, J.P.; Bocchi, E.; Bohm, M.; Brunner-La Rocca, H.-P.; Choi, D.J.; Chopra, V.; Chuquiure-Valenzuela, E.; et al. Empagliflozin in Heart Failure with a Preserved Ejection Fraction. *N. Engl. J. Med.* **2021**, *385*, 1451–1461. [CrossRef] [PubMed]

76. Mancia, G.; Cannon, C.P.; Tikkanen, I.; Zeller, C.; Ley, L.; Woerle, H.J.; Broedl, U.C.; Johansen, O.E. Impact of Empagliflozin on Blood Pressure in Patients With Type 2 Diabetes Mellitus and Hypertension by Background Antihypertensive Medication. *Hypertension* **2016**, *68*, 1355–1364. [CrossRef]
77. Baker, W.L.; Buckley, L.F.; Kelly, M.S.; Bucheit, J.D.; Parod, E.D.; Brown, R.; Carbone, S.; Abbate, A.; Dixon, D.L. Effects of Sodium-Glucose Cotransporter 2 Inhibitors on 24-Hour Ambulatory Blood Pressure: A Systematic Review and Meta-Analysis. *J. Am. Heart Assoc.* **2017**, *6*, e005686. [CrossRef]
78. Mazidi, M.; Rezaie, P.; Gao, H.K.; Kengne, A.P. Effect of Sodium-Glucose Cotransport-2 Inhibitors on Blood Pressure in People With Type 2 Diabetes Mellitus: A Systematic Review and Meta-Analysis of 43 Randomized Control Trials With 22 528 Patients. *J. Am. Heart Assoc.* **2017**, *6*, e004007. [CrossRef]
79. Vasilakou, D.; Karagiannis, T.; Athanasiadou, E.; Mainou, M.; Liakos, A.; Bekiari, E.; Sarigianni, M.; Matthews, D.R.; Tsapas, A. Sodium-glucose cotransporter 2 inhibitors for type 2 diabetes: A systematic review and meta-analysis. *Ann. Intern. Med.* **2013**, *159*, 262–274. [CrossRef]
80. Heerspink, H.J.; Perkins, B.A.; Fitchett, D.H.; Husain, M.; Cherney, D.Z. Sodium Glucose Cotransporter 2 Inhibitors in the Treatment of Diabetes Mellitus: Cardiovascular and Kidney Effects, Potential Mechanisms, and Clinical Applications. *Circulation* **2016**, *134*, 752–772. [CrossRef]
81. Di Bona, G.F. Neural control of renal function in health and disease. *Clin. Auton. Res.* **1994**, *4*, 69–74. [CrossRef] [PubMed]
82. Di Bona, G.F.; Kopp, U.C. Neural control of renal function. *Physiol. Rev.* **1997**, *77*, 75–197. [CrossRef] [PubMed]
83. Singh, R.R.; Denton, K.M. Renal Denervation. *Hypertension* **2018**, *72*, 528–536. [CrossRef] [PubMed]
84. Di Bona, G.F.; Esler, M. Translational medicine: The antihypertensive effect of renal denervation. *Am. J. Physiol. Regul. Integr. Comp. Physiol.* **2010**, *298*, R245–R253. [CrossRef] [PubMed]
85. Symplicity HTN-2 Investigators; Esler, M.D.; Krum, H.; Sobotka, P.A.; Schlaich, M.P.; Schmieder, R.E.; Bohm, M. Renal sympathetic denervation in patients with treatment-resistant hypertension (The Symplicity HTN-2 Trial): A randomised controlled trial. *Lancet* **2010**, *376*, 1903–1909. [CrossRef]
86. Bhatt, D.L.; Kandzari, D.E.; O'Neill, W.W.; D'Agostino, R.; Flack, J.M.; Katzen, B.T.; Leon, M.B.; Liu, M.; Mauri, L.; Negoita, M.; et al. A controlled trial of renal denervation for resistant hypertension. *N. Engl. J. Med.* **2014**, *370*, 1393–1401. [CrossRef]
87. Azizi, M.; Schmieder, R.E.; Mahfoud, F.; Weber, M.A.; Daemen, J.; Davies, J.; Basile, J.; Kirtane, A.J.; Wang, Y.; Lobo, M.D.; et al. Endovascular ultrasound renal denervation to treat hypertension (RADIANCE-HTN SOLO): A multicentre, international, single-blind, randomised, sham-controlled trial. *Lancet* **2018**, *391*, 2335–2345. [CrossRef]
88. Bohm, M.; Kario, K.; Kandzari, D.E.; Mahfoud, F.; Weber, M.A.; Schmieder, R.E.; Tsioufis, K.; Pocock, S.; Konstantinidis, D.; Choi, J.W.; et al. Efficacy of catheter-based renal denervation in the absence of antihypertensive medications (SPYRAL HTN-OFF MED Pivotal): A multicentre, randomised, sham-controlled trial. *Lancet* **2020**, *395*, 1444–1451. [CrossRef]
89. Kandzari, D.E.; Bohm, M.; Mahfoud, F.; Townsend, R.R.; Weber, M.A.; Pocock, S.; Tsioufis, K.; Tousoulis, D.; Choi, J.W.; East, C.; et al. Effect of renal denervation on blood pressure in the presence of antihypertensive drugs: 6-month efficacy and safety results from the SPYRAL HTN-ON MED proof-of-concept randomised trial. *Lancet* **2018**, *391*, 2346–2355. [CrossRef]
90. Schlaich, M.P.; Sobotka, P.A.; Krum, H.; Lambert, E.; Esler, M.D. Renal sympathetic-nerve ablation for uncontrolled hypertension. *N. Engl. J. Med.* **2009**, *361*, 932–934. [CrossRef]
91. Azizi, M.; Pereira, H.; Bobrie, G.; Gosse, P.; Renal Denervation for Hypertension (DENERHTN) Investigators. Renal denervation for resistant hypertension-Authors' reply. *Lancet* **2015**, *386*, 1240. [CrossRef]
92. Mahfoud, F.; Bohm, M.; Schmieder, R.; Narkiewicz, K.; Ewen, S.; Ruilope, L.; Schlaich, M.; Williams, B.; Fahy, M.; Mancia, G. Effects of renal denervation on kidney function and long-term outcomes: 3-year follow-up from the Global SYMPLICITY Registry. *Eur. Heart J.* **2019**, *40*, 3474–3482. [CrossRef] [PubMed]
93. Fengler, K.; Rommel, K.P.; Blazek, S.; Besler, C.; Hartung, P.; von Roeder, M.; Petzold, M.; Winkler, S.; Hollriegel, R.; Desch, S.; et al. A Three-Arm Randomized Trial of Different Renal Denervation Devices and Techniques in Patients With Resistant Hypertension (RADIOSOUND-HTN). *Circulation* **2019**, *139*, 590–600. [CrossRef] [PubMed]
94. Mahfoud, F.; Azizi, M.; Ewen, S.; Pathak, A.; Ukena, C.; Blankestijn, P.J.; Bohm, M.; Burnier, M.; Chatellier, G.; Zaleski, I.D.; et al. Proceedings from the 3rd European Clinical Consensus Conference for clinical trials in device-based hypertension therapies. *Eur. Heart J.* **2020**, *41*, 1588–1599. [CrossRef] [PubMed]
95. Bruno, R.M.; Taddei, S.; Borghi, C.; Colivicchi, F.; Desideri, G.; Grassi, G.; Mazza, A.; Muiesan, M.L.; Parati, G.; Pontremoli, R.; et al. Italian Society of Arterial Hypertension (SIIA) Position Paper on the Role of Renal Denervation in the Management of the Difficult-to-Treat Hypertensive Patient. *High Blood Press. Cardiovasc. Prev.* **2020**, *27*, 109–117. [CrossRef] [PubMed]
96. Sarathy, H.; Cohen, J.B. Renal Denervation for the Treatment of Hypertension: Unnerving or Underappreciated? *Clin. J. Am. Soc. Nephrol.* **2021**, *16*, 1426–1428. [CrossRef] [PubMed]
97. Mahfoud, F.; Luscher, T.F.; Andersson, B.; Baumgartner, I.; Cifkova, R.; Dimario, C.; Doevendans, P.; Fagard, R.; Fajadet, J.; Komajda, M.; et al. Expert consensus document from the European Society of Cardiology on catheter-based renal denervation. *Eur. Heart J.* **2013**, *34*, 2149–2157. [CrossRef] [PubMed]
98. Bacaksiz, A.; Uyarel, H.; Jafarov, P.; Kucukbuzcu, S. Iatrogenic renal artery stenosis after renal sympathetic denervation. *Int. J. Cardiol.* **2014**, *172*, e389–e390. [CrossRef]
99. Celik, I.E.; Acar, B.; Kurtul, A.; Murat, S.N. De novo renal artery stenosis after renal sympathetic denervation. *J. Clin. Hypertens.* **2015**, *17*, 242–243. [CrossRef]

100. Diego-Nieto, A.; Cruz-Gonzalez, I.; Martin-Moreiras, J.; Rama-Merchan, J.C.; Rodriguez-Collado, J.; Sanchez-Fernandez, P.L. Severe Renal Artery Stenosis After Renal Sympathetic Denervation. *JACC Cardiovasc. Interv.* **2015**, *8*, e193–e194. [CrossRef]
101. Kaltenbach, B.; Id, D.; Franke, J.C.; Sievert, H.; Hennersdorf, M.; Maier, J.; Bertog, S.C. Renal artery stenosis after renal sympathetic denervation. *J. Am. Coll. Cardiol.* **2012**, *60*, 2694–2695. [CrossRef] [PubMed]
102. Wang, Y. What is the true incidence of renal artery stenosis after sympathetic denervation? *Front. Physiol.* **2014**, *5*, 311. [CrossRef]
103. Vonend, O.; Antoch, G.; Rump, L.C.; Blondin, D. Secondary rise in blood pressure after renal denervation. *Lancet* **2012**, *380*, 778. [CrossRef]
104. Mahfoud, F.; Luscher, T.F. Renal denervation: Symply trapped by complexity? *Eur. Heart J.* **2015**, *36*, 199–202. [CrossRef] [PubMed]
105. Bhudia, R.P. Treatment of the hypertensive patient in 2030. *J. Hum. Hypertens.* **2021**, *35*, 818–820. [CrossRef]

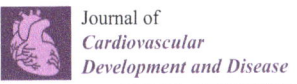

Review

Hypertension and Arrhythmias: A Clinical Overview of the Pathophysiology-Driven Management of Cardiac Arrhythmias in Hypertensive Patients

Jacopo Marazzato [1], Federico Blasi [1], Michele Golino [1], Paolo Verdecchia [2,3], Fabio Angeli [1,4] and Roberto De Ponti [1,*]

1. Department of Medicine and Surgery, University of Insubria, 21100 Varese, Italy; j.marazzato88@gmail.com (J.M.); federico.blasi.md@gmail.com (F.B.); micheleg1390@gmail.com (M.G.); angeli.internet@gmail.com (F.A.)
2. Fondazione Umbra Cuore e Ipertensione-ONLUS, 06100 Perugia, Italy; verdecchiapaolo@gmail.com
3. Division of Cardiology, Hospital S. Maria della Misericordia, 06100 Perugia, Italy
4. Department of Medicine and Cardiopulmonary Rehabilitation, Maugeri Care and Research Institute, IRCCS Tradate, 21049 Tradate, Italy
* Correspondence: roberto.deponti@uninsubria.it; Tel.: +39-0332278934

Abstract: Because of demographic aging, the prevalence of arterial hypertension (HTN) and cardiac arrhythmias, namely atrial fibrillation (AF), is progressively increasing. Not only are these clinical entities strongly connected, but, acting with a synergistic effect, their association may cause a worse clinical outcome in patients already at risk of ischemic and/or haemorrhagic stroke and, consequently, disability and death. Despite the well-known association between HTN and AF, several pathogenetic mechanisms underlying the higher risk of AF in hypertensive patients are still incompletely known. Although several trials reported the overall clinical benefit of renin–angiotensin–aldosterone inhibitors in reducing incident AF in HTN, the role of this class of drugs is greatly reduced when AF diagnosis is already established, thus hinting at the urgent need for primary prevention measures to reduce AF occurrence in these patients. Through a thorough review of the available literature in the field, we investigated the basic mechanisms through which HTN is believed to promote AF, summarising the evidence supporting a pathophysiology-driven approach to prevent this arrhythmia in hypertensive patients, including those suffering from primary aldosteronism, a non-negligible and under-recognised cause of secondary HTN. Finally, in the hazy scenario of AF screening in hypertensive patients, we reviewed which patients should be screened, by which modality, and who should be offered oral anticoagulation for stroke prevention.

Keywords: hypertension; atrial fibrillation; primary hyperaldosteronism; antihypertensive agents; artificial pacemakers; anticoagulants

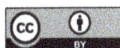

1. Introduction

The overall prevalence of hypertension (HTN) in adults is roughly 30–45% [1] and becomes even more common with advancing age [2]. HTN is also a well-known risk factor for atrial fibrillation (AF) [3–5], which may even occur when borderline values of blood pressure (BP) are recorded [6–10]. Moreover, AF exerts an important prognostic role in hypertensive patients, thus potentially leading to ischaemic and haemorrhagic stroke, hospitalisations for heart failure, and, in the worst circumstances, death [10–12]. Therefore, it stands to reason that primary prevention measures devoted to reducing incident AF are required to avoid potentially troublesome cardiac and cerebrovascular events which may occur in this clinical scenario. Moreover, increasing age and the associated burden of other comorbidities such as diabetes mellitus, heart failure, coronary artery disease, chronic kidney disease, obesity, and obstructive sleep apnea would synergistically act with HTN as major contributors to AF development and progression [10].

Through a review of the available literature, we investigated the pathophysiological mechanisms responsible for incident AF in hypertensive patients. The aim of this review was therefore to summarise a pathophysiology-driven, patient-tailored approach to prevent the onset of cardiac arrhythmias, namely atrial fibrillation, in the general population affected by HTN. To underscore the importance of a pathophysiological approach to HTN, a dedicated focus has also been reported on which hypertensive patients would greatly benefit from specific treatment options in the setting of primary hyperaldosteronism, a non-negligible cause of secondary HTN.

Moreover, when AF nonetheless develops as an unavoidable consequence of atrial myopathy, it should be recognised in a timely manner to avoid potentially harmful consequences. Although several issues do exist about the possibility of AF screening in hypertensive patients, in this hazy scenario, we investigated the available modalities to detect silent/subclinical AF episodes in hypertensive patients and which patients should be offered oral anticoagulation for stroke prevention.

2. Materials and Methods

We performed a bibliographic research on Medline considering manuscripts published up to 2021, according to the following Boolean research strings: "Arterial hypertension AND arrhythmias", "Arterial hypertension AND atrial fibrillation", "Arterial hypertension AND supraventricular arrhythmias". The literature research was independently conducted by two authors (FB and JM) and then revised by JM, FB, and MG, who reached a shared decision by consensus in case of discordance.

3. Common Pathophysiological Aspects Explaining the Link between Hypertension and Cardiac Arrhythmias

As observed in animal models, HTN per se is associated with ion channel imbalance and the progressive development of myocardial fibrosis in hypertensive hearts [13–15]. The ensuing molecular and structural alterations would therefore represent a fertile substrate for arrhythmogenesis. On the one hand, HTN-related shear stress would lead to both a long outward potassium (K^+) current (Kv1.5) [13] and the altered release of intracellular calcium (Ca^{2+}) from the sarcoplasmic reticulum [14], thus leading to a shorter action potential duration and delayed afterdepolarizations (DAD) in myocardial cells, respectively. In fact, a shorter action potential duration would predispose to enhanced automatism and re-entrant mechanisms [16]. In addition to ion channel abnormalities, HTN is also associated with maladaptive gap junction remodelling due to the abnormal expression of gap junction proteins such as connexin 43 and 40 [15,17] which would determine the abnormal conduction properties and fibrotic evolution of myocardial tissue, thus prompting nonuniform anisotropy, slow conduction, and, therefore, arrhythmogenesis in hypertensive hearts. In addition to this, cardiovascular risk factors, HTN included, are accompanied by low-grade inflammation and oxidative stress, which further promote ion channels and connexin downregulation/dysfunction, abnormal Ca^{2+} handling, and, finally, the activation of profibrotic signaling, which would all promote arrhythmogenesis [18].

Furthermore, as displayed on Figure 1, the HTN-related activation of the renin–angiotensin–aldosterone (RAA) cascade and sympathetic nervous system (SNS), in addition to myocardial ischemia in hypertrophic hearts, would also play a major role in the pathogenesis of cardiac arrhythmias in HTN [19,20]. All these mechanisms are discussed in the next sections of this article.

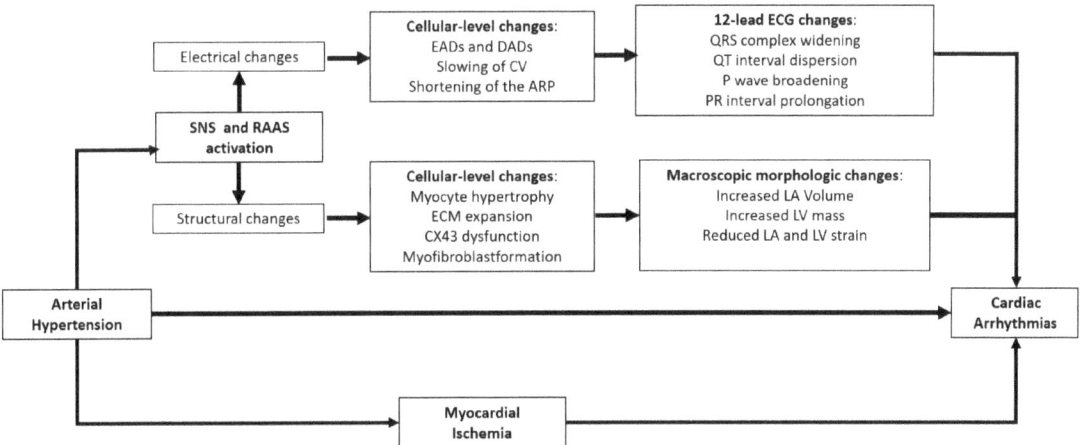

Figure 1. Electro-pathological and clinical changes occurring in hypertensive hearts. ARP, atrial refractory period; SNS, sympathetic nervous system; CV, conduction velocity; CX43, connexin 43; DADs, delayed afterdepolarizations; EADs, early afterdepolarizations; ECM, extracellular matrix; LA, left atrial; LA Vol, left atrial volume; LV, left ventricular; RAAS, renin–angiotensin–aldosterone system. See text for further details.

3.1. Myocardial Electro-Pathological Remodelling in Arterial Hypertension: The Key Role of Renin–Angiotensin–Aldosterone and Sympathetic Nervous Systems

Different hormone systems are involved in this complex scenario. On the one hand, angiotensin II, a mediator of RAAS, does modulate specific ion currents in cardiac myocytes, including L- and T-type inward Ca^{2+} [21,22] and K^+ currents [23]. Moreover, in a murine model, aldosterone seems to increase the molecular expression of L-type Ca^{2+} channels while reducing the activity of both delayed rectifier (IKr) and transient outward K^+ currents (Ito1) [24]. Aldosterone has also been shown to induce Ca^{2+} overload due to the opening of ryanodine receptors in the sarcoplasmic reticulum [25], which may increase delayed afterdepolarizations (DAD), thereby raising the chance of cardiac arrhythmias mediated by triggered activity [26]. In this regard, Pluteanu et al. [27] demonstrated the existence of subcellular alterations in Ca^{2+} handling in spontaneous hypertensive rats, which were associated with an increased propensity of atrial myocytes to develop frequency-dependent and arrhythmogenic Ca^{2+} alternans, a mechanism potentially triggering cardiac arrhythmias.

In addition to ion channel modifications, the RAAS plays a key role in the progression of atrial and ventricular fibrosis through the proliferation of fibroblasts in the extracellular matrix [19,20]. In fact, myocardial fibrosis, associated with connexin dysregulation, generally leads to slow and heterogeneous conduction velocity, nonhomogenous impulse propagation, and re-entrant atrial and ventricular arrhythmias [11,28]. HTN, as well as the ensuing LV hypertrophy, may also cause an abnormal expression of junctional complexes, which have been associated with greater myocardium vulnerability [15,29]. Moreover, the imbalance between oxygen demand and supply occurring in this setting would further activate myofibroblasts and induce hypertrophic modifications in vascular smooth muscle cells [29,30], thus leading to a vicious cycle made up of collagen deposition [31], progressive myocyte hypertrophy, and diastolic dysfunction [32], which is regarded as the first compensatory pathophysiological response in hypertensive hearts [33]. In addition to these mechanisms, SNS would also lead to enhanced RAAS activity and HTN-induced LV afterload, with a remarkable synergistic effect on arrhythmia onset in hypertrophic hearts [20].

From a pathophysiological perspective, diastolic dysfunction generally causes a reduction in LA passive emptying, thus increasing LA pressures during atrial diastole and eventually causing LA enlargement [34]. Over time, the progressive distension and stretching of the LA and pulmonary veins may induce an electrical remodelling of these anatomical chambers, thus leading to shorter atrial effective refractory periods [35], the greater dispersion of atrial repolarisation and, therefore, vulnerability to AF [36,37]. LA stretching would also prompt electrical dissociation among muscle bundles, which would further facilitate the initiation and maintenance of multiple small re-entrant wavelets to sustain this cardiac arrhythmia [20].

As to the clinical implication of these pathophysiological mechanisms, AF episodes in hypertensive patients are greatly associated with the severity of LV myocardial stiffness or, in other words, the extent of diastolic dysfunction [38]. In this regard, as assessed on a vast patient cohort undergoing echocardiographic evaluation [38], Tsang et al. showed how the greater the degree of diastolic dysfunction, the higher the probability of AF episodes occurring [38]. Therefore, as shown on Figure 1, the increased LV mass, LV myocardial stiffness, and ensuing diastolic dysfunction and LA enlargement would all play a great role in the genesis of cardiac arrhythmias, namely AF, in hypertensive patients [39,40].

3.2. The Role of Myocardial Ischemia

Myocardial ischemia may lead to arrhythmogenesis in HTN due to mechanisms inherently connected to LVH or atherosclerotic disease involving the major epicardial coronary arteries. On the one hand, changes in arteriolar wall thickening and relative capillary density may lead to reduced microvascular flow in hypertrophic hearts [41–43]. However, HTN-mediated ischemia is not limited to small vessels only, and the global involvement of the coronary artery tree in hypertensive hearts well explains the overall risk of myocardial ischemia and scar formation in these patients [29]. In this regard, a strong connection between the obstruction of atrial coronary branches and AF occurrence in the setting of acute myocardial infarction has been described [44,45]. As observed in studies conducted on animal models [46], atrial ischemia and the ensuing LA stretching synergistically interact in leading to a reduced myocardial conduction velocity and an increased conduction heterogeneity, which would elicit myocardial vulnerability and AF. Of note, not only could atrial ischemia be the result of atherosclerotic heart disease, but pulmonary hypertension and the ensuing combination of hypoxia with increased atrial pressure may prompt AF by means of ischemic mechanisms [47].

Moreover, Kolvekar et al. described an association between atrial ischemia and the sclerosis of sinus node and atrioventricular node branches [48], and, as pointed out in a retrospective study conducted by Ciulla et al. [49], the prevalence of AF seems higher in patients with a diseased sinus node artery (41.2% vs. 7.4% $p < 0.001$). Hence, the ischemic damage caused by flow abnormality in the sinus node artery may undermine the structural integrity of the sinus node itself, thus determining a widespread structural and electrical atrial remodelling, which represents the underlying substrate to AF development in this clinical setting.

However, not only AF could be the result of ischemic mechanisms involving atrial branches of epicardial coronary arteries (i.e., primary atrial ischemia), but ventricular ischemia could also be responsible for this cardiac arrhythmia (i.e., ventricular-induced or secondary atrial ischemia). On the one hand, atrial stretching occurring in the setting of myocardial infarction would increase the LA surface area, thus prolonging electrical conduction and facilitating AF initiation and maintenance [50]. However, the greater the ischemic involvement of the LV, the higher the incidence of AF. In a subanalysis of the CULPRIT-SHOCK (Culprit Lesion Only PCI versus Multivessel PCI in Cardiogenic Shock) trial, compared with patients with LV myocardial infarction and no cardiogenic shock (CS), the authors observed a significant incidence of AF in patients with CS: global ischemia induced by extensive LV involvement in CS, the ensuing extensive myocardial injury, and the increased LA size and pressure would all explain the remarkable prevalence of AF observed in this high-risk population [51]. Moreover, myocardial ischemia may also lead to the transmural dispersion of ventricular repolarization, which may favour early after depolarizations (EAD) and polymorphic ventricular tachycardias in the affected patients [20,21,29,52,53].

4. Arterial Hypertension and Atrial Fibrillation: Pathophysiology-Based Strategies to Prevent a Hazardous Association

Given the remarkable prevalence of AF in hypertensive patients, the clinical impact of blood pressure in relation to the occurrence of AF deserves special analysis. A pathophysiology-based approach to HTN in AF patients and a proposed algorithm for the early detection of AF in HTN are provided in the next sections of this article.

4.1. Clinical Implications of High Blood Pressure in Patients with Atrial Fibrillation

The presence of uncontrolled HTN in AF patients promotes the already described electro-anatomical atrial remodelling, which is responsible for AF evolution from paroxysmal to more persistent clinical forms of arrhythmia with an overall dismal prognosis in this patient population [54–61]. Indeed, in a large Swedish registry of AF patients on oral anticoagulants, Friberg et al. found that HTN was not only an independent predictor for thromboembolic complications but also of intracranial [HR 1.32, 95% CI (1.15–1.52)] and major bleedings [HR 1.25, 95% CI (1.16–1.33)] [62]. These results are indeed reflected by the integration of HTN in both CHA2DS2-VASc and HAS-BLED scores to estimate the thromboembolic and haemorrhagic hazard, as recommended by current guidelines on AF management [63,64]. However, it is still debated which, between a long-standing history of increased blood pressure and high systolic blood pressure values per se, portends a greater risk of ischemic and haemorrhagic events in hypertensive patients. In a vast community-based prospective registry, Ishii et al. showed that, in AF patients, only systolic blood pressure values beyond 150 mmHg were significantly associated with a higher risk of ischemic [HR 1.74, 95% CI (1.08–2.72)] and bleeding events [HR 2.01, 95% CI (1.21–3.23)] as compared with adequately matched normotensive cases [65]. Similar results were provided by a subanalysis of the Japanese J-RHYTHM AF registry, including more than 7046 patients with nonvalvular AF [66], suggesting that every clinician should aim at an adequate blood pressure control to improve outcome in AF patients.

Moreover, HTN seems responsible for cardioembolic stroke through mechanisms which would act independently from AF. Although the SPRINT (Systolic Blood Pressure Intervention Trial) reported an exceedingly high risk of thromboembolic events in patients with pre-existent and new-onset AF, despite adequate blood pressure control [67], on the other hand, a body of evidence suggests that HTN per se could also directly promote left atrial thrombosis. In this regard, Zabalgoitia et al. [68] demonstrated a lower flow velocity and a higher risk of thrombosis in the left atrial appendix in hypertensive patients regardless of AF, with results confirmed by a subanalysis of the SPAF-III (Stroke Prevention in Atrial Fibrillation III) trial [69]. In hypertensive patients, endocardial thrombogenesis seems promoted by oxidative stress [70–73], which is increased by RAAS activation and by the subsequent inflammation occurring in diseased atria and in the left atrial appendage [74–76].

Therefore, blood pressure control is paramount to minimize the risk of myocardial ischemia, stroke, and oral-anticoagulant-related bleedings in AF cases. Until more data are available, blood pressure values in AF patients on oral anticoagulants should be at least <130 mmHg and <80 mmHg for systolic and diastolic blood pressure values, respectively [1,9,77], and oral anticoagulants should be used with caution in patients with persistent uncontrolled hypertension [10]. Moreover, in case of any clinical suspicion of myocardial ischemia, the prompt assessment of the atherosclerotic involvement of epicardial coronary arteries is mandatory in these patients.

Therefore, it stands to reason that primary prevention measures to prevent AF occurrence and the early detection of this arrhythmia [68] are paramount in patients diagnosed with HTN to avoid the described life-threatening major cerebral and cardiovascular events.

4.2. Primary Prevention of Atrial Fibrillation: A Pathophysiology-Based Approach in Patients with Essential Hypertension

Given the predominant role of RAAS in the pathogenesis of AF, ACE inhibitors (ACEi) and angiotensin receptor blockers (ARB) seem a reasonable first-line treatment option in hypertensive patients. Moreover, LVH has been shown to be partially reversible after treatment with RAAS blockers, with studies demonstrating improved electrical and structural parameters and reduced AF burden following treatment with these agents [78–80].

In the Losartan Intervention For Endpoint reduction in hypertension (LIFE) study, 9193 hypertensive patients were randomized to once-daily losartan- or atenolol-based antihypertensive therapy to detect outcome differences regarding the long-term occurrence of new-onset AF. Compared with Atenolol, Losartan was associated with significantly fewer AF episodes and a better overall outcome [RR 0.67, 95% CI 0.55–0.83] [81].

ACEi or ARB could have an even greater role in avoiding AF occurrence in patients with LVH and systolic heart failure [82–84]. Although this effect has been attributed to the antifibrotic and antiapoptotic effect of these drugs, this superiority over betablockers is nonetheless quite surprising. Therefore, despite the intrinsic antiarrhythmic effect of betablockers, both cardiac fibrosis and negative remodelling play a central role in AF onset in hypertensive patients. Even when tested versus calcium antagonists, RAAS blockers showed a lower risk of AF development in a similar patient population [85].

Although RAAS blockers showed a net superiority over beta-blockers for AF prevention in HTN patients, their combined use seems beneficial in hypertensive patients suffering from heart failure. In a meta-analysis including 11,952 patients, Nasr et al. reported that betablockers significantly reduced the incidence of AF onset in heart failure, provided that a background treatment with ACEi was warranted, and similar outcomes were observed for MRA in similar patients [86]. Another clear benefit of betablockers is the well-known protection against sudden cardiac death [53,87].

In light of this evidence, betablockers seem to further support the action of RAAS blockers in AF prevention in hypertensive patients; however, they should not be regarded as a first-line therapy for HTN unless there is a specific indication for their use, such as heart failure, angina symptoms, or established AF [1].

In conclusion, although RAAS inhibitors do not seem to prevent AF recurrence in patients with an already established diagnosis of this cardiac arrhythmia [88–90], ACEi and ARB should be first offered to patients with essential hypertension to prevent incident AF. Although betablockers and MRA should be generally used in addition to ACEi and ARB in specific settings, MRA are to be first considered in specific subsets, such as patients suffering from primary aldosteronism (PA), a non-negligible cause of secondary hypertension.

Finally, there is strong evidence from preclinical research and clinical studies that targeting inflammation and oxidative stress may provide a path to ameliorate cardiac arrhythmia burden. Indeed, cardioprotective SGLT2 inhibitors, statins, and omega-3 fatty acids exhibit potent antioxidative and anti-inflammatory properties. These agents most likely affect the proarrhythmia primary mechanisms, such as triggered activity as well as profibrotic signalling. However, the causal relationship is missing, and further studies are required to assess the real impact of these drugs on arrhythmogenesis in hypertensive patients [18].

4.3. Focus on Primary Aldosteronism: An Under-Recognized Cause of Secondary Hypertension Prompting a Targeted Medical and Surgical Treatment

PA, also known as primary hyperaldosteronism or Conn's syndrome, refers to the excess production of aldosterone essentially caused by hyperplasia or tumors involving adrenal glands and resulting in high blood pressure in the affected patients [91]. It is the most common endocrine cause of secondary hypertension, with a prevalence spanning from 4.3–9.5% in hypertensive patients to 17–23% in those with resistant HTN [92]. Moreover, a body of evidence suggests that PA confers a greater risk of stroke, AF, and cardiovascular disease than similar patient cohorts with essential hypertension [93].

As to associated cardiac arrhythmias, AF is by far the most observed rhythm disorder (7.2% prevalence on average), with other cardiac arrhythmias occurring in up to 5.2% of cases [94,95].

PA could promote arrhythmogenesis through different mechanisms [96]. On the one hand, aldosterone hypersecretion induces inflammation by producing reactive oxygen species which activate proinflammatory transcription factors in macrophages [74–76], causing cardiac interstitial macrophage infiltration with subsequent fibrosis [97]. On the other hand, through resting membrane hyperpolarization, Na^+-K^+ ATPase inhibition, and the suppression of K^+ channel conductance, aldosterone-mediated hypokalemia further explains the mechanisms of arrhythmogenesis occurring in PA patients [98–100]. Accordingly, a study from the German Conn's Registry confirmed that AF was more commonly found in patients with the hypokalemic variant of PA than in those with normal values of serum potassium levels [95].

Therefore, PA has targeted medical treatment and potentially curative surgical solutions, which may ameliorate the associated cardiovascular risks as well as the rate of incident AF.

Figure 2 shows a flowchart helping the clinician to diagnose and manage PA when clinically suspected [101]. Broadly speaking, patients who demonstrate a suppressed renin, markedly elevated aldosterone (i.e., when plasma aldosterone concentration is greater than 550 pmol/L or 15 ng/dL), and spontaneous hypokalemia can also be diagnosed with PA without confirmatory testing [102]. When PA diagnosis is confirmed, dietary sodium restriction and medical treatment with MRA should be immediately offered, not only to reduce blood pressure but also to lower the overall risk of AF occurrence [103]. However, surgical adrenalectomy seems associated with even better long-term cardiovascular outcomes [101], a further reduction in AF occurrence, and other major cardiovascular comorbidities in these patients [104]. Therefore, in the case of PA diagnosis, cross-sectional imaging is required to localise the adrenal mass, thus prompting further surgical evaluation in selected PA cases (Figure 3).

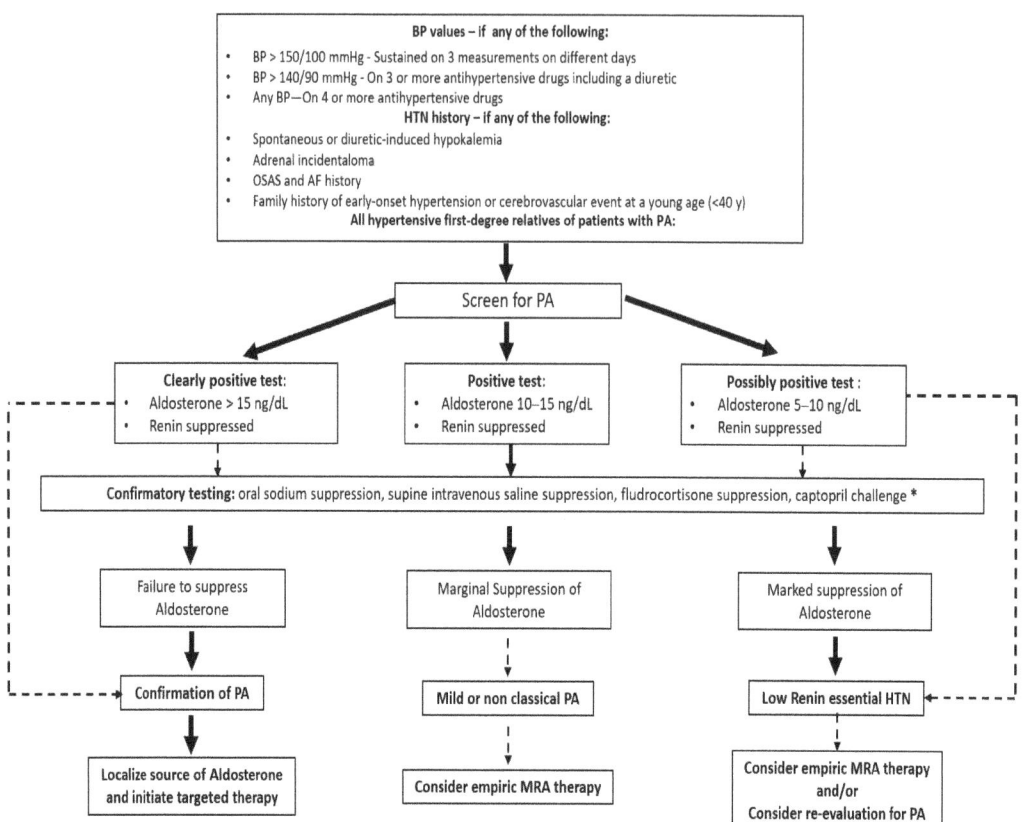

Figure 2. Screening and diagnostic approach for primary aldosteronism. A positive screen for primary aldosteronism should suggest high aldosterone levels and a suppressed renin activity. Confirmatory testing can be used in this setting. Solid arrows indicate recommended decision pathways; dashed arrows indicate other possible diagnostic alternatives in appropriate clinical contexts. * Confirmatory testing suggesting aldosterone hypersecretion: (1) oral sodium suppression (positive if 24 h urinary aldosterone excretion rate is greater than 12–14 mg/die); (2) supine intravenous saline suppression (positive if aldosterone levels are greater than 10 ng/dL after 2 L of saline infusion); (3) fludrocortisone suppression (positive if seated aldosterone greater than 6 ng/dL with plasma renin activity lower than 1.0 ng/mL/h); and, finally, (4) captopril challenge (positive if less than 30% suppression of aldosterone from baseline while plasma renin activity remains suppressed post 25 mg of oral captopril). AF, atrial fibrillation; BP, blood pressure; HTN, hypertension; MRA, mineralcorticoid-receptor antagonists; OSAS, obstructive sleep apnea syndrome; PA, primary aldosteronism. (Modified and adapted from document of The Endocrine Society [101]).

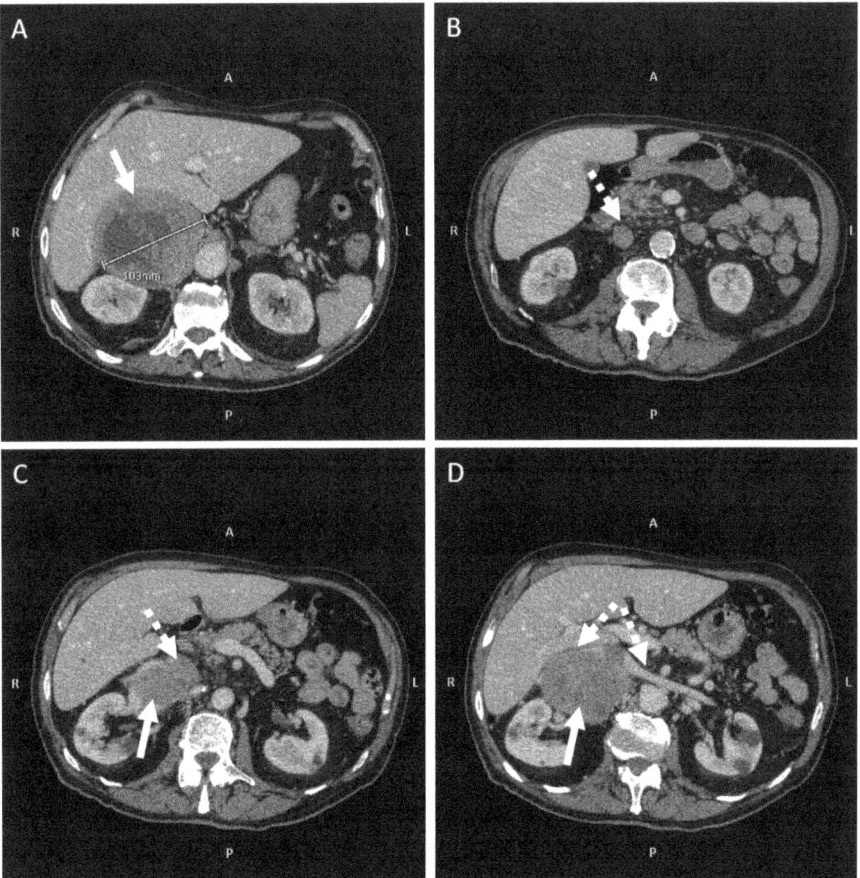

Figure 3. (**A–D**). Computed tomography of the abdomen in a patient with suspected primary aldosteronism. A 78-year-old patient referred to medical attention for dysregulated hypertension, irregular heartbeat, and remarkable peripheral oedema. Upon admission, 12-lead ECG showed atrial fibrillation with high ventricular rate. Transthoracic echocardiogram displayed signs of moderate left ventricular hypertrophy only. Laboratory tests showed remarkably low potassium levels together with high levels of serum aldosterone and suppressed renin activity. Therefore, computed tomography scan of the abdomen with iodine contrast administration was then carried out to identify any adrenal mass (**A–D**). A 10 cm, bulky adrenal tumor is well evident from cross-sectional imaging acquired during the arterial phase (**A**). The mass (white arrows) shows hypodense foci and colliquative areas with signs of compression of the neighboring anatomical structures. From a caudal to a more cranial perspective, the inferior vena cava and renal veins are progressively compressed and anteriorly dislodged by the adrenal mass (dashed arrows, **B–D**), thus explaining the remarkable peripheral oedema clinically observed in this patient. The patient is currently scheduled for abdominal video laparoscopy for adrenal mass excision and the ensuing histopathologic characterization.

5. Early Detection of Atrial Fibrillation in Hypertensive Patients: A Proposed Algorithm

Despite all efforts to prevent AF in hypertensive patients, structural heart disease and atrial cardiomyopathy in this setting would nonetheless cause progressive atrial derangement and electrical vulnerability, thus promoting a vicious cycle known as "atrial failure", which is intimately connected with AF development [105].

It is well known that AF is a potentially life-threatening cause of cerebral thromboembolism, and clinically silent forms might wreak even greater havoc if not recognised in a timely manner. For these reasons, hypertensive patients with an uncertain history of AF and evidence of prior cerebrovascular events should be accurately studied to differentiate strokes of cardioembolic origin from those secondary to atherosclerotic disease or cerebral haemorrhage [106]. In these cases, ECG monitoring can be helpful to identify patients with clinically silent AF [107,108], and, in the case of cryptogenic stroke, an implantable cardiac monitor (ICM) should be considered [10]. Over the last decade, cardiac implantable electronic devices (CIEDs) [109], ICM included [110], have proved extremely helpful in the early detection of subclinical AF episodes, but it is still debated which arrhythmic burden should prompt immediate oral anticoagulation in these patients. For the sake of clarity, clinically silent AF is defined for asymptomatic arrhythmia episodes detected on 12-lead ECG or an ECG strip; conversely, subclinical AF is represented by arrhythmia detected by CIEDs [10]. However, differentiating clinical from subclinical AF is not a matter of mere speculation. In fact, subclinical AF seems to portend a lower thromboembolic risk compared with clinical AF [111], and no clear cause–effect relationship between subclinical AF and ischemic stroke has been clearly proven in this setting [109]. However, the longer the duration of subclinical AF episodes, the greater their association with thromboembolic events [112]. For this reason, a recent European Heart Rhythm Association (EHRA) consensus document suggested oral anticoagulation administration for subclinical AF episodes longer than 5.5 h/day only when a significant risk of cerebral thromboembolism is established (i.e, CHA2DS2Vasc scores $\geq$ 2 and 3 in men and women, respectively) [111]. Whether this strategy pays off in terms of better clinical outcome is unclear. In fact, by randomising elderly patients with stroke risk factors and no AF history to the ICM strategy or usual care, the LOOP study did not prove the superiority of ICM over controls in terms of better clinical outcome after early AF detection [110]. Several issues raised by the same investigators might explain the overall negative results of this trial, such as the inadequate estimate of the primary outcome event rate, the relatively short duration of follow-up, and the initiation of oral anticoagulation for subclinical episodes lasting as low as 6 min. In keeping with prior observations [112], these results would suggest that not all subclinical AF episodes may benefit from early anticoagulation, and two ongoing randomized controlled trials might provide clearer answers in patients with CIEDs [113,114].

Moreover, in this already hazy scenario, it is all but crystal-clear which hypertensive patients with neither stroke history nor CIEDs/ICM should be screened for silent AF, and, not least, through which modality. On the one hand, the burden of cardiovascular comorbidities and blood biomarkers might play an important role in identifying people at a sufficient risk to warrant AF screening [115]. The thorough assessment of the P wave morphology on surface ECG may also be useful in identifying potential risk markers for AF, such as prolonged P wave duration, left atrial enlargement, and advanced interatrial (i.e., Bachmann bundle) block. [116]. Similar observation can be made for LVH, diastolic dysfunction, and left atrial enlargement as assessed on transthoracic echocardiogram [116]. However, what would be the best approach for AF screening in high-risk patients? On one side of the spectrum of the available modalities for AF screening, on account of the low cost and the great sensitivity yield, radial pulse taking should be regarded as the first option to be offered in patients aged $\geq$65 years and deemed at high risk of developing AF. Surface ECG analysis in the case of arrhythmic pulse is therefore warranted, and, if clinical AF is confirmed, oral anticoagulation should be promptly administered according to the patient's thromboembolic risk profile [10]. Furthermore, a variety of screening technologies have been developed over the years and with progressively better AF detection accuracy [117], but no comparative trials have been carried out so far with any of these devices. Accordingly, European guidelines on AF diagnosis and management [10] strongly recommend a single-lead ECG tracing of $\geq$30 s or 12-lead ECG to confirm a diagnosis of clinical AF when detected by screening tools. Although similar observation can be applied to the use of ICM in the same setting, the positive clinical interaction observed in the LOOP trial between high blood pressure values and better clinical outcome in early anticoagulated patients in the ICM arm may prompt the use of an implantable loop recorder (ILR) as a screening tool in selected patients with HTN.

In conclusion, AF detection in its early stage is paramount, and an appropriate therapy might eschew severe complications potentially leading to disability and death in the affected patients. However, it should be ascertained which patients portend a greater risk of AF and thereby who should be screened for this arrhythmia and by which modality. While waiting for sounder results from ongoing clinical trials, Figure 4 provides a proposed algorithm for silent/subclinical AF detection and management in hypertensive patients.

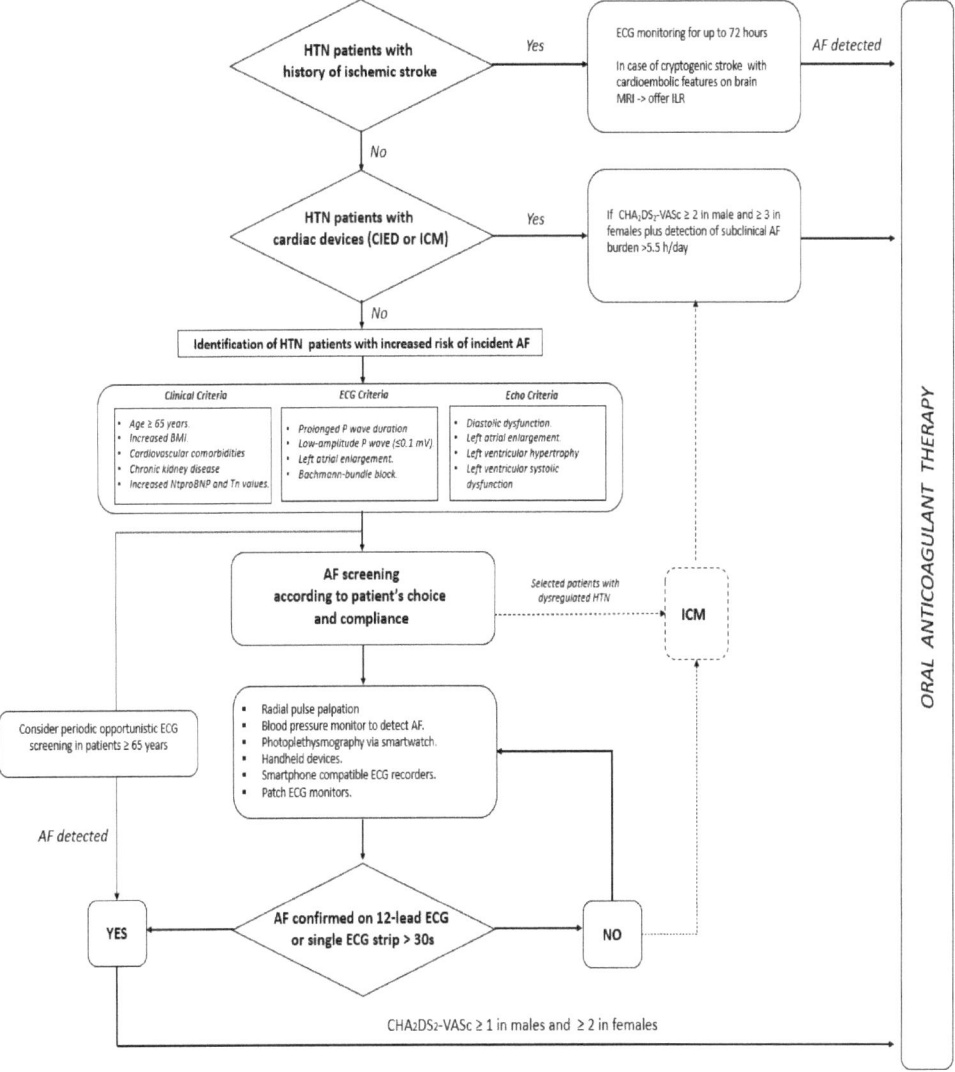

Figure 4. Proposed algorithm for early detection and management of silent and subclinical atrial fibrillation episodes. AF = atrial fibrillation; CIED = cardiac implantable electronic devices; ICM = internal cardiac monitor; ILR = internal loop recorder; HTN = hypertension.

6. Conclusions and Future Directions

Through enhanced RAAS and the ensuing pathophysiological mechanisms, HTN represents a well-known substrate for cardiac arrhythmias. Although several trials reported the overall clinical benefit of RAAS inhibitors in reducing AF onset in essential HTN, the role of this class of drugs is greatly reduced when AF diagnosis is already established. Therefore, primary prevention measures are strongly recommended to avoid the potential occurrence of AF in a population already at risk of ischemic and/or haemorrhagic cerebral stroke and, consequently, of disability and death. On the one hand, a patient-tailored, pathophysiology-driven strategy is mandatory in all hypertensive patients, from the administration of RAAS inhibitors in essential HTN to the early detection of secondary HTN causes, namely PA, warranting a specific medical and surgical treatment which has proved to ameliorate the overall outcome in this specific population.

Finally, although several issues still exist as to the possibility of AF screening in the general population affected by HTN, the early detection of silent/subclinical episodes of AF should be nonetheless carried out while waiting for sounder evidence from ongoing randomised controlled trials in the field.

Author Contributions: Conceptualization, J.M. and F.B.; methodology, J.M.; validation, R.D.P., F.A. and P.V.; investigation, F.B. and M.G.; writing—original draft preparation, J.M.; writing—review and editing, F.B. and M.G.; visualization, M.G.; supervision, F.A. and P.V.; project administration, R.D.P. All authors have read and agreed to the published version of the manuscript. All authors contributed to the study conception and design.

Funding: This research received no external funding.

Institutional Review Board Statement: Not applicable.

Informed Consent Statement: Not applicable.

Conflicts of Interest: The authors declare no conflict of interest.

References

1. Williams, B.; Mancia, G.; Spiering, W.; Agabiti Rosei, E.; Azizi, M.; Burnier, M.; Clement, D.L.; Coca, A.; de Simone, G.; Dominiczak, A.; et al. ESC/ESH Guidelines for the Management of Arterial Hypertension, The Task Force for the Management of Arterial Hypertension of the European Society of Cardiology and the European Society of Hypertension, The Task Force for the Management of Arterial Hypertension of the European Society of Cardiology and the European Society of Hypertension. *J. Hypertens.* **2018**, *36*, 1953–2041. [CrossRef] [PubMed]
2. Chow, C.K.; Teo, K.K.; Rangarajan, S.; Islam, S.; Gupta, R.; Avezum, A.; Bahonar, A.; Chifamba, J.; Dagenais, G.; Diaz, R.; et al. PURE Study Investigators. Prevalence, awareness, treatment, and control of hypertension in rural and urban communities in high-, middle-, and low-income countries. *JAMA* **2013**, *310*, 959–968. [CrossRef] [PubMed]
3. Lip, G.Y.H.; Coca, A.; Kahan, T.; Boriani, G.; Manolis, A.S.; Olsen, M.H.; Oto, A.; Potpara, T.S.; Steffel, J.; Marín, F.; et al. Hypertension and cardiac arrhythmias, A consensus document from the European Heart Rhythm Association (EHRA) and ESC Council on Hypertension, endorsed by the Heart Rhythm Society (HRS), Asia-Pacific Heart Rhythm Society (APHRS) and Sociedad Latinoamericana de Estimulacion Cardiaca y Electrofisiologia (SOLEACE). *Europace* **2017**, *19*, 891–911. [PubMed]
4. Laukkanen, J.A.; Khan, H.; Kurl, S.; Willeit, P.; Karppi, J.; Ronkainen, K.; Di Angelantonio, E. Left ventricular mass and the risk of sudden cardiac death, A population based study. *J. Am. Heart Assoc.* **2014**, *3*, e001285. [CrossRef] [PubMed]
5. Manolis, A.; Doumas, M.; Poulimenos, L.; Kallistratos, M.; Mancia, G. The unappreciated importance of blood pressure in recent and older atrial fibrillation trials. *J. Hypertens.* **2013**, *31*, 2109–2117. [CrossRef] [PubMed]
6. Conen, D.; Tedrow, U.B.; Koplan, B.A.; Glynn, R.J.; Buring, J.E.; Albert, C.M. Influence of systolic and diastolic blood pressure on the risk of incident atrial fibrillation in women. *Circulation* **2009**, *119*, 2146–2152. [CrossRef] [PubMed]
7. Grundvold, I.; Skretteberg, P.T.; Liestøl, K.; Erikssen, G.; Kjeldsen, S.E.; Arnesen, H.; Erikssen, J.; Bodegard, J. Upper normal blood pressures predict incident atrial fibrillation in healthy middle-aged men, A 35-year follow-up study. *Hypertension* **2012**, *59*, 198–204. [CrossRef] [PubMed]
8. Nalliah, C.J.; Sanders, P.; Kalman, J.M. The impact of diet and lifestyle on atrial fibrillation. *Curr. Cardiol. Rep.* **2018**, *20*, 137. [CrossRef] [PubMed]
9. Dzeshka, M.S.; Shantsila, A.; Shantsila, E.; Lip, G.Y.H. Atrial fibrillation and hypertension. *Hypertension* **2017**, *70*, 854–861. [CrossRef] [PubMed]

10. Hindricks, G.; Potpara, T.; Dagres, N.; Arbelo, E.; Bax, J.J.; Blomström-Lundqvist, C.; Boriani, G.; Castella, M.; Dan, G.A.; Dilaveris, P.E.; et al. 2020 ESC Guidelines for the diagnosis and management of atrial fibrillation developed in collaboration with the European Association for Cardio-Thoracic Surgery (EACTS). *Eur. Heart J.* **2021**, *42*, 373–498. [CrossRef] [PubMed]
11. Lip, G.Y.; Andreotti, F.; Fauchier, L.; Huber, K.; Hylek, E.; Knight, E.; Lane, D.; Levi, M.; Marín, F.; Palareti, G.; et al. European Heart Rhythm Association. Bleeding risk assessment and management in atrial fibrillation patients. Executive summary of a position document from the European Heart Rhythm Association [EHRA], endorsed by the European Society of Cardiology [ESC] working group on thrombosis. *Thromb. Haemost.* **2011**, *106*, 997–1011. [CrossRef] [PubMed]
12. Palareti, G.; Cosmi, B. Bleeding with anticoagulation therapy—who is at risk, and how best to identify such patients. *Thromb. Haemost.* **2009**, *102*, 268–278. [CrossRef]
13. Boycott, H.E.; Barbier, C.S.; Eichel, C.A.; Costa, K.D.; Martins, R.P.; Louault, F.; Dilanian, G.; Coulombe, A.; Hatem, S.N.; Balse, E. Shear stress triggers insertion of voltage-gated potassium channels from intracellular compartments in atrial myocytes. *Proc. Natl. Acad. Sci. USA* **2013**, *110*, E3955–E3964. [CrossRef] [PubMed]
14. Woo, S.H.; Risius, T.; Morad, M. Modulation of local Ca2+ release sites by rapid fluid puffing in rat atrial myocytes. *Cell Calcium* **2007**, *41*, 397–403. [CrossRef]
15. Fialova, M.; Dlugosova, K.; Okruhlicová, L.; Kristek, F.; Manoach, M.; Tribulová, N. Adaptation of the heart to hypertension is associated with maladaptive gap junction connexin-43 remodeling. *Physiol. Res.* **2008**, *57*, 7–11. [CrossRef]
16. Lau, D.H.; Mackenzie, L.; Kelly, D.J.; Psaltis, P.J.; Brooks, A.G.; Worthington, M.; Rajendram, A.; Kelly, D.R.; Zhang, Y.; Kuklik, P.; et al. Hypertension and atrial fibrillation, Evidence of progressive atrial remodeling with electrostructural correlate in a conscious chronically instrumented ovine model. *Heart Rhythm.* **2010**, *7*, 1282–1290. [CrossRef]
17. Tribulova, N.; Bacova, B.S.; Benova, T.; Viczenczova, C. Can we protect from malignant arrhythmias by modulation of cardiac cell-to-cell coupling? *J Electrocardiol.* **2015**, *48*, 434–440. [CrossRef]
18. Andelova, K.; Bacova, B.S.; Sykora, M.; Hlivak, P.; Barancik, M.; Tribulova, N. Mechanisms Underlying Antiarrhythmic Properties of Cardioprotective Agents Impacting Inflammation and Oxidative Stress. *Int. J. Mol. Sci.* **2022**, *23*, 1416. [CrossRef] [PubMed]
19. Verdecchia, P.; Angeli, F.; Reboldi, G. Hypertension and Atrial Fibrillation. Doubts and Certainties from Basic and Clinical Studies. *Circ Res.* **2018**, *122*, 352–368. [CrossRef] [PubMed]
20. Afzal, M.R.; Savona, S.; Mohamed, O.; Mohamed-Osman, A.; Kalbfleisch, S.J. Hypertension and Arrhythmias. *Heart Failure Clin.* **2019**, *15*, 543–550. [CrossRef]
21. De Mello, W.C. Intracellular angiotensin II regulates the inward calcium current in cardiac myocytes. *Hypertension* **1998**, *32*, 976–982. [CrossRef]
22. Ferron, L.; Capuano, V.; Ruchon, Y.; Deroubaix, E.; Coulombe, A.; Renaud, J.F. Angiotensin II signaling pathways mediate expression of cardiac T-type calcium channels. *Circ. Res.* **2003**, *93*, 1241–1248. [CrossRef] [PubMed]
23. Daleau, P.; Turgeon, J. Angiotensin II modulates the delayed rectifier potassium current of guinea pig ventricular myocytes. *Pflugers Arch.* **1994**, *427*, 553–555. [CrossRef] [PubMed]
24. Ouvrard-Pascaud, A.; Sainte-Marie, Y.; Bénitah, J.P.; Perrier, R.; Soukaseum, C.; Nguyen Dinh Cat, A.; Royer, A.; Le Quang, K.; Charpentier, F.; Demolombe, S.; et al. Conditional mineralocorticoid receptor expression in the heart leads to life-threatening arrhythmias. *Circulation* **2005**, *111*, 3025–3033. [CrossRef]
25. Tsai, C.T.; Chiang, F.T.; Tseng, C.D.; Hwang, J.J.; Kuo, K.T.; Wu, C.K.; Yu, C.C.; Wang, Y.C.; Lai, L.P.; Lin, J.L. Increased expression of mineralo-corticoid receptor in human atrial fibrillation and a cellular model of atrial fibrillation. *J. Am. Coll. Cardiol.* **2010**, *55*, 758–770. [CrossRef] [PubMed]
26. Gomez, A.M.; Rueda, A.; Sainte-Marie, Y.; Pereira, L.; Zissimopoulos, S.; Zhu, X.; Schaub, R.; Perrier, E.; Perrier, R.; Latouche, C.; et al. Mineralocorticoid modulation of cardiac ryanodine receptor activity is associated with downregulation of FK506-binding proteins. *Circulation* **2009**, *119*, 2179–2187. [CrossRef]
27. Pluteanu, F.; Heß, J.; Plackic, J.; Nikonova, Y.; Preisenberger, J.; Bukowska, A.; Schotten, U.; Rinne, A.; Kienitz, M.C.; Schäfer, M.K.; et al. Early subcellular Ca^{2+} remodelling and increased propensity for Ca^{2+} alternans in left atrial myocytes from hypertensive rats. *Cardiovasc. Res.* **2015**, *106*, 87–97. [CrossRef] [PubMed]
28. Nattel, S.; Heijman, J.; Zhou, L.; Dobrev, D. Molecular Basis of Atrial Fibrillation Pathophysiology and Therapy, A translational perspective. *Circ. Res.* **2020**, *127*, 51–72. [CrossRef] [PubMed]
29. Kahan, T.; Bergfeldt, L. Left ventricular hypertrophy in hypertension, Its arrhythmogenic potential. *Heart* **2005**, *91*, 250–256. [CrossRef] [PubMed]
30. Gonzalez, A.; Lopez, B.; Ravassa, S.; San José, G.; Díez, J. The complex dynamics of myocardial interstitial fibrosis in heart failure. Focus on collagen cross-linking. *Biochim. Biophys. Acta Mol. Cell. Res.* **2019**, *1866*, 1421–1432. [CrossRef]
31. Camici, P.G.; Crea, F. Coronary microvascular dysfunction. *N. Engl. J. Med.* **2007**, *356*, 830–840. [CrossRef] [PubMed]
32. Goette, A.; Kalman, J.M.; Aguinaga, L.; Akar, J.; Cabrera, J.A.; Chen, S.A.; Chugh, S.S.; Corradi, D.; D'Avila, A.; Dobrev, D.; et al. EHRA/HRS/APHRS/SOLAECE expert consensus on atrial cardiomyopathies, Definition, characterization, and clinical implication. *Europace* **2016**, *18*, 1455–1490. [CrossRef] [PubMed]
33. Redfield, M.M. Heart failure with preserved ejection fraction. *N. Engl. J. Med.* **2016**, *375*, 1868–1877. [CrossRef]
34. Triposkiadis, F.; Tentolouris, K.; Androulakis, A.; Trikas, A.; Toutouzas, K.; Kyriakidis, M.; Gialafos, J.; Toutouzas, P. Left atrial mechanical function in the healthy elderly, New insights from a combined assessment of changes in atrial volume and transmitral flow velocity. *J. Am. Soc. Echocardiogr.* **1995**, *8*, 801–809. [CrossRef]

35. Ravelli, F.; Allessie, M. Effects of atrial dilatation on refractory period and vulnerability to atrial fibrillation in the isolated Langendorff perfused rabbit heart. *Circulation* **1997**, *96*, 1686–1695. [CrossRef]
36. Satoh, T.; Zipes, D.P. Unequal atrial stretch in dogs increases dispersion of refractoriness conductive to developing atrial fibrillation. *J. Cardiovasc. Electrophysiol.* **1996**, *7*, 833–842. [CrossRef] [PubMed]
37. Jais, P.; Peng, J.T.; Shah, D.C.; Garrigue, S.; Hocini, M.; Yamane, T.; Haïssaguerre, M.; Barold, S.S.; Roudaut, R.; Clémenty, J. Left ventricular diastolic dysfunction in patients with so-called lone atrial fibrillation. *J. Cardiovasc. Electrophysiol.* **2000**, *11*, 623–625. [CrossRef] [PubMed]
38. Tsang, T.S.M.; Gersh, B.J.; Appleton, C.P.; Tajik, A.J.; Barnes, M.E.; Bailey, K.R.; Oh, J.K.; Leibson, C.; Montgomery, S.C.; Seward, J.B. Left Ventricular Diastolic Dysfunction as a Predictor of the First Diagnosed Nonvalvular Atrial Fibrillation in 840 Elderly Men and Women. *JACC* **2002**, *40*, 1636–1644. [CrossRef]
39. Verdecchia, P.; Reboldi, G.; Gattobigio, R.; Bentivoglio, M.; Borgioni, C.; Angeli, F.; Carluccio, E.; Sardone, M.G.; Porcellati, C. Atrial fibrillation in hypertension, Predictors and outcome. *Hypertension* **2003**, *41*, 218–223. [CrossRef] [PubMed]
40. Ciaroni, S.; Cuenoud, L.; Bloch, A. Clinical study to investigate the predictive parameters for the onset of atrial fibrillation in patients with essential hypertension. *Am. Heart J.* **2000**, *139*, 814–819. [CrossRef]
41. Duncker, D.J.; Zhang, J.; Bache, R.J. Coronary pressure-flow relation in left ventricular hypertrophy. Importance of changes in back pressure versus changes in minimum resistance. *Circ. Res.* **1993**, *72*, 579–587. [CrossRef]
42. Duncker, D.J.; Ishibashi, Y.; Bache, R.J. Effect of treadmill exercise on transmural distribution of blood flow in hypertrophied left ventricle. *Am. J. Physiol.* **1998**, *275*, H1274–H1282. [CrossRef]
43. Vatner, S.F.; Hittinger, L. Coronary vascular mechanisms involved in decompensation from hypertrophy to heart failure. *J. Am. Coll. Cardiol.* **1993**, *22*, 34A–40A. [CrossRef]
44. Kyriakidis, M.; Barbetseas, J.; Antonopoulos, A.; Skouros, C.; Tentolouris, C.; Toutouzas, P. Early atrial arrhythmias in acute myocardial infarction. Role of the sinus node artery. *Chest* **1992**, *101*, 944–947. [CrossRef] [PubMed]
45. Hod, H.; Lew, A.S.; Keltai, M.; Cercek, B.; Geft, I.L.; Shah, P.K.; Ganz, W. Early atrial fibrillation during evolving myocardial infarction, A consequence of impaired left atrial perfusion. *Circulation* **1987**, *75*, 146–150. [CrossRef] [PubMed]
46. Lu Marvin, L.R.; De Venecia, T.; Patnaik, S.; Figueredo, V.M. Atrial myocardial infarction, A tale of the forgotten chamber. *Int. J. Cardiol.* **2015**, *202*, 904–909. [CrossRef]
47. Alasady, M.; Shipp, N.J.; Brooks, A.G.; Lim, H.S.; Lau, D.H.; Barlow, D.; Kuklik, P.; Worthley, M.I.; Roberts-Thomson, K.C.; Saint, D.A.; et al. Myocardial infarction and atrial fibrillation, Importance of atrial ischemia. *Circ. Arrhythm. Electrophysiol.* **2013**, *6*, 738–745. [CrossRef]
48. Kolvekar, S.; D'Souza, A.; Akhtar, P.; Reek, C.; Garratt, C.; Spyt, T. Role of atrial ischaemia in development of atrial fibrillation following coronary artery bypass surgery. *Eur. J. Cardiothorac. Surg.* **1997**, *11*, 70–75. [CrossRef]
49. Ciulla, M.; Astuti, M.; Carugo, S. The atherosclerosis of the sinus node artery is associated with an increased history of supraventricular arrhythmias, A retrospective study on 541 standard coronary angiograms. *PeerJ* **2015**, *3*, e1156. [CrossRef]
50. Bikou, O.; Kho, C.; Ishikawa, K. Atrial stretch and arrhythmia after myocardial infarction. *Aging* **2018**, *11*, 11–12. [CrossRef] [PubMed]
51. Feistritzer, H.J.; Desch, S.; Zeymer, U.; Fuernau, G.; de Waha-Thiele, S.; Dudek, D.; Huber, K.; Stepinska, J.; Schneider, S.; Ouarrak, T.; et al. Prognostic Impact of Atrial Fibrillation in Acute Myocardial Infarction and Cardiogenic Shock. *Circ. Cardiovasc. Interv.* **2019**, *12*, e007661. [CrossRef]
52. Jebberi, Z.; Marazzato, J.; De Ponti, R.; Bagliani, G.; Leonelli, F.M.; Boveda, S. Polymorphic Wide QRS Complex Tachycardia, Differential Diagnosis. *Card. Electrophysiol. Clin.* **2019**, *11*, 333–344. [CrossRef]
53. Marazzato, J.; Angeli, F.; De Ponti, R.; Di Pasquale, G.; Verdecchia, P. Atrial fibrillation and sudden cardiac death, A mystery to unravel? *GIC* **2021**, *22*, 544–553. [CrossRef]
54. Cosentino, F.; Grant, P.J.; Aboyans, V.; Bailey, C.J.; Ceriello, A.; Delgado, V.; Federici, M.; Filippatos, G.; Grobbee, D.E.; Hansen, T.B.; et al. ESC Scientific Document Group, 2019 ESC Guidelines on diabetes, pre-diabetes, and cardiovascular diseases developed in collaboration with the EASD, The Task Force for diabetes, pre-diabetes, and cardiovascular diseases of the European Society of Cardiology (ESC) and the European Association for the Study of Diabetes (EASD). *Eur. Heart J.* **2020**, *41*, 255–323. [CrossRef]
55. Prystowsky, E.N.; Halperin, J.; Kowey, P. Atrial fibrillation, atrial flutter and atrial tachycardia. In *Hurst's the Heart, 14e*; McGraw-Hill: New York, NY, USA, 2017; pp. 1950–1966.
56. De Vos, C.B.; Pisters, R.; Nieuwlaat, R.; Prins, M.H.; Tieleman, R.G.; Coelen, R.J.; van den Heijkant, A.C.; Allessie, M.A.; Crijns, H.J. Progression from paroxysmal to persistent atrial fibrillation clinical correlates and prognosis. *J. Am. Coll. Cardiol.* **2010**, *55*, 725–731. [CrossRef]
57. Potpara, T.S.; Stankovic, G.R.; Beleslin, B.D.; Polovina, M.M.; Marinkovic, J.M.; Ostojic, M.C.; Lip, G.Y.H. A 12-year follow-up study of patients with newly diagnosed lone atrial fibrillation, Implications of arrhythmia progression on prognosis, The Belgrade Atrial Fibrillation study. *Chest* **2012**, *141*, 339–347. [CrossRef] [PubMed]
58. Potpara, T.S.; Polovina, M.M.; Marinkovic, J.M.; Lip, G.Y. A comparison of clinical characteristics and long-term prognosis in asymptomatic and symptomatic patients with first-diagnosed atrial fibrillation, The Belgrade Atrial Fibrillation study. *Int. J. Cardiol.* **2013**, *168*, 4744–4749. [CrossRef] [PubMed]

59. Rapsomaniki, E.; Timmis, A.; George, J.; Pujades-Rodriguez, M.; Shah, A.D.; Denaxas, S.; White, I.R.; Caulfield, M.J.; Deanfield, J.E.; Smeeth, L.; et al. Blood pressure and incidence of twelve cardiovascular diseases, Lifetime risks, healthy life-years lost, and age-specific associations in 1.25 million people. *Lancet* **2014**, *383*, 1899–1911. [CrossRef]
60. Li, C.; Engström, G.; Hedblad, B.; Hedblad, B.; Berglund, G.; Janzon, L. Blood pressure control and risk of stroke, A population-based prospective cohort study. *Stroke* **2005**, *36*, 725–730. [CrossRef]
61. Wolf, P.A.; Abbott, R.D.; Kannel, W.B. Atrial fibrillation, A major contributor to stroke in the elderly. The Framingham Study. *Arch. Intern. Med.* **1987**, *147*, 1561–1564. [CrossRef] [PubMed]
62. Friberg, L.; Rosenqvist, M.; Lip, G.Y. Evaluation of risk stratification schemes for ischaemic stroke and bleeding in 182 678 patients with atrial fibrillation, The Swedish Atrial Fibrillation cohort study. *Eur. Heart J.* **2012**, *33*, 1500–1510. [CrossRef]
63. Paciaroni, M.; Agnelli, G.; Ageno, W.; Caso, V. Timing of anticoagulation therapy in patients with acute ischaemic stroke and atrial fibrillation. *Thromb. Haemost.* **2016**, *116*, 410–416. [CrossRef] [PubMed]
64. Gage, B.F.; Waterman, A.D.; Shannon, W.; Boechler, M.; Rich, M.W.; Radford, M.J. Validation of clinical classification schemes for predicting stroke, Results from the national registry of atrial fibrillation. *JAMA* **2001**, *285*, 2864–2870. [CrossRef] [PubMed]
65. Ishii, M.; Ogawa, H.; Unoki, T.; An, Y.; Iguchi, M.; Masunaga, N.; Esato, M.; Chun, Y.H.; Tsuji, H.; Wada, H.; et al. Relationship of Hypertension and Systolic Blood Pressure with the Risk of Stroke or Bleeding in Patients with Atrial Fibrillation, The Fushimi AF Registry. *Am. J. Hypertens.* **2017**, *30*, 1073–1082. [CrossRef] [PubMed]
66. Kodani, E.; Inoue, H.; Atarashi, H.; Okumura, K.; Yamashita, T.; Otsuka, T.; Origasa, H. Impact of Blood Pressure Visit-to-Visit Variability on Adverse Events in Patients With Nonvalvular Atrial Fibrillation, Subanalysis of the J-RHYTHM Registry. *J. Am. Heart Assoc.* **2021**, *10*, e018585. [CrossRef] [PubMed]
67. Parcha, V.; Patel, N.; Kalra, R.; Kim, J.; Gutiérrez, O.M.; Arora, G.; Arora, P. Incidence and Implications of Atrial Fibrillation/Flutter in Hypertension Insights From the SPRINT Trial. *Hypertension* **2020**, *75*, 1483–1490. [CrossRef] [PubMed]
68. Zabalgoitia, M.; Halperin, J.L.; Pearce, L.A.; Blackshear, J.L.; Asinger, R.W.; Hart, R.G. Transesophageal echocardiographic correlates of clinical risk of thromboembolism in nonvalvular atrial fibrillation. Stroke Prevention in Atrial Fibrillation III Investigators. *J. Am. Coll. Cardiol.* **1998**, *31*, 1622–1626. [CrossRef]
69. Goldman, M.E.; Pearce, L.A.; Hart, R.G.; Zabalgoitia, M.; Asinger, R.W.; Safford, R.; Halperin, J.L. Pathophysiologic correlates of thromboembolism in nonvalvular atrial fibrillation, I. reduced flow velocity in the left atrial appendage (the Stroke Prevention in Atrial Fibrillation [SPAF-III] study). *J. Am. Soc. Echocardiogr.* **1999**, *12*, 1080–1087. [CrossRef]
70. Bukowska, A.; Zacharias, I.; Weinert, S.; Skopp, K.; Hartmann, C.; Huth, C.; Goette, A. Coagulation factor Xa induces an inflammatory signalling by activation of protease-activated receptors in human atrial tissue. *Eur. J. Pharmacol.* **2013**, *718*, 114–123. [CrossRef] [PubMed]
71. Bukowska, A.; Rocken, C.; Erxleben, M.; Röhl, F.W.; Hammwöhner, M.; Huth, C.; Ebert, M.P.; Lendeckel, U.; Goette, A. Atrial expression of endothelial nitric oxide synthase in patients with and without atrial fibrillation. *Cardiovasc. Pathol.* **2010**, *19*, e51–e60. [CrossRef] [PubMed]
72. Goette, A.; Bukowska, A.; Lendeckel, U.; Erxleben, M.; Hammwöhner, M.; Strugala, D.; Pfeiffenberger, J.; Röhl, F.W.; Huth, C.; Ebert, M.P.; et al. Angiotensin II receptor blockade reduces tachycardia-induced atrial adhesion molecule expression. *Circulation* **2008**, *117*, 732–742. [CrossRef] [PubMed]
73. Hammwohner, M.; Ittenson, A.; Dierkes, J.; Bukowska, A.; Klein, H.U.; Lendeckel, U.; Goette, A. Platelet expression of CD40/CD40 ligand and its relation to inflammatory markers and adhesion molecules in patients with atrial fibrillation. *Exp. Biol. Med.* **2007**, *232*, 581–589.
74. Fiebeler, A.; Schmidt, F.; Müller, D.N.; Park, J.K.; Dechend, R.; Bieringer, M.; Shagdarsuren, E.; Breu, V.; Haller, H.; Luft, F.C. Mineralocorticoid receptor affects AP-1 and nuclear factor-kappab activation in angiotensin II-induced cardiac injury. *Hypertension* **2001**, *37*, 787–793. [CrossRef] [PubMed]
75. Keidar, S.; Kaplan, M.; Pavlotzky, E.; Coleman, R.; Hayek, T.; Hamoud, S.; Aviram, M. Aldosterone administration to mice stimulates macrophage NADPH oxidase and increases atherosclerosis development, A possible role for angiotensin-convert-ing enzyme and the receptors for angiotensin II and aldosterone. *Circulation* **2004**, *109*, 2213–2220. [CrossRef] [PubMed]
76. Sun, Y.; Zhang, J.; Lu, L.; Chen, S.S.; Quinn, M.T.; Weber, K.T. Aldosterone-induced inflammation in the rat heart, Role of oxidative stress. *Am. J. Pathol.* **2002**, *161*, 1773–1781. [CrossRef]
77. Kim, D.; Yang, P.S.; Kim, T.H.; Jang, E.; Shin, H.; Kim, H.Y.; Yu, H.T.; Uhm, J.S.; Kim, J.Y.; Pak, H.N.; et al. Ideal blood pressure in patients with atrial fibrillation. *J. Am. Coll. Cardiol.* **2018**, *72*, 1233–1245. [CrossRef] [PubMed]
78. Kimura, S.; Ito, M.; Tomita, M.; Hoyano, M.; Obata, H.; Ding, L.; Chinushi, M.; Hanawa, H.; Kodama, M.; Aizawa, Y. Role of mineralocorticoid receptor on atrial structural remodeling and inducibility of atrial fibrillation in hypertensive rats. *Hypertens. Res.* **2011**, *34*, 584–591. [CrossRef] [PubMed]
79. Matsuyama, N.; Tsutsumi, T.; Kubota, N.; Nakajima, T.; Suzuki, H.; Takeyama, Y. Direct action of an angiotensin II receptor blocker on angiotensin II-induced left atrial conduction delay in spontaneously hypertensive rats. *Hypertens. Res.* **2009**, *32*, 721–726. [CrossRef] [PubMed]
80. Fogari, R.; Zoppi, A.; Maffioli, P.; Mugellini, A.; Preti, P.; Perrone, T.; Derosa, G. Effect of telmisartan on paroxysmal atrial fibrillation recurrence in hypertensive patients with normal or increased left atrial size. *Clin. Cardiol.* **2012**, *35*, 359–364. [CrossRef] [PubMed]

81. Wachtell, K.; Lehto, M.; Gerdts, E.; Olsen, M.H.; Hornestam, B.; Dahlöf, B.; Ibsen, H.; Julius, S.; Kjeldsen, S.E.; Lindholm, L.H.; et al. Angiotensin II receptor blockade reduces new-onset atrial fibrillation and subsequent stroke compared to atenolol, The Losartan Intervention For End Point Reduction in Hypertension (LIFE) study. *J. Am. Coll. Cardiol.* **2005**, *45*, 712–719. [CrossRef] [PubMed]
82. Cohn, J.N.; Tognoni, G. Valsartan Heart Failure Trial Investigators. A randomized trial of the angiotensin-receptor blocker valsartan in chronic heart failure. *N. Engl. J. Med.* **2001**, *345*, 1667–1675. [CrossRef] [PubMed]
83. Ducharme, A.; Swedberg, K.; Pfeffer, M.A.; Cohen-Solal, A.; Granger, C.B.; Maggioni, A.P.; Michelson, E.L.; McMurray, J.J.V.; Olsson, L.; Rouleau, J.L.; et al. Prevention of atrial fibrillation in patients with symptomatic chronic heart failure by candesartan in the Candesartan in Heart failure, Assessment of Reduction in Mortality and morbidity (CHARM) program. *Am. Heart J.* **2006**, *152*, 86–92. [CrossRef] [PubMed]
84. Vermes, E.; Tardif, J.C.; Bourassa, M.G.; Racine, N.; Levesque, S.; White, M.; Guerra, P.G.; Ducharme, A. Enalapril decreases the incidence of atrial fibrillation in patients with left ventricular dysfunction, Insight from the Studies of Left Ventricular Dysfunction (SOLVD) trials. *Circulation.* **2003**, *107*, 2926–2931. [CrossRef] [PubMed]
85. Schaer, B.A.; Schneider, C.; Jick, S.S.; Conen, D.; Osswald, S.; Meier, C.R. Risk for incident atrial fibrillation in patients who receive antihypertensive drugs, A nested case-control study. *Ann. Intern. Med.* **2010**, *152*, 78–84. [CrossRef] [PubMed]
86. Swedberg, K.; Zannad, F.; McMurray, J.J.; Krum, H.; van Veldhuisen, D.J.; Shi, H.; Vincent, J.; Pitt, B. Eplerenone and atrial fibrillation in mild systolic heart failure, Results from the EMPHASIS-HF (Eplerenone in Mild Patients Hospitalization and SurvIval Study in Heart Failure) study. *J. Am. Coll. Cardiol.* **2012**, *59*, 1598–1603. [CrossRef] [PubMed]
87. Al-Gobariet, M.; El Khatib, C.; Pillon, F.; Gueyffier, F. Beta-blockers for the prevention of sudden cardiac death in heart failure patients, A meta-analysis of randomized controlled trials. *BMC Cardiovasc Disord.* **2013**, *13*, 52. [CrossRef]
88. Disertori, M.; Latini, R.; Barlera, S.; Franzosi, M.G.; Staszewsky, L.; Maggioni, A.P.; Lucci, D.; Di Pasquale, G.; Tognoni, G. Valsartan for prevention of recurrent atrial fibrillation. *N. Engl. J. Med.* **2009**, *360*, 1606–1617. [PubMed]
89. Goette, A.; Schon, N.; Kirchhof, P.; Breithardt, G.; Fetsch, T.; Häusler, K.G.; Klein, H.U.; Steinbeck, G.; Wegscheider, K.; Meinertz, T. Angiotensin II-antagonist in paroxysmal atrial fibrillation (ANTIPAF) trial. *Circ. Arrhythm. Electrophysiol.* **2012**, *5*, 43–51. [CrossRef] [PubMed]
90. Tveit, A.; Grundvold, I.; Olufsen, M.; Seljeflot, I.; Abdelnoor, M.; Arnesen, H.; Smith, P. Candesartan in the prevention of relapsing atrial fibrillation. *Int. J. Cardiol.* **2007**, *120*, 85–91. [CrossRef]
91. Schirpenbach, C.; Reincke, M. Primary aldosteronism, Current knowledge and controversies in Conn's syndrome. *Nat. Rev. Endocrinol.* **2007**, *3*, 220–227. [CrossRef] [PubMed]
92. Funder, J.W.; Carey, R.M.; Mantero, F.; Murad, M.H.; Reincke, M.; Shibata, H.; Stowasser, M.; Young, W.F., Jr. The management of primary aldosteronism, Case detection, diagnosis, and treatment, An endocrine society clinical practice guideline. *J. Clin. Endocrinol. Metab.* **2016**, *101*, 1889–1916. [CrossRef] [PubMed]
93. Hundemer, G.L.; Curhan, G.C.; Yozamp, N.; Wang, M.; Vaidya, A. Cardiometabolic outcomes and mortality in medically treated primary aldosteronism, A retrospective cohort study. *Lancet Diabetes Endocrinol.* **2018**, *6*, 51–59. [CrossRef]
94. Milliez, P.; Girerd, X.; Plouin, P.F.; Blacher, J.; Safar, M.E.; Mourad, J.J. Evidence for an increased rate of cardiovascular events in patients with primary aldosteronism. *J. Am. Coll. Cardiol.* **2005**, *45*, 1243–1248. [CrossRef] [PubMed]
95. Born-Frontsberg, E.; Reincke, M.; Rump, L.C.; Hahner, S.; Diederich, S.; Lorenz, R.; Allolio, B.; Seufert, J.; Schirpenbach, C.; Beuschlein, F.; et al. Cardiovascular and cerebrovascular comorbidities of hypokalemic and normokalemic primary aldosteronism, Results of the German Conn's Registry. *J. Clin. Endocrinol. Metab.* **2009**, *94*, 1125–1130. [CrossRef]
96. Pan, C.-T.; Tsai, C.; Chen, Z.W.; Chang, Y.Y.; Wu, V.C.; Hung, C.S.; Lin, Y.H. Atrial Fibrillation in Primary Aldosteronism. *Horm. Metab. Res.* **2020**, *52*, 357–365. [CrossRef]
97. Oestreicher, E.M.; Martinez-Vasquez, D.; Stone, J.R.; Jonasson, L.; Roubsanthisuk, W.; Mukasa, K.; Adler, G.K. Aldosterone and not plasminogen activator inhibitor-1 is a critical mediator of early angiotensin II/NG-nitro-L-arginine methyl ester-induced myocardial injury. *Circulation* **2003**, *108*, 2517–2523. [CrossRef]
98. Krijthe, B.P.; Heeringa, J.; Kors, J.A.; Hofman, A.; Franco, O.H.; Witteman, J.C.; Stricker, B.H. Serum potassium levels and the risk of atrial fibrillation, The Rotterdam Study. *Int. J. Cardiol.* **2013**, *168*, 5411–5415. [CrossRef] [PubMed]
99. Auer, J.; Weber, T.; Berent, R.; Lamm, G.; Eber, B. Serum potassium level and risk of postoperative atrial fibrillation in patients undergoing cardiac surgery. *J. Am. Coll. Cardiol.* **2004**, *44*, 938–939. [CrossRef] [PubMed]
100. Weiss, J.N.; Qu, Z.; Shivkumar, K. Electrophysiology of hypokalemia and hyperkalemia. *Circ. Arrhyth. Electrophysiol.* **2017**, *10*, e004667. [CrossRef]
101. Vaidya, A.; Mulatero, P.; Baudrand, R.; Adler, G.K. The Expanding Spectrum of Primary Aldosteronism, Implications for Diagnosis, Pathogenesis, and Treatment. *Endocr. Rev.* **2018**, *39*, 1057–1088. [CrossRef]
102. Wang, K.; Hu, J.; Yang, J.; Song, Y.; Fuller, P.J.; Hashimura, H.; He, W.; Feng, Z.; Cheng, Q.; Du, Z.; et al. Development and Validation of Criteria for Sparing Confirmatory Tests in Diagnosing Primary Aldosteronism. *J. Clin. Endocrinol. Metab.* **2020**, *105*, dgaa282. [CrossRef] [PubMed]
103. Hundemer, G.L.; Curhan, G.C.; Yozamp, N.; Wang, M.; Vaidya, A. Incidence of Atrial Fibrillation and Mineralocorticoid Receptor Activity in Patients With Medically and Surgically Treated Primary Aldosteronism. *JAMA Cardiol.* **2018**, *3*, 768–774. [CrossRef] [PubMed]

104. Rossi, G.P.; Maiolino, G.; Flego, A.; Belfiore, A.; Bernini, G.; Fabris, B.; Ferri, C.; Giacchetti, G.; Letizia, C.; Maccario, M.; et al. PAPY Study Investigators. Adrenalectomy Lowers Incident Atrial Fibrillation in Primary Aldosteronism Patients at Long Term. *Hypertension* **2018**, *71*, 585–591. [CrossRef] [PubMed]
105. Boriani, G.; Imberti, J.F.; Vitolo, M. The challenge to improve knowledge on the interplay between subclinical atrial fibrillation, atrial cardiomyopathy, and atrial remodeling. *J. Cardiovasc. Electrophysiol.* **2021**, *32*, 1364–1366. [CrossRef]
106. Rabkin, S.W.; Moe, G. The case against using hypertension as the only criterion for oral anticoagulation in atrial fibrillation. *Can. J. Cardiol.* **2015**, *31*, 576–579. [CrossRef] [PubMed]
107. Freedman, B.; Camm, J.; Calkins, H.; Healey, J.S.; Rosenqvist, M.; Wang, J.; Albert, C.M.; Anderson, C.S.; Antoniou, S.; Benjamin, E.J.; et al. AF-Screen Collaborators. Screening for atrial fibrillation, A report of the AF-SCREEN International Collaboration. *Circulation* **2017**, *135*, 1851–1867. [CrossRef] [PubMed]
108. Healey, J.S.; Alings, M.; Ha, A.; Leong-Sit, P.; Birnie, D.H.; de Graaf, J.J.; Freericks, M.; Verma, A.; Wang, J.; Leong, D.; et al. ASSERT-II Investigators. Subclinical atrial fibrillation in older patients. *Circulation* **2017**, *136*, 1276–1283. [CrossRef] [PubMed]
109. Healey, J.S.; Connolly, S.J.; Gold, M.R.; Israel, C.W.; Van Gelder, I.C.; Capucci, A.; Lau, C.P.; Fain, E.; Yang, S.; Bailleul, C.; et al. ASSERT Investigators. Subclinical atrial fibrillation and the risk of stroke. *N. Engl. J. Med.* **2012**, *366*, 120–129, Erratum in *N. Engl. J. Med.* **2016**, *374*, 998. [CrossRef]
110. Svendsen, J.H.; Diederichsen, S.Z.; Højberg, S.; Krieger, D.W.; Graff, C.; Kronborg, C.; Olesen, M.S.; Nielsen, J.B.; Holst, A.G.; Brandes, A.; et al. Implantable loop recorder detection of atrial fibrillation to prevent stroke (The LOOP Study), A randomised controlled trial. *Lancet* **2021**, *398*, 1507–1516, Erratum in *Lancet* **2021**, *398*, 1486. [CrossRef]
111. Gorenek, B.; Bax, J.; Boriani, G.; Chen, S.A.; Dagres, N.; Glotzer, T.V.; Healey, J.S.; Israel, C.W.; Kudaiberdieva, G.; Levin, L.Å.; et al. ESC Scientific Document Group. Device-detected subclinical atrial tachyarrhythmias, Definition, implications and management-an European Heart Rhythm Association (EHRA) consensus document, endorsed by Heart Rhythm Society (HRS), Asia Pacific Heart Rhythm Society (APHRS) and Sociedad Latinoamericana de Estimulación Cardíaca y Electrofisiología (SOLEACE). *Europace* **2017**, *19*, 1556–1578, Erratum in *Europace* **2017**, *19*, 1507; Erratum in *Europace* **2018**, *20*, 658. [CrossRef]
112. Van Gelder, I.C.; Healey, J.S.; Crijns, H.J.G.M.; Wang, J.; Hohnloser, S.H.; Gold, M.R.; Capucci, A.; Lau, C.P.; Morillo, C.A.; Hobbel, A.H.; et al. Duration of device-detected subclinical atrial fibrillation and occurrence of stroke in ASSERT. *Eur. Heart J.* **2017**, *38*, 1339–1344. [CrossRef] [PubMed]
113. Lopes, R.D.; Alings, M.; Connolly, S.J.; Beresh, H.; Granger, C.B.; Mazuecos, J.B.; Boriani, G.; Nielsen, J.C.; Conen, D.; Hohnloser, S.H.; et al. Rationale and design of the Apixaban for the Reduction of Thrombo-Embolism in Patients With Device-Detected Sub-Clinical Atrial Fibrillation (ARTESiA) trial. *Am. Heart J.* **2017**, *189*, 137–145. [CrossRef] [PubMed]
114. Paulus, K.; Blank, B.F.; Calvert, M.; Camm, A.J.; Chlouverakis, G.; Diener, H.C.; Goette, A.; Huening, A.; Lip, G.Y.H.; Simantirakis, E.; et al. Probing oral anticoagulation in patients with atrial high rate episodes. Rationale and design of the Non vitamin K antagonist Oral anticoagulants in patients with Atrial High rate episodes (NOAH—AFNET 6) trial. *Am. Heart J.* **2017**, *190*, 12–18. [CrossRef]
115. Diederichsen, S.; Haugan, K.J.; Brandes, A.; Graff, C.; Krieger, D.; Kronborg, C.; Holst, A.G.; Nielsen, J.B.; Køber, L.; Højberg, S.; et al. Incidence and predictors of atrial fibrillation episodes as detected by implantable loop recorder in patients at risk From the LOOP study. *Am. Heart J.* **2019**, *219*, 117–127. [CrossRef] [PubMed]
116. Pérez-Riera, A.R.; Barbosa-Barros, R.; Pereira-Rejálaga, L.E.; Nikus, K.; Shenasa, M. Electrocardiographic and Echocardiographic Abnormalities in Patients with Risk Factors for Atrial Fibrillation. *Card. Electrophysiol. Clin.* **2021**, *13*, 211–219. [CrossRef] [PubMed]
117. Jones, N.R.; Taylor, C.J.; Hobbs, F.D.R.; Bowman, L.; Casadei, B. Screening for atrial fibrillation, A call for evidence. *Eur. Heart J.* **2020**, *41*, 1075–1085. [CrossRef] [PubMed]

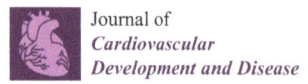

Review

Tight Blood Pressure Control in Chronic Kidney Disease

Giorgio Gentile [1,2], Kathryn Mckinney [3] and Gianpaolo Reboldi [4,*]

1. College of Medicine and Health, University of Exeter, Exeter EX1 2LU, UK; g.gentile2@exeter.ac.uk
2. Department of Nephrology, Royal Cornwall Hospitals NHS Trust, Truro TR1 3LQ, UK
3. Faculty of Biology, College of Letters and Science, University of Wisconsin-Madison, Madison, WI 53706, USA; kmckinney3@wisc.edu
4. Centro di Ricerca Clinica e Traslazionale (CERICLET), Department of Medicine, University of Perugia, 06156 Perugia, Italy
* Correspondence: paolo.reboldi@unipg.it

Abstract: Hypertension affects over a billion people worldwide and is the leading cause of cardiovascular disease and premature death worldwide, as well as one of the key determinants of chronic kidney disease worldwide. People with chronic kidney disease and hypertension are at very high risk of renal outcomes, including progression to end-stage renal disease, and, even more importantly, cardiovascular outcomes. Hence, blood pressure control is crucial in reducing the human and socio-economic burden of renal and cardiovascular outcomes in those patients. However, current guidelines from hypertension and renal societies have issued different and sometimes conflicting recommendations, which risk confusing clinicians and potentially contributing to a less effective prevention of renal and cardiovascular outcomes. In this review, we critically appraise existing evidence and key international guidelines, and we finally formulate our own opinion that clinicians should aim for a blood pressure target lower than 130/80 in all patients with chronic kidney disease and hypertension, unless they are frail or with multiple comorbidities. We also advocate for an even more ambitious systolic blood pressure target lower than 120 mmHg in younger patients with a lower burden of comorbidities, to minimise their risk of renal and cardiovascular events during their lifetime.

Keywords: hypertension; chronic kidney disease; blood pressure targets; intensive blood pressure control; renal outcomes; cardiovascular outcomes

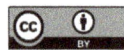

1. Introduction

Hypertension affects 1.39 billion people worldwide (25% of the total adult population) and is the leading cause of cardiovascular disease, including stroke and myocardial infarction, and premature death [1]. Hypertension causes 7,500,000 premature deaths per year (12.8% of global casualties), outnumbering both diabetes (3,400,000 deaths, 3.4%) and obesity (2,800,000 deaths, 4.8%) [2]. As the rise in blood pressure (BP) with age is a universal feature of human aging, and as the global population is getting older, hypertension will likely become even more prevalent by 2040 [3].

Hypertension is also a leading cause of chronic kidney disease (CKD) through its harmful effects on kidney vasculature; in turn, worsening CKD leads to increased sympathetic tone and salt sensitivity, upregulation of the renin–angiotensin–aldosterone system (RAAS), endothelial dysfunction, and worsening arterial stiffness, eventually driving the further progression of hypertension [4]. This vicious cycle ultimately causes a progression towards end-stage renal disease (ESRD) requiring renal replacement therapy (RRT) [5], and even worse, a dramatic increase in cardiovascular (CV) morbidity and mortality [6]. For hypertensive people with stage 3 or 4 CKD (estimated glomerular filtration rate (eGFR) of 30–59 mL/min/1.73 m^2 or 15–29 mL/min/1.73 m^2, respectively), as defined by the Kidney Disease: Improving Global Outcomes (KDIGO) guidelines [7], the risk of dying of CV disease far exceeds the risk of developing ESRD [8].

Hence, blood pressure control is crucial to slow the progression of CKD and reduce the catastrophic socio-economic burden of CV events in this high-risk population [9,10]. Possible therapeutic strategies include the choice of certain drugs, isolated or in combination, which might theoretically provide additional reno- or cardioprotective benefits (e.g., ACE inhibitors, angiotensin receptor blockers (ARBs), calcium channel blockers (CCBs), etc.), or achieving specific BP targets, which are often tighter in the presence of significant albuminuria (albumin-to-creatinine ratio (ACR) > 70 mg/mmol) [11] or proteinuria (i.e., >0.3 g/24 h) [12]. However, there is still a considerable and heated debate regarding the 'optimal' blood pressure target in hypertensive patients with CKD. At one extreme of the spectrum are international societies such as the American College of Cardiology (ACC), which recommends a BP target lower than 130/80 mmHg independently of the level of proteinuria [13], or the International Society of Nephrology (ISN), with an even more ambitious systolic BP target of <120 mmHg. On the other side of the spectrum, the 2018 European Society of Cardiology/European Society of Hypertension (ESC/ESH) guideline recommends to lower systolic BP to a range of 130–139 mmHg, irrespective of proteinuria [14], and the 2021 NICE guidelines are even more cautious by advocating for a BP target lower than 140/90 in CKD patients with an ACR < 70 mg/mmol, and lower than 130/80 only in the presence of an ACR $\geq$ 70.

The current review will critically appraise all existing evidence used to create the different and subtly divergent guidelines for hypertension control in CKD patients and try to formulate a balanced opinion on the role of tight BP control in CKD by specifically focusing on BP targets rather than specific drug classes. However, for the sake of clarity we will also briefly consider the evidence on the specific reno- and cardioprotective role of some antihypertensive agents independently of the degree of BP control.

2. Current Guidelines on BP Targets in Non-Dialysis CKD Patients

Key guidelines from hypertension and renal societies are summarised in Table 1.

Table 1. Current guidelines on BP targets in non-dialysis CKD patients.

Guideline Agency	Country	Year	Target Recommendation (mmHg)	First-Line Agents Recommended
Hypertension societies				
Joint National Commission on Prevention, Detection, Assessment and Treatment of Hypertension (JNC-VIII) [15]	United States	2014	<140/90 (people aged 18–69 with CKD or diabetes) No recommendation for CKD patients aged 70 or above ("treatment should be individualized taking into consideration factors such as frailty, comorbidities, and albuminuria")	ACEi or ARB (regardless of ethnicity or diabetic status)
American College of Cardiology (ACC) [13]	United States	2017	<130/80 in all adults with hypertension and CKD, regardless of proteinuria	ACEi (ARB if the ACEi is not tolerated)
European Society of Hypertension/European Society of Cardiology (ESH/ESC) [14]	Europe	2018	Systolic BP between 130 and 139	ACEi or ARB (regardless of diabetic status)
Renal societies				
European Best Practice Guidelines (EBPG) [16]	Europe	2013	<140/90 (no albuminuria/proteinuria) <130/80 (ACR $\geq$ 30 mg/g, i.e., at least moderately increased albuminuria, or UPCR $\geq$ 150)	ACEi or ARB

Table 1. *Cont.*

Guideline Agency	Country	Year	Target Recommendation (mmHg)	First-Line Agents Recommended
Italian Society of Nephrology [17]	Italy	2013	<140/90 (normoalbuminuria) <130/80 (albuminuria >30 mg/24 h, i.e., at least moderately increased albuminuria)	ACEi or ARB
Kidney Health Australia- Caring for Australasians with Renal Impairment (KHA-CARI) [18]	Australia	2014	<140/90 (normoalbuminuria or moderately increased albuminuria) <130/80 (severely increased albuminuria)	ACEi or ARB
Canadian Society of Nephrology (CSN) [19]	Canada	2015	<140/90 (regardless of diabetes or proteinuria)	ACEi or ARB
UK Kidney Association (UKKA) [20]	UK	2021	<130/80 (if, following a shared decision-making discussion, it is tolerated by the individual)	No explicit recommendation
National Institute for Health and Care Excellence (NICE) [11]	UK	2021	<140/90 (if ACR < 70 mg/mmol) <130/80 (if ACR ≥ 70 mg/mmol; target range 120 to 129 mmHg)	ACEi or ARB (titrated at the highest tolerated dose, for any patient with ACR > 30 mg/mmol)
Kidney Disease: Improving Global Outcomes (KDIGO) [21]	Global (International Society of Nephrology)	2021	Systolic BP <120 (if tolerated)	ACEi or ARB (for any patient with moderately or severely increased albuminuria)

Abbreviations: ACEi—Angiotensin converting enzyme inhibitor; ARB—angiotensin receptor blocker; ACR—albumin-to-creatinine ratio; UPCR—urine protein-to-creatinine ratio; UK—United Kingdom.

2.1. Hypertension Guidelines

Amongst the hypertension guidelines published over the last decade, the JNC-VIII guideline initially suggested a BP target <140/90 mmHg in CKD patients aged 18–69. In patients aged 70 or above, no specific recommendations were issued, apart from a generic advice that "treatment should be individualized taking into consideration factors such as frailty, comorbidities, and albuminuria" [15]. The JNC-VIII committee issued its recommendations after reviewing three studies: the Modification of Diet in Renal Disease (MDRD) study [22], the African American Study of Kidney Disease and Hypertension (AASK) [23] and the Blood-Pressure Control for Renoprotection in Patients with Non-Diabetic Chronic Renal Disease (REIN-2) study [24].

The MDRD study [25] was designed as two separate randomised trials; the first one in 585 patients with a GFR between 25 and 55 mL/min/1.73 m^2 (study A) and the second one in 255 patients with a GFR of 13–24 mL/min/1.73 m^2 (study B). Although in both trials tight BP control (mean arterial pressure (MAP) ≤92 mmHg, i.e., 125/75 mmHg) did not improve the primary composite outcome of ESRD, time of doubling of serum creatinine or GFR reduction compared to standard BP control over 2.2 years of follow-up, a post-hoc analysis indicated a benefit from tight BP control in patients with baseline proteinuria levels >1 g/24 h [26]. However, this might be explained by the fact that ACEis were used much more frequently in patients randomised to a tighter BP control compared to a standard control, which might have led to greater renoprotective benefits in the subgroup of patients with higher baseline proteinuria [26].

The AASK trial [23] enrolled 1094 African Americans aged 18 to 70 years with hypertensive renal disease and no marked proteinuria and used a 3 × 2 factorial design to compare the effects of intensive (target MAP 92 mmHg) versus standard (102–107 mmHg) BP control, as well as ACEis, CCBs and β-blockers, on a composite outcome of death,

ESRD or reduction in the GFR of ≥50%. Despite a significant difference in achieved BP amongst the two arms (128/78 vs. 141/85 mmHg) over 4.1 years of follow-up, tighter BP control did not reduce the risk of the primary composite outcome or the GFR slope (−2.21 vs. 1.95 mL/min/1.73 m^2/year in the standard BP control group). During the 4.1 years of follow-up, the achieved BP averaged 128/78 mmHg in the lower BP group and 141/85 mmHg in the standard BP group. Interestingly, ACEis allowed a significant reduction in the risk of the primary outcome compared to CCBs and β-blockers. However, ramipril allowed a 22% and 38% greater reduction in the composite outcome compared to metoprolol and amlodipine, respectively.

The REIN-2 trial [24] enrolled 338 patients with non-diabetic CKD, randomised to either tight BP control (diastolic BP < 90 mm Hg) or standard BP control. Tighter BP control did not lead to any improvement in the primary outcome of time to ESRD over 3 years of follow-up (hazard ratio (HR) 1, 95% confidence interval [CI] 0.61–1.64; p = 0.99).

After three years from the publication of the JNC-VIII guidelines, in 2017, the ACC took a very different stance by suggesting a much more ambitious BP target of <130/80 mmHg in all hypertensive adults with CKD, regardless of the levels of proteinuria [13]. The main reason for this new position was the publication of the landmark Systolic Blood Pressure Intervention Trial (SPRINT) in 2015 [27]. In this trial, 9361 non-diabetic patients at high CV risk (previous CV event or with at least one risk factor, including smoking, dyslipidemia or CKD) were randomised to either intensive (systolic BP < 120 mmHg) or standard (<140 mmHg) BP control. The primary endpoint was a composite of myocardial infarction, other acute coronary syndromes, stroke, heart failure or CV death. At 1 year, achieved BP was 121.4 versus 136.2 mmHg in the intensive and standard BP control groups, respectively. The study was stopped earlier than anticipated (after a median follow-up time of 3.26 years) because of clear evidence of a significant benefit of intensive BP control on the primary composite outcome compared to standard BP control (HR 0.75, 95% CI 0.64–0.89, p < 0.001). Additionally, intensive BP control allowed a significant reduction in all-cause mortality (HR 0.73, 95% CI 0.6–0.9, p = 0.003). Similar benefits were observed in the subgroup of patients with stage 3 or 4 CKD (approximately 28% of the study population), which was considered as strong evidence in favour of a BP target lower than 130/80, especially because most patients with CKD die due to CV complications [8].

In 2018, the ESH/ESC issued updated guidance on BP control in CKD patients, which seems to be a compromise between the JNC-VIII and the ACC guidelines. In fact, the ESH/ESC guideline suggests that "in patients with CKD, BP should be lowered to <140/90 mmHg and towards 130/80 mmHg" [14]. In particular, the guidance recommends to lower systolic BP to a range of 130–139 mmHg in patients with diabetic or non-diabetic CKD [28–30]. The ESH/ESC committee acknowledged that a tighter BP control can significantly reduce all-cause mortality in CKD patients, as highlighted by a meta-analysis of Malhotra et al., which extracted mortality data from 18 trials that enrolled 15,924 CKD patients assigned to a more versus less intensive BP control [31]. Baseline mean systolic BP was 146 mmHg in both groups, but it dropped to 132 mmHg with tighter BP control versus 140 mmHg with a less intensive control. This 8-mmHg difference amongst the two groups translated into a 14% reduction in all-cause mortality with more intensive BP control (odds ratio (OR) 0.86; 95% CI, 0.76–0.97; p = 0.01), a finding without significant heterogeneity that was consistent across multiple subgroups. However, the committee also noted that achieved systolic BP was 132 mmHg in the "intensive" BP control group, and expressed some concerns on pursuing an even tighter control (i.e., <130/80). They mentioned that a systematic review by Upadhyay et al. failed to show any clinical benefit to the risk of death, CV events, ESRD or change in renal function with a BP target of <130/80 compared to <140/90 in non-diabetic CKD [32]. The ESC/ESH committee did not seem to acknowledge, however, that this meta-analysis also mentioned that "a lower target may be beneficial in persons with proteinuria greater than 300 to 1000 mg/day", or the fact that only the MDRD, AASK and REIN-2 studies were included, for a total of just 2272 patients [22–24]. To further support the recommendation of a systolic BP target of 130–139 mmHg, the ESH/ESH guideline also mentioned a large retrospective study in 398,419 hypertensive patients (30% with diabetes), which showed that the lowest risk of ESRD and mortality was achieved by a systolic BP of 137 mmHg, whereas a clear increase in the risk of mortality was shown in patients with systolic BP lower than 120 mmHg [29]. However, observational studies are particularly prone to confounding and bias, and reverse causation might easily distort true causal relationships. Hence, in our opinion the ESC/ESH guideline has been influenced by the adoption of the "J-curve phenomenon", which suggests that overaggressive BP control might actually increase the risk of fatal and non-fatal CV events, as well as renal complications, whenever systolic or diastolic BP is reduced below a certain threshold [33]. However, no evidence in favour of the J-curve emerged from meta-regression analyses of randomised studies, in which potential determinants of reverse causality (i.e., older age, heart failure and cancer) were equally distributed by randomisation between the treatment groups [34]. This is a frequently forgotten but important point against the clinical relevance of the J-curve phenomenon in regard to BP levels usually observed in trials and clinical practice.

All hypertension guidelines concur that either ACEis or ARBs should be first-line drugs in CKD patients regardless of diabetic status, although the ACC states that ACEis should be tried first, whereas ARBs should only be used in patients who are intolerant to ACEis.

2.2. Renal Guidelines

The critical appraisal of major renal guidelines published over the last decade allows the immediate identification of a clear turning point, namely the publication of the SPRINT trial in 2015 [27]. In the pre-SPRINT era, renal guidelines typically recommended a BP target of <140/90 in all CKD patients without albuminuria or proteinuria (in line with JNC-VIII recommendations, issued in 2014), whereas a tighter BP control of <130/80 mmHg was recommended in patients with moderately or severely increased albuminuria, or UPCR $\geq$ 150 g/g creatinine [16–19]. The recommendations issued by the older renal guidelines were based on a few prospective cohort studies [35,36], randomised clinical trials [22,23,26] and meta-analyses [32,37]. In particular, the recommendation for a BP target < 140/90 mmHg in CKD patients with no albuminuria or proteinuria seemed to be perfectly in line with the findings of a meta-analysis from the Cochrane Collaboration [37], which included four studies and more than 22,000 patients. [22–24, 38]. Over 3.8 years of follow-up, intensive BP control (achieved BP: 128.6/78.3 mmHg) did not decrease the risk of all-cause death (relative risk [RR] 0.89, 99% CI 0.52–1.52, p = 0.93) or ESRD (RR 1.01, 99% CI 0.75–1.36, p = 0.92) compared to standard BP control (achieved BP: 139.2/84.5 mmHg). On the other hand, the recommendation for intensive BP control (<130/80) in patients with abnormal albuminuria or proteinuria mainly relied on observational data from the Multiple Risk Factor Intervention Trial (MRFIT) and the Okinawa mass screening program [35,36]. In MRFIT, BP values above 127/82 mmHg were associated with a significant increase in the risk of ESRD in 332,554 men (age: 35–57) [35]. Along the same line, BP readings above 131/79 in men and 131/78 in women significantly increased the risk of ESRD in 98,759 patients of the Okinawa mass screening program, even after adjusting for proteinuria [36]. The findings of those large cohort studies seemed to reconcile with the data from the MDRD and AASK studies [22,23,26] and the meta-analysis from Upadhyay et al., which considered a number of clinical outcomes, including all-cause death, CV death and ESRD [32]. Although tighter BP control (<125/75–130/80 mmHg) did not show any benefit on any CV or renal outcomes compared to standard BP control (<140/90), some possible benefits with a more intensive BP control were observed in the subgroup of patients with proteinuria > 300 mg/day (AASK) or 1000 mg/day (MDRD).

After the publication of the SPRINT trial in 2015 [27], which included a significant proportion of patients with stage 3 or 4 CKD (almost 30% of the study population), the renal community has started to debate the opportunity of adopting a BP target lower than 130/80 mmHg regardless of the levels of albuminuria or proteinuria, given the spectacular effectiveness of intensive versus standard BP control in reducing the risk of the primary composite outcome of myocardial infarction, other acute coronary syndromes, stroke, heart failure or CV death. Surprisingly, especially given the fact that most CKD patients will actually develop a fatal or non-fatal cardiovascular event rather than progressing to ESRD [8], the lively debate on BP targets in CKD did not translate into the rapid creation of new guidelines. For instance, the 2019 NICE guideline "Hypertension in adults: diagnosis and management" [39] did not incorporate the evidence from SPRINT, whereas readers were referred to the old 2014 NICE guideline for the general management of CKD [40]. From a "nephrological" perspective, and especially after the publication of the ACC [13] and ESC/ESH [14] guidelines, in March 2021 the UK Kidney Association, one of most influential renal associations worldwide, felt compelled to issue some urgent guidance for British clinicians, and decided to largely align to the ACC guideline [13] in recommending a BP target of <130/80 mmHg in all patients with CKD to improve CV outcomes, if tolerated by the individual and following a shared decision-making discussion with the patient [20]. In the same month (March 2021), the eagerly awaited KDIGO 2021 Clinical Practice Guideline for the management of BP in CKD was finally released [21]. In fairness, the KDIGO working group started to create a new guideline in 2017, following the Controversies Conference in Edinburgh, which was convened to "identify emerging evidence, ongoing controversies, and unsettled questions" [41], but the updated guideline was only released in 2021, partly because of the impact of the Coronavirus (COVID-19) pandemic. The 2021 KDIGO guideline is even bolder than the UK Kidney Association guideline and suggests that all adults with CKD (not receiving dialysis) and hypertension should be treated to reach a target systolic BP < 120 mmHg, if tolerated. This recommendation is largely based on the cardioprotective, survival and potential cognitive benefits of intensive BP control in the SPRINT trial and its ancillary studies, including the SPRINT MIND and a pre-specified subgroup analysis of CKD patients by Cheung et al. [27,42,43]

In August 2021, NICE finally released their updated guidance for CKD patients [11]. However, this guidance puts much emphasis on ACR values ≥70 mg/mmol to identify higher-risk CKD patients that would benefit from tighter BP control (<130/80 mmHg), whereas the "traditional" BP target of <140/90 mmHg is still recommended in people with an ACR < 70 mg/mmol.

3. Benefits and Harms of Specific Antihypertensive Drugs in CKD Patients

3.1. Non-Diabetic Kidney Disease

At each level of achieved BP, ACEis guarantee additional renoprotective benefits compared to other antihypertensive drugs that do not block the RAAS in patients with non-diabetic kidney disease. Those class-specific renoprotective benefits do not simply translate into an additional reduction in urinary protein excretion despite identical BP reduction [44], but into a significant reduction in the risk of ESRD or a combined outcome of ESRD and the doubling of serum creatinine compared to other antihypertensive drugs that do not inhibit the RAAS, as highlighted by a meta-analysis on patient-level data, which included two landmark trials [45–47]. However, these additional BP-independent renoprotective effects were only evident in the subgroup of patients with baseline proteinuria >500 mg/24 h (or an ACR > 30 mg/mmol). Similar findings come from another meta-analysis showing a 40% decrease in the risk of ESRD or the doubling of serum creatinine with ACEis compared to a placebo [48], and from a randomised trial enrolling non-diabetic patients with advanced CKD [49]. On the other hand, there is no clear evidence of any BP-lowering independent reno- or cardioprotective effects with ACEi treatment in patients with non-diabetic kidney disease and proteinuria lower than 500 mg/24 h [50–52]. Hence, ACEis are mainly beneficial in people with higher baseline levels of albuminuria or proteinuria, [53–55] a key point reflected in recent renal guidelines [11,21].

ARBs reduce proteinuria over the short- (1–4 months) and long-term (5 to 12 months) to a similar degree as ACE inhibitors, whereas a dual RAAS blockade with ACE inhibitors and ARBs reduces proteinuria even further compared to either agent alone [56], although this did not translate into an improvement in the GFR in a meta-analysis that included 109 patients with IgA nephropathy from six randomised controlled trials [57].

ACEis or ARBs significantly reduced a composite CV outcome of myocardial infarction, coronary revascularisation, unstable angina, stroke and other adverse cardiovascular events compared to the control treatment in patients with non-diabetic kidney disease (RR 0.56, 95% CI 0.47–0.67, $p < 0.001$), but those benefits were not evident in individual outcomes of the composite endpoint [58].

3.2. Diabetic Kidney Disease

Alongside intensive glycemic control [59–61], BP control is a cornerstone of the prevention and treatment of diabetic kidney disease. In a meta-analysis of randomised trials enrolling diabetic patients with or without CKD, ARBs significantly improved several renal outcomes, including ESRD, doubling of serum creatinine, progression from moderately increased albuminuria to severely increased albuminuria and regression from moderately increased albuminuria to normoalbuminuria, compared to a placebo. However, ARBs did not improve all-cause mortality, while ACEis decreased all-cause mortality and the progression from moderately to severely increased albuminuria, but failed to reduce the risk of ESRD or the doubling of serum creatinine [62]. A subsequent meta-analysis from Sarafidis et al. [63] reached very similar conclusions, although ACEis did not reduce the risk of all-cause mortality, likely due to the inclusion of the large Non-Insulin-Dependent Diabetes, Hypertension, Microalbuminuria or Proteinuria, Cardiovascular Events, and Ramipril (DIABHYCAR) trial, which did not show any benefit of ramipril versus a placebo on the risk of all-cause mortality [64]. However, the dose of ramipril used in the DIABHYCAR trial was really small (1.25 mg) compared to the dosage used in studies where the ACEis had much more encouraging results on all-cause mortality, including the micro-HOPE [65]. ACEis or ARBs can also reduce the risk of heart failure and other CV outcomes, including myocardial infarction and stroke, in patients with diabetic kidney disease [58]. Finally, a network meta-analysis including 119 randomised controlled trials and 64,768 CKD patients with or without diabetes showed that both ACEis and ARBs can decrease the risk of major CV events and renal failure, although only ACEis also decreased the risk of all-cause mortality compared to the active control [66].

Patients with type 2 diabetes and moderately increased albuminuria treated with higher doses of ARBs show a sustained reduction in albumin excretion rate, less progression to severely increased albuminuria and increased regression to normoalbuminuria, compared to lower doses of the same drugs, although there are no data on the effects of different doses of ARBs on all-cause mortality of CV outcomes [67]. ACEi/ARB combination treatment is not routinely recommended in diabetic kidney disease, and to the best of our knowledge, it is not endorsed by any recent hypertension or renal guidelines. The main reason for this stance is that a dual RAAS blockade (ramipril plus telmisartan), compared to monotherapy, did not decrease the risk of the primary composite outcome of all-cause death, ESRD or the doubling of serum creatinine in the Ongoing Telmisartan Alone and in Combination with Ramipril Global Endpoint Trial (ONTARGET) [68], a finding consistent with a meta-analysis from Kunz et al. [56].

4. Blood Pressure Targets in Special Populations

4.1. Children

The main evidence on BP targets in children with CKD derives from the Effect of Strict Blood Pressure Control and ACE inhibition on the Progression of CKD in Pediatric Patients (ESCAPE) trial [69], which randomised 385 children (aged 3–18) with CKD, all treated with ACEis, to either intensive BP control (target 24-h MAP below the 50th percentile) or standard BP control (MAP between the 50th and the 99th percentile), and added additional medications that did not block the RAAS. Over 5 years of follow-up, intensive BP control significantly decreased the risk of the primary composite renal endpoint of progression to ESRD or the time to 50% decline in the GFR compared to standard BP control (HR 0.65;

95% CI, 0.44 to 0.94; $p = 0.02$). Those benefits were even higher in children with higher baseline proteinuria. The findings from the ESCAPE trial have been recently appraised by the NICE committee, which agreed that the therapeutic target in children and young people with CKD and proteinuria is to keep systolic BP below the 50th percentile for their corresponding height [70]. This recommendation is also endorsed by the 2021 KDIGO guideline, which suggests that "24-h MAP measured using ambulatory blood pressure monitoring (ABPM) should be lowered to one that is at ≤50th percentile of normal children with corresponding age, sex, and height" [21].

4.2. Elderly

In 2021, the NICE committee critically appraised the scant evidence on specific BP targets in the elderly and concluded that none of the available data are useful for formulating a specific recommendation in those patients [70]. The committee also discussed the possible increase in adverse events potentially associated with tighter BP control in the elderly, especially dizziness and falls. Although it was noted that this concern was opinion-based rather than evidence-based, the committee agreed to cross-reference the recommendations in the 2019 NICE hypertension guideline for people who are frail or with multiple health concerns [39]. Specifically, the guideline says that "the use of clinical judgement should be highlighted in decision making for people with frailty or multimorbidity" and that "a number of factors should be considered when discussing treatment options in this group". This advice is actually very close to the one originally included in the JNC-VIII guideline in 2014 (i.e., in patients aged 70 or above, "treatment should be individualized taking into consideration factors such as frailty, comorbidities, and albuminuria") [15].

The 2021 KDIGO guideline supported the idea that, in most CKD patients and hypertension, the CV benefits of a target systolic BP < 120 mmHg versus <140 mmHg outweigh the risk of harm, even in the frail and elderly [21]. However, although over 40% of the 2646 CKD patients of the SPRINT trial were aged 75 or above, the median frailty index (FI) was 0.18 in the 1159 participants aged 80 or older [71]. As the FI needs to be >0.21 to classify a patient as 'frail', this means that the typical elderly patient enrolled in the SPRINT trial was an ambulatory patient likely to attend mostly outpatient clinical care practices, as well as the appointments for the study itself. Also, diabetic patients were excluded from SPRINT. This means that the KDIGO recommendation on the benefits of a systolic BP target <120 mmHg "even in the frail and elderly" is questionable, as only 27.6% of the SPRINT patients were actually frail [71], whereas the remaining three quarters were unlikely to represent the "typical" elderly patients seen in daily clinical practice who might well have a much higher burden of comorbidities. This is a very relevant point in our opinion, as a 1% increase in the FI is associated with increased risk for self-reported falls, injurious falls, and all-cause hospitalisations [71].

4.3. Dialysis Patients

In patients with ESRD undergoing haemodialysis or peritoneal dialysis, there is a staggering increase in CV morbidity and mortality, which can be 10- to 100-fold higher than in the general population [72]. Unsurprisingly, given the fact that up to 80% of dialysis patients are also hypertensives, and often with poor BP control [73], antihypertensive treatment can significantly decrease their CV morbidity and mortality, as well as all-cause mortality [74]. However, to the best of our knowledge there is a single randomised controlled trial comparing the CV benefits of different BP targets in patients on dialysis treatment, the Blood Pressure in Dialysis (BID) pilot study [75,76]. In this trial, 126 dialysis patients with a 2-week average predialysis systolic BP of ≥155 mmHg were randomised to either a predialysis SBP target of 110–140 mm Hg or 155–165 mmHg. The mean difference in systolic BP achieved between the two arms was 12.9 mmHg. At 12 months, there was no significant difference in the median change to the left ventricular mass from the baseline amongst participants assigned to intensive or standard BP control (median difference: -0.84 g/m^2 (interquartile range, IQR: -17.1 to 10.0) in the intensive arm, versus 1.4 g/m^2, (IQR: −11.6 to 10.4) in the standard arm, p = 0.43). A non-statistically significant increase in the risk of hospitalisation and vascular access thrombosis was observed in the intensive arm. Unfortunately, no major CV events were assessed in this pilot trial [77]. Although some very outdated guidelines, including the 2005 K/DOQI [78], the 2006 haemodialysis guideline from the Canadian Society of Nephrology [79] and the 2012 guideline from the Japanese Society for Dialysis Therapy [80] consistently suggest a predialysis BP target <140/90 mmHg in such patients, there is a deafening silence on the topic in all recent renal guidelines, including the 2021 KDIGO guideline, which specifically talks about "BP management in patients with CKD, with or without diabetes, not receiving dialysis" [21]. This is hardly surprising, given the lack of any evidence on the effects of intensive versus standard BP control on hard CV outcomes, including CV mortality, in dialysis patients. Hence, nephrologists are forced to rely on observational data for some guidance on the desirable BP targets in ESRD patients on dialysis treatment, but those data epidemiological findings are conflicting [81–86] as they are biased by reverse causality issues [87] or simply disregard the significant differences in comorbidities, age, ethnicity, and socio-economic status in such patients [88]. Hence, following the publication of the BID pilot study, additional high-quality randomised controlled trials assessing the effect of different BP targets on CV outcomes in dialysis patients are warranted to shed some light on this grey area of the literature.

5. Conclusions

Despite many years of heated debate in the hypertension and nephrology communities, the jury is still out on the desirable BP target in CKD patients. Undoubtedly, the publication of the SPRINT trial in 2015 [27] has been a seismic event to which hypertension societies [13,14] have reacted more promptly (three years earlier) than the renal ones [11,20,21]. On the other hand, the new renal guidelines issued in 2021 are in some cases as bold as the ACC guideline in suggesting a tighter BP control of <130/80 mmHg regardless of the levels of proteinuria, such as the UK Kidney Association guideline [20], and in some cases even bolder, such as the eagerly anticipated 2021 KDIGO guideline [21], which pushed the "optimal" systolic BP target in CKD patients to an unprecedented <120 mmHg. In stark contrast, the 2021 NICE guideline seems to adopt a much more conservative approach by recommending a more traditional BP target of <140/90 in CKD patients with an ACR of <70 mg/mmol and <130/80 in the presence of an ACR of ≥70 mg/mmol. Those targets are strikingly similar to pre-2015 renal guidelines [16–18].

Thus, what kind of BP target should be adopted by clinicians in daily clinical practice for their patients with CKD and hypertension? Our attempt to provide a balanced answer to this clinical dilemma will start from what we consider to be a critical point: in CKD patients, the risk of dying from CV disease widely exceeds the risk of developing ESRD [8]. Shockingly, a post-hoc analysis of the CV and renal outcomes in the Antihypertensive and Lipid-Lowering Treatment to Prevent Heart Attack Trial (ALLHAT) showed that 1337 out of 5545 patients with a baseline-estimated GFR lower than 60 mL/min/1.73 m^2 died from CV disease over the extended follow-up period (4.9 years of randomised trials plus 4 years of extension), whereas only 461/5545 developed ESRD [89]. In other words, if we imagine three patients with stage 3 or 4 CKD and we follow them up over a period of 8.9 years, we will observe that two patients will die from a CV event, whereas only one will develop ESRD. Hence, our efforts should pragmatically prioritize the prevention of CV events rather than the prevention of ESRD in CKD patients, and the adoption of a pragmatical target BP should never neglect this unquestionable reality. To ascertain the benefits of more versus less intensive BP control, we recently published an updated trial sequential analysis on 16 randomised controlled trials which compared different BP targets and reported specific CV outcomes, including CV death, myocardial infarction, stroke and heart failure [90]. Our trial sequential analysis aimed at estimating whether the evidence progressively accrued on the aforementioned outcomes can be considered strong and conclusive; the logic of "early stopping rules" used during randomised controlled trials to establish whether it is still ethical to continue the study on the basis of data accrued thus far can be applied to the trial sequential analysis to understand if the accrued data are conclusive and no further randomised controlled studies are needed [91,92]. Notably, at least eight studies included in our analysis targeted a systolic BP lower than 130 mmHg and a diastolic BP lower than 80 mmHg in the more intensive arm. Our cumulative trial sequential analysis showed firm and conclusive evidence of the benefit of intensive BP control (i.e., <130/80 mmHg) for myocardial infarction, stroke, and heart failure. For CV death, the efficacy monitoring boundary was touched, but not crossed, after the inclusion of the Strategy of Blood Pressure Intervention in the Elderly Hypertensive Patients (STEP) trial [93], which means that albeit statistically significant, the benefit of intensive BP control on CV death might not be considered as conclusive at present. Our results are consistent with a recent meta-analysis of 10 randomised controlled trials by Zhang et al., which showed that intensive BP control reduces the risk of all-cause mortality, CV mortality and composite CV events in CKD patients [94].

Based on our recent trial sequential analysis and the meta-analysis from Zhang et al., we feel that clinicians should preferably follow the ACC guideline [13] and the UK Kidney Association guideline [20], which both recommend a target BP lower than 130/80 mmHg in all adults with CKD and hypertension, regardless of the level of proteinuria, provided that intensive BP control is well tolerated [20].

Although we commend the KDIGO working group for their courageous position on the systolic BP target of <120 mmHg, we are reluctant to endorse their statement that such a target should be routinely pursued "even in the frail and elderly". In fact, the large majority of patients enrolled in the SPRINT trial were not frail [71], and we are somewhat concerned that this target can be difficult to achieve in daily clinical practice [21], especially in "real world" CKD patients who are very elderly (aged 80–85 or older), frail and with multiple comorbidities, wherein a BP target of <150/90 mmHg seems to be reasonable and in line with several international guidelines [39,95–99]. Indeed, CKD is often associated with resistance to antihypertensive treatment and failure to achieve the intensive BP target, as highlighted by a post-hoc analysis of the SPRINT study [99]. On the other hand, we also feel that clinicians should not be excessively concerned about the so-called "J-curve phenomenon" if they decide to pursue this more ambitious target in younger patients with a longer life expectancy with the objective of preventing major CV events and CV deaths. In fact, post-hoc analyses of the ONTARGET trial [100] and the Valsartan Antihypertensive Long-Term Use Evaluation trial [101] did not show any evidence of an excess risk of CV events at lower-achieved BP values, suggesting that the J-curve phenomenon is mainly explained by reverse causality due to coexisting diseases (e.g., cancer, heart failure, etc.) associated with low BP and poor outcome.

In terms of first-line drugs for CKD patients, current hypertension and renal guidelines consistently recommend the usage of either ACEis or ARBs in both diabetic and non-diabetic kidney disease for their clear reno- and cardiovascular benefits [66,102–108], and a full dose should be used whenever possible and well tolerated. However, clinicians should bear in mind that the majority of CKD patients will require a combination treatment with two or more antihypertensive agents to achieve a satisfactory degree of BP control (i.e., at least <130/80 mmHg if tolerated), and that additional renoprotective drugs are available, including third-generation dihydropyridine CCBs [108–110]. An ACEi/ARB combination treatment is not recommended by any available guideline and should be avoided because of the increased risk of acute kidney injury and hyperkalaemia. Combination treatments (e.g., ACEi or ARB plus CCB) should be tailored to the individual patient, trying to balance the need for an intensive BP control, the risk of side effects and the need to ensure long-term adherence, and concomitant CV risk factors (smoking, dyslipidemia, diabetes, etc.) should be aggressively tackled to further reduce CV and renal outcomes.

In conclusion, we recommend that clinicians pursue a target BP of <130/80 mmHg in all CKD patients with hypertension, unless they are frail (36-item FI > 0.21) [71], or very elderly (aged 80–85 or older) and with multiple comorbidities (e.g., heart failure, cancer, malnutrition, chronic infections, etc.) [111]. We also advocate for a more ambitious systolic BP target of <120 mmHg, as per the 2021 KDIGO guideline [21], in younger patients with a lower burden of comorbidities to minimise CV morbidity and mortality over their lifetime and obtain longer survival times, while avoiding unnecessary excess risk of adverse events with overaggressive BP control in very elderly patients with a significant number of comorbidities and a lower residual life expectancy.

Author Contributions: Conceptualization, G.G., K.M. and G.R.; writing—original draft preparation, G.G., K.M. and G.R.; writing—review and editing, G.G., K.M. and G.R.; visualization, G.G., K.M. and G.R.; supervision, G.R.; project administration, G.R. All authors have read and agreed to the published version of the manuscript.

Funding: This research received no external funding.

Institutional Review Board Statement: Not applicable.

Informed Consent Statement: Not applicable.

Data Availability Statement: Not applicable.

Conflicts of Interest: The authors declare no conflict of interest.

References

1. Mills, K.T.; Stefanescu, A.; He, J. The global epidemiology of hypertension. *Nat. Rev. Nephrol.* **2020**, *16*, 223–237. [CrossRef] [PubMed]
2. World Health Organization. Global Health Risks. Mortality and Burden of Disease Attributable To selected Major Risks. 2009. Available online: http://www.who.int/healthinfo/global_burden_disease/GlobalHealthRisks_report_full.pdf (accessed on 7 April 2022).
3. Foreman, K.J.; Marquez, N.; Dolgert, A.; Fukutaki, K.; Fullman, N.; McGaughey, M.; Pletcher, M.A.; Smith, A.E.; Tang, K.; Yuan, C.-W.; et al. Forecasting life expectancy, years of life lost, and all-cause and cause-specific mortality for 250 causes of death: Reference and alternative scenarios for 2016–40 for 195 countries and territories. *Lancet* **2018**, *392*, 2052–2090. [CrossRef]
4. Pugh, D.; Gallacher, P.J.; Dhaun, N. Management of Hypertension in Chronic Kidney Disease. *Drugs* **2019**, *79*, 365–379. [CrossRef] [PubMed]
5. Bakris, G.L.; Ritz, E. The message for World Kidney Day 2009: Hypertension and kidney disease–a marriage that should be prevented. *J. Hypertens.* **2009**, *27*, 666–669. [CrossRef] [PubMed]
6. Gansevoort, R.T.; Correa-Rotter, R.; Hemmelgarn, B.R.; Jafar, T.H.; Heerspink, H.J.; Mann, J.F.; Matsushita, K.; Wen, C.P. Chronic kidney disease and cardiovascular risk: Epidemiology, mechanisms, and prevention. *Lancet* **2013**, *382*, 339–352. [CrossRef]
7. Stevens, P.E.; Levin, A. Evaluation and management of chronic kidney disease: Synopsis of the kidney disease: Improving global outcomes 2012 clinical practice guideline. *Ann. Intern. Med.* **2013**, *158*, 825–830. [CrossRef]
8. Foley, R.N.; Murray, A.M.; Li, S.; Herzog, C.A.; McBean, A.M.; Eggers, P.W.; Collins, A.J. Chronic kidney disease and the risk for cardiovascular disease, renal replacement, and death in the United States Medicare population, 1998 to 1999. *J. Am. Soc. Nephrol.* **2005**, *16*, 489–495. [CrossRef]
9. Lee, J.Y.; Park, J.T.; Joo, Y.S.; Lee, C.; Yun, H.R.; Yoo, T.H.; Kang, S.W.; Choi, K.H.; Ahn, C.; Oh, K.H.; et al. Association of Blood Pressure With the Progression of CKD: Findings From KNOW-CKD Study. *Am. J. Kidney Dis.* **2021**, *78*, 236–245. [CrossRef]
10. Lee, Y.B.; Lee, J.S.; Hong, S.H.; Kim, J.A.; Roh, E.; Yoo, H.J.; Baik, S.H.; Choi, K.M. Optimal blood pressure for patients with chronic kidney disease: A nationwide population-based cohort study. *Sci. Rep.* **2021**, *11*, 1538. [CrossRef]
11. National Institute for Health and Care Excellence (NICE). Chronic Kidney Disease: Assessment and Management. 2021. Available online: https://www.nice.org.uk/guidance/ng203/resources/chronic-kidney-disease-assessment-and-management-pdf-66143713055173 (accessed on 7 April 2022).
12. Taler, S.J.; Agarwal, R.; Bakris, G.L.; Flynn, J.T.; Nilsson, P.M.; Rahman, M.; Sanders, P.W.; Textor, S.C.; Weir, M.R.; Townsend, R.R. KDOQI US commentary on the 2012 KDIGO clinical practice guideline for management of blood pressure in CKD. *Am. J. Kidney Dis.* **2013**, *62*, 201–213. [CrossRef]
13. Whelton, P.K.; Carey, R.M.; Aronow, W.S.; Casey, D.E., Jr.; Collins, K.J.; Dennison Himmelfarb, C.; DePalma, S.M.; Gidding, S.; Jamerson, K.A.; Jones, D.W.; et al. 2017 ACC/AHA/AAPA/ABC/ACPM/AGS/APhA/ASH/ASPC/NMA/PCNA Guideline for the Prevention, Detection, Evaluation, and Management of High Blood Pressure in Adults: A Report of the American College of Cardiology/American Heart Association Task Force on Clinical Practice Guidelines. *J. Am. Coll. Cardiol.* **2018**, *71*, e127–e248. [CrossRef] [PubMed]

14. Williams, B.; Mancia, G.; Spiering, W.; Agabiti Rosei, E.; Azizi, M.; Burnier, M.; Clement, D.L.; Coca, A.; de Simone, G.; Dominiczak, A.; et al. 2018 ESC/ESH Guidelines for the management of arterial hypertension: The Task Force for the management of arterial hypertension of the European Society of Cardiology and the European Society of Hypertension: The Task Force for the management of arterial hypertension of the European Society of Cardiology and the European Society of Hypertension. *J. Hypertens.* **2018**, *36*, 1953–2041. [CrossRef] [PubMed]
15. James, P.A.; Oparil, S.; Carter, B.L.; Cushman, W.C.; Dennison-Himmelfarb, C.; Handler, J.; Lackland, D.T.; LeFevre, M.L.; MacKenzie, T.D.; Ogedegbe, O.; et al. 2014 Evidence-Based Guideline for the Management of High Blood Pressure in Adults: Report From the Panel Members Appointed to the Eighth Joint National Committee (JNC 8). *JAMA* **2014**, *311*, 507–520. [CrossRef] [PubMed]
16. Verbeke, F.; Lindley, E.; Van Bortel, L.; Vanholder, R.; London, G.; Cochat, P.; Wiecek, A.; Fouque, D.; Van Biesen, W. A European Renal Best Practice (ERBP) position statement on the Kidney Disease: Improving Global Outcomes (KDIGO) Clinical Practice Guideline for the Management of Blood Pressure in Non-dialysis-dependent Chronic Kidney Disease: An endorsement with some caveats for real-life application. *Nephrol. Dial. Transplant.* **2013**, *29*, 490–496. [CrossRef]
17. Del Vecchio, L.; Boero, R.; Losito, A.; Minutolo, R.; Pontremoli, R.; Zuccala', A.; Ravani, P.; Cagnoli, B.; Quintaliani, G.; Strippoli, G.F.; et al. Ipertensione arteriosa in CKD: Suggerimenti di pratica clinica e di applicazione delle linee guida. *G Italy Nefrol.* **2013**, *30*, 1–17.
18. Pilmore, H.; Dogra, G.; Roberts, M.; Lambers Heerspink, H.J.; Ninomiya, T.; Huxley, R.; Perkovic, V. Cardiovascular disease in patients with chronic kidney disease. *Nephrology* **2014**, *19*, 3–10. [CrossRef]
19. Akbari, A.; Clase, C.M.; Acott, P.; Battistella, M.; Bello, A.; Feltmate, P.; Grill, A.; Karsanji, M.; Komenda, P.; Madore, F.; et al. Canadian Society of Nephrology Commentary on the KDIGO Clinical Practice Guideline for CKD Evaluation and Management. *Am. J. Kidney Dis.* **2015**, *65*, 177–205. [CrossRef]
20. Fish, R.; Chitalia, N.; Doulton, T.; Durman, K.; Lamerton, E.; Lioudaki, E.; MacDiarmaid-Gordon, A.; Mark, P.; Ratcliffe, L.; Tomson, C.; et al. Commentary on NICE Guideline (NG136) 'Hypertension in Adults: Diagnosis and Management' Including Proposals for Blood Pressure Management in Patients with Chronic Kidney Disease. 2021. Available online: https://ukkidney.org/sites/renal.org/files/Commentary%20on%20NICE%20guideline%20%28NG136%29%20HypertensionFINAL.pdf (accessed on 5 April 2022).
21. The Kidney Disease: Improving Kidney Outcomes (KDIGO). KDIGO 2021 Clinical Practice Guideline for the Management of Blood Pressure in Chronic Kidney Disease. *Kidney Int.* **2021**, *99*, S1–S87. [CrossRef]
22. Klahr, S.; Levey, A.S.; Beck, G.J.; Caggiula, A.W.; Hunsicker, L.; Kusek, J.W.; Striker, G. The effects of dietary protein restriction and blood-pressure control on the progression of chronic renal disease. Modification of Diet in Renal Disease Study Group. *N. Engl. J. Med.* **1994**, *330*, 877–884. [CrossRef]
23. Wright, J.T., Jr.; Bakris, G.; Greene, T.; Agodoa, L.Y.; Appel, L.J.; Charleston, J.; Cheek, D.; Douglas-Baltimore, J.G.; Gassman, J.; Glassock, R.; et al. Effect of blood pressure lowering and antihypertensive drug class on progression of hypertensive kidney disease: Results from the AASK trial. *JAMA* **2002**, *288*, 2421–2431. [CrossRef]
24. Ruggenenti, P.; Perna, A.; Loriga, G.; Ganeva, M.; Ene-Iordache, B.; Turturro, M.; Lesti, M.; Perticucci, E.; Chakarski, I.N.; Leonardis, D.; et al. Blood-pressure control for renoprotection in patients with non-diabetic chronic renal disease (REIN-2): Multicentre, randomised controlled trial. *Lancet* **2005**, *365*, 939–946. [CrossRef]
25. Beck, G.J.; Berg, R.L.; Coggins, C.H.; Gassman, J.J.; Hunsicker, L.G.; Schluchter, M.D.; Williams, G.W. Design and statistical issues of the Modification of Diet in Renal Disease Trial. The Modification of Diet in Renal Disease Study Group. *Control Clin. Trials* **1991**, *12*, 566–586. [CrossRef]
26. Peterson, J.C.; Adler, S.; Burkart, J.M.; Greene, T.; Hebert, L.A.; Hunsicker, L.G.; King, A.J.; Klahr, S.; Massry, S.G.; Seifter, J.L. Blood pressure control, proteinuria, and the progression of renal disease. The Modification of Diet in Renal Disease Study. *Ann. Intern. Med.* **1995**, *123*, 754–762. [CrossRef] [PubMed]
27. Wright, J.T., Jr.; Williamson, J.D.; Whelton, P.K.; Snyder, J.K.; Sink, K.M.; Rocco, M.V.; Reboussin, D.M.; Rahman, M.; Oparil, S.; Lewis, C.E.; et al. A Randomized Trial of Intensive versus Standard Blood-Pressure Control. *N. Engl. J. Med.* **2015**, *373*, 2103–2116. [CrossRef] [PubMed]
28. Jafar, T.H.; Stark, P.C.; Schmid, C.H.; Landa, M.; Maschio, G.; de Jong, P.E.; de Zeeuw, D.; Shahinfar, S.; Toto, R.; Levey, A.S. Progression of chronic kidney disease: The role of blood pressure control, proteinuria, and angiotensin-converting enzyme inhibition: A patient-level meta-analysis. *Ann. Intern. Med.* **2003**, *139*, 244–252. [CrossRef] [PubMed]
29. Sim, J.J.; Shi, J.; Kovesdy, C.P.; Kalantar-Zadeh, K.; Jacobsen, S.J. Impact of achieved blood pressures on mortality risk and end-stage renal disease among a large, diverse hypertension population. *J. Am. Coll. Cardiol.* **2014**, *64*, 588–597. [CrossRef] [PubMed]
30. Tsai, W.C.; Wu, H.Y.; Peng, Y.S.; Yang, J.Y.; Chen, H.Y.; Chiu, Y.L.; Hsu, S.P.; Ko, M.J.; Pai, M.F.; Tu, Y.K.; et al. Association of Intensive Blood Pressure Control and Kidney Disease Progression in Nondiabetic Patients With Chronic Kidney Disease: A Systematic Review and Meta-analysis. *JAMA Intern. Med.* **2017**, *177*, 792–799. [CrossRef] [PubMed]
31. Malhotra, R.; Nguyen, H.A.; Benavente, O.; Mete, M.; Howard, B.V.; Mant, J.; Odden, M.C.; Peralta, C.A.; Cheung, A.K.; Nadkarni, G.N.; et al. Association Between More Intensive vs Less Intensive Blood Pressure Lowering and Risk of Mortality in Chronic Kidney Disease Stages 3 to 5: A Systematic Review and Meta-analysis. *JAMA Intern. Med.* **2017**, *177*, 1498–1505. [CrossRef]

32. Upadhyay, A.; Earley, A.; Haynes, S.M.; Uhlig, K. Systematic review: Blood pressure target in chronic kidney disease and proteinuria as an effect modifier. *Ann. Intern. Med.* **2011**, *154*, 541–548. [CrossRef]
33. Mancia, G.; Grassi, G. Aggressive Blood Pressure Lowering Is Dangerous: The J-Curve. *Hypertension* **2014**, *63*, 29–36. [CrossRef]
34. Reboldi, G.; Gentile, G.; Angeli, F.; Ambrosio, G.; Mancia, G.; Verdecchia, P. Blood pressure lowering in diabetic patients. *J. Hypertens.* **2012**, *30*, 438–439. [CrossRef] [PubMed]
35. Klag, M.J.; Whelton, P.K.; Randall, B.L.; Neaton, J.D.; Brancati, F.L.; Ford, C.E.; Shulman, N.B.; Stamler, J. Blood pressure and end-stage renal disease in men. *N. Engl. J. Med.* **1996**, *334*, 13–18. [CrossRef] [PubMed]
36. Tozawa, M.; Iseki, K.; Iseki, C.; Kinjo, K.; Ikemiya, Y.; Takishita, S. Blood pressure predicts risk of developing end-stage renal disease in men and women. *Hypertension* **2003**, *41*, 1341–1345. [CrossRef] [PubMed]
37. Arguedas, J.A.; Perez, M.I.; Wright, J.M. Treatment blood pressure targets for hypertension. *Cochrane Database Syst. Rev.* **2009**. Art. No.: CD0043. [CrossRef] [PubMed]
38. Toto, R.D.; Mitchell, H.C.; Smith, R.D.; Lee, H.C.; McIntire, D.; Pettinger, W.A. "Strict" blood pressure control and progression of renal disease in hypertensive nephrosclerosis. *Kidney Int.* **1995**, *48*, 851–859. [CrossRef] [PubMed]
39. National Institute for Health and Care Excellence (NICE). Hypertension in Adults: Diagnosis and Management. 2019. Available online: https://www.nice.org.uk/guidance/ng136/resources/hypertension-in-adults-diagnosis-and-management-pdf-6614 1722710213 (accessed on 6 April 2022).
40. National Institute for Health and Care Excellence (NICE). Chronic Kidney Disease in Adults: Assessment and Management. 2014. Available online: https://www.nice.org.uk/guidance/cg182 (accessed on 7 April 2022).
41. Drawz, P.E.; Beddhu, S.; Bignall, O.N.R., 2nd; Cohen, J.B.; Flynn, J.T.; Ku, E.; Rahman, M.; Thomas, G.; Weir, M.R.; Whelton, P.K. KDOQI US Commentary on the 2021 KDIGO Clinical Practice Guideline for the Management of Blood Pressure in CKD. *Am. J. Kidney Dis.* **2022**, *79*, 311–327. [CrossRef]
42. Cheung, A.K.; Rahman, M.; Reboussin, D.M.; Craven, T.E.; Greene, T.; Kimmel, P.L.; Cushman, W.C.; Hawfield, A.T.; Johnson, K.C.; Lewis, C.E.; et al. Effects of Intensive BP Control in CKD. *J. Am. Soc. Nephrol.* **2017**, *28*, 2812–2823. [CrossRef]
43. Williamson, J.D.; Pajewski, N.M.; Auchus, A.P.; Bryan, R.N.; Chelune, G.; Cheung, A.K.; Cleveland, M.L.; Coker, L.H.; Crowe, M.G.; Cushman, W.C.; et al. Effect of Intensive vs Standard Blood Pressure Control on Probable Dementia: A Randomized Clinical Trial. *JAMA* **2019**, *321*, 553–561. [CrossRef]
44. Gansevoort, R.T.; Sluiter, W.J.; Hemmelder, M.H.; de Zeeuw, D.; de Jong, P.E. Antiproteinuric effect of blood-pressure-lowering agents: A meta-analysis of comparative trials. *Nephrol. Dial. Transpl.* **1995**, *10*, 1963–1974.
45. Jafar, T.H.; Schmid, C.H.; Landa, M.; Giatras, I.; Toto, R.; Remuzzi, G.; Maschio, G.; Brenner, B.M.; Kamper, A.; Zucchelli, P.; et al. Angiotensin-converting-enzyme inhibitors and progression of nondiabetic renal disease. A meta-analysis of patient-level data. *Ann. Intern. Med.* **2001**, *135*, 73–87. [CrossRef]
46. Maschio, G.; Alberti, D.; Janin, G.; Locatelli, F.; Mann, J.F.; Motolese, M.; Ponticelli, C.; Ritz, E.; Zucchelli, P. Effect of the angiotensin-converting-enzyme inhibitor benazepril on the progression of chronic renal insufficiency. The Angiotensin-Converting-Enzyme Inhibition in Progressive Renal Insufficiency Study Group. *N. Engl. J. Med.* **1996**, *334*, 939–945. [CrossRef] [PubMed]
47. Gisen, S.G. Randomised placebo-controlled trial of effect of ramipril on decline in glomerular filtration rate and risk of terminal renal failure in proteinuric, non-diabetic nephropathy. The GISEN Group (Gruppo Italiano di Studi Epidemiologici in Nefrologia). *Lancet* **1997**, *349*, 1857–1863.
48. Kshirsagar, A.V.; Joy, M.S.; Hogan, S.L.; Falk, R.J.; Colindres, R.E. Effect of ACE inhibitors in diabetic and nondiabetic chronic renal disease: A systematic overview of randomized placebo-controlled trials. *Am. J. Kidney Dis.* **2000**, *35*, 695–707. [CrossRef]
49. Hou, F.F.; Zhang, X.; Zhang, G.H.; Xie, D.; Chen, P.Y.; Zhang, W.R.; Jiang, J.P.; Liang, M.; Wang, G.B.; Liu, Z.R.; et al. Efficacy and safety of benazepril for advanced chronic renal insufficiency. *N. Engl. J. Med.* **2006**, *354*, 131–140. [CrossRef] [PubMed]
50. Mann, J.F.; Gerstein, H.C.; Pogue, J.; Bosch, J.; Yusuf, S. Renal insufficiency as a predictor of cardiovascular outcomes and the impact of ramipril: The HOPE randomized trial. *Ann. Intern. Med.* **2001**, *134*, 629–636. [CrossRef] [PubMed]
51. Asselbergs, F.W.; Diercks, G.F.; Hillege, H.L.; van Boven, A.J.; Janssen, W.M.; Voors, A.A.; de Zeeuw, D.; de Jong, P.E.; van Veldhuisen, D.J.; van Gilst, W.H. Effects of fosinopril and pravastatin on cardiovascular events in subjects with microalbuminuria. *Circulation* **2004**, *110*, 2809–2816. [CrossRef] [PubMed]
52. Rahman, M.; Pressel, S.; Davis, B.R.; Nwachuku, C.; Wright, J.T., Jr.; Whelton, P.K.; Barzilay, J.; Batuman, V.; Eckfeldt, J.H.; Farber, M.; et al. Renal outcomes in high-risk hypertensive patients treated with an angiotensin-converting enzyme inhibitor or a calcium channel blocker vs a diuretic: A report from the Antihypertensive and Lipid-Lowering Treatment to Prevent Heart Attack Trial (ALLHAT). *Arch. Intern. Med.* **2005**, *165*, 936–946. [CrossRef]
53. Maki, D.D.; Ma, J.Z.; Louis, T.A.; Kasiske, B.L. Long-term effects of antihypertensive agents on proteinuria and renal function. *Arch. Intern. Med.* **1995**, *155*, 1073–1080. [CrossRef]
54. Jafar, T.H.; Stark, P.C.; Schmid, C.H.; Landa, M.; Maschio, G.; Marcantoni, C.; de Jong, P.E.; de Zeeuw, D.; Shahinfar, S.; Ruggenenti, P.; et al. Proteinuria as a modifiable risk factor for the progression of non-diabetic renal disease. *Kidney Int.* **2001**, *60*, 1131–1140. [CrossRef]
55. Ruggenenti, P.; Schieppati, A.; Remuzzi, G. Progression, remission, regression of chronic renal diseases. *Lancet* **2001**, *357*, 1601–1608. [CrossRef]
56. Kunz, R.; Friedrich, C.; Wolbers, M.; Mann, J.F. Meta-analysis: Effect of monotherapy and combination therapy with inhibitors of the renin angiotensin system on proteinuria in renal disease. *Ann. Intern. Med.* **2008**, *148*, 30–48. [CrossRef] [PubMed]

57. Cheng, J.; Zhang, X.; Tian, J.; Li, Q.; Chen, J. Combination therapy an ACE inhibitor and an angiotensin receptor blocker for IgA nephropathy: A meta-analysis. *Int. J. Clin. Pract.* **2012**, *66*, 917–923. [CrossRef] [PubMed]
58. Balamuthusamy, S.; Srinivasan, L.; Verma, M.; Adigopula, S.; Jalandhara, N.; Hathiwala, S.; Smith, E. Renin angiotensin system blockade and cardiovascular outcomes in patients with chronic kidney disease and proteinuria: A meta-analysis. *Am. Heart J.* **2008**, *155*, 791–805. [CrossRef] [PubMed]
59. Dcct, S.G. The effect of intensive treatment of diabetes on the development and progression of long-term complications in insulin-dependent diabetes mellitus. The Diabetes Control and Complications Trial Research Group. *N. Engl. J. Med.* **1993**, *329*, 977–986.
60. Ukpds, S.G. Intensive blood-glucose control with sulphonylureas or insulin compared with conventional treatment and risk of complications in patients with type 2 diabetes (UKPDS 33). UK Prospective Diabetes Study (UKPDS) Group. *Lancet* **1998**, *352*, 837–853. [CrossRef]
61. Edic, S.G. Retinopathy and nephropathy in patients with type 1 diabetes four years after a trial of intensive therapy. The Diabetes Control and Complications Trial/Epidemiology of Diabetes Interventions and Complications Research Group. *N. Engl. J. Med.* **2000**, *342*, 381–389.
62. Strippoli, G.F.; Craig, M.C.; Schena, F.P.; Craig, J.C. Role of blood pressure targets and specific antihypertensive agents used to prevent diabetic nephropathy and delay its progression. *J. Am. Soc. Nephrol.* **2006**, *17*, S153–S155. [CrossRef]
63. Sarafidis, P.A.; Stafylas, P.C.; Kanaki, A.I.; Lasaridis, A.N. Effects of renin-angiotensin system blockers on renal outcomes and all-cause mortality in patients with diabetic nephropathy: An updated meta-analysis. *Am. J. Hypertens.* **2008**, *21*, 922–929. [CrossRef]
64. Marre, M.; Lievre, M.; Chatellier, G.; Mann, J.F.; Passa, P.; Menard, J. Effects of low dose ramipril on cardiovascular and renal outcomes in patients with type 2 diabetes and raised excretion of urinary albumin: Randomised, double blind, placebo controlled trial (the DIABHYCAR study). *BMJ* **2004**, *328*, 495. [CrossRef]
65. Hope, S.G. Effects of ramipril on cardiovascular and microvascular outcomes in people with diabetes mellitus: Results of the HOPE study and MICRO-HOPE substudy. Heart Outcomes Prevention Evaluation Study Investigators. *Lancet* **2000**, *355*, 253–259. [CrossRef]
66. Xie, X.; Liu, Y.; Perkovic, V.; Li, X.; Ninomiya, T.; Hou, W.; Zhao, N.; Liu, L.; Lv, J.; Zhang, H.; et al. Renin-Angiotensin System Inhibitors and Kidney and Cardiovascular Outcomes in Patients With CKD: A Bayesian Network Meta-analysis of Randomized Clinical Trials. *Am. J. Kidney Dis.* **2016**, *67*, 728–741. [CrossRef] [PubMed]
67. Blacklock, C.L.; Hirst, J.A.; Taylor, K.S.; Stevens, R.J.; Roberts, N.W.; Farmer, A.J. Evidence for a dose effect of renin-angiotensin system inhibition on progression of microalbuminuria in Type 2 diabetes: A meta-analysis. *Diabet. Med.* **2011**, *28*, 1182–1187. [CrossRef] [PubMed]
68. Mann, J.F.; Schmieder, R.E.; McQueen, M.; Dyal, L.; Schumacher, H.; Pogue, J.; Wang, X.; Maggioni, A.; Budaj, A.; Chaithiraphan, S.; et al. Renal outcomes with telmisartan, ramipril, or both, in people at high vascular risk (the ONTARGET study): A multicentre, randomised, double-blind, controlled trial. *Lancet* **2008**, *372*, 547–553. [CrossRef]
69. Wuhl, E.; Trivelli, A.; Picca, S.; Litwin, M.; Peco-Antic, A.; Zurowska, A.; Testa, S.; Jankauskiene, A.; Emre, S.; Caldas-Afonso, A.; et al. Strict blood-pressure control and progression of renal failure in children. *N. Engl. J. Med.* **2009**, *361*, 1639–1650. [CrossRef] [PubMed]
70. National Institute for Health and Care Excellence (NICE). Evidence Review for Optimal Blood Pressure Targets for Adults, Children and Young People with CKD. 2021. Available online: https://www.ncbi.nlm.nih.gov/books/NBK574726/ (accessed on 6 April 2022).
71. Pajewski, N.M.; Williamson, J.D.; Applegate, W.B.; Berlowitz, D.R.; Bolin, L.P.; Chertow, G.M.; Krousel-Wood, M.A.; Lopez-Barrera, N.; Powell, J.R.; Roumie, C.L.; et al. Characterizing Frailty Status in the Systolic Blood Pressure Intervention Trial. *J. Gerontol. Ser. A* **2016**, *71*, 649–655. [CrossRef] [PubMed]
72. Coppolino, G.; Lucisano, G.; Bolignano, D.; Buemi, M. Acute cardiovascular complications of hemodialysis. *Minerva Urol. Nefrol.* **2010**, *62*, 67–80.
73. Bucharles, S.G.E.; Wallbach, K.K.S.; Moraes, T.P.d.; Pecoits-Filho, R. Hypertension in patients on dialysis: Diagnosis, mechanisms, and management. *J. Bras Nefrol.* **2019**, *41*, 400–411. [CrossRef]
74. Heerspink, H.J.; Ninomiya, T.; Zoungas, S.; de Zeeuw, D.; Grobbee, D.E.; Jardine, M.J.; Gallagher, M.; Roberts, M.A.; Cass, A.; Neal, B.; et al. Effect of lowering blood pressure on cardiovascular events and mortality in patients on dialysis: A systematic review and meta-analysis of randomised controlled trials. *Lancet* **2009**, *373*, 1009–1015. [CrossRef]
75. Gul, A.; Miskulin, D.; Gassman, J.; Harford, A.; Horowitz, B.; Chen, J.; Paine, S.; Bedrick, E.; Kusek, J.W.; Unruh, M.; et al. Design of the Blood Pressure Goals in Dialysis pilot study. *Am. J. Med. Sci.* **2014**, *347*, 125–130. [CrossRef]
76. Miskulin, D.C.; Gassman, J.; Schrader, R.; Gul, A.; Jhamb, M.; Ploth, D.W.; Negrea, L.; Kwong, R.Y.; Levey, A.S.; Singh, A.K.; et al. BP in Dialysis: Results of a Pilot Study. *J. Am. Soc. Nephrol.* **2018**, *29*, 307–316. [CrossRef]
77. McCallum, W.; Sarnak, M.J. Blood pressure target for the dialysis patient. *Semin. Dial.* **2019**, *32*, 35–40. [CrossRef] [PubMed]
78. National Kidney Foundation, S.G. K/DOQI clinical practice guidelines for cardiovascular disease in dialysis patients. *Am. J. Kidney Dis. Off. J. Natl. Kidney Found.* **2005**, *45*, S1–S153.
79. Jindal, K.; Chan, C.T.; Deziel, C.; Hirsch, D.; Soroka, S.D.; Tonelli, M.; Culleton, B.F. Hemodialysis clinical practice guidelines for the Canadian Society of Nephrology. *J. Am. Soc. Nephrol.* **2006**, *17*, S1–S27. [CrossRef] [PubMed]

80. Hirakata, H.; Nitta, K.; Inaba, M.; Shoji, T.; Fujii, H.; Kobayashi, S.; Tabei, K.; Joki, N.; Hase, H.; Nishimura, M.; et al. Japanese Society for Dialysis Therapy guidelines for management of cardiovascular diseases in patients on chronic hemodialysis. *Ther. Apher. Dial.* **2012**, *16*, 387–435. [CrossRef] [PubMed]
81. Port, F.K.; Hulbert-Shearon, T.E.; Wolfe, R.A.; Bloembergen, W.E.; Golper, T.A.; Agodoa, L.Y.; Young, E.W. Predialysis blood pressure and mortality risk in a national sample of maintenance hemodialysis patients. *Am. J. Kidney Dis. Off. J. Natl. Kidney Found.* **1999**, *33*, 507–517. [CrossRef]
82. Mazzuchi, N.; Carbonell, E.; Fernandez-Cean, J. Importance of blood pressure control in hemodialysis patient survival. *Kidney Int.* **2000**, *58*, 2147–2154. [CrossRef]
83. Foley, R.N.; Herzog, C.A.; Collins, A.J. Blood pressure and long-term mortality in United States hemodialysis patients: USRDS Waves 3 and 4 Study. *Kidney Int.* **2002**, *62*, 1784–1790. [CrossRef]
84. Klassen, P.S.; Lowrie, E.G.; Reddan, D.N.; DeLong, E.R.; Coladonato, J.A.; Szczech, L.A.; Lazarus, J.M.; Owen, W.F., Jr. Association between pulse pressure and mortality in patients undergoing maintenance hemodialysis. *JAMA J. Am. Med. Assoc.* **2002**, *287*, 1548–1555. [CrossRef]
85. Stidley, C.A.; Hunt, W.C.; Tentori, F.; Schmidt, D.; Rohrscheib, M.; Paine, S.; Bedrick, E.J.; Meyer, K.B.; Johnson, H.K.; Zager, P.G. Changing relationship of blood pressure with mortality over time among hemodialysis patients. *J. Am. Soc. Nephrol. JASN* **2006**, *17*, 513–520. [CrossRef]
86. Myers, O.B.; Adams, C.; Rohrscheib, M.R.; Servilla, K.S.; Miskulin, D.; Bedrick, E.J.; Zager, P.G. Age, race, diabetes, blood pressure, and mortality among hemodialysis patients. *J. Am. Soc. Nephrol. JASN* **2010**, *21*, 1970–1978. [CrossRef]
87. Jhee, J.H.; Park, J.; Kim, H.; Kee, Y.K.; Park, J.T.; Han, S.H.; Yang, C.W.; Kim, N.-H.; Kim, Y.S.; Kang, S.-W.; et al. The Optimal Blood Pressure Target in Different Dialysis Populations. *Sci. Rep.* **2018**, *8*, 14123. [CrossRef] [PubMed]
88. Crews, D.C.; Powe, N.R. Blood pressure and mortality among ESRD patients: All patients are not created equal. *J. Am. Soc. Nephrol. JASN* **2010**, *21*, 1816–1818. [CrossRef] [PubMed]
89. Rahman, M.; Ford, C.E.; Cutler, J.A.; Davis, B.R.; Piller, L.B.; Whelton, P.K.; Wright, J.T., Jr.; Barzilay, J.I.; Brown, C.D.; Colon, P.J., Sr.; et al. Long-term renal and cardiovascular outcomes in Antihypertensive and Lipid-Lowering Treatment to Prevent Heart Attack Trial (ALLHAT) participants by baseline estimated GFR. *Clin. J. Am. Soc. Nephrol.* **2012**, *7*, 989–1002. [CrossRef] [PubMed]
90. Reboldi, G.; Angeli, F.; Gentile, G.; Verdecchia, P. Benefits of more intensive versus less intensive blood pressure control. Updated trial sequential analysis. *Eur. J. Intern. Med.* **2022**, Online ahead of print. [CrossRef] [PubMed]
91. Wetterslev, J.; Thorlund, K.; Brok, J.; Gluud, C. Trial sequential analysis may establish when firm evidence is reached in cumulative meta-analysis. *J. Clin. Epidemiol.* **2008**, *61*, 64–75. [CrossRef] [PubMed]
92. Wetterslev, J.; Thorlund, K.; Brok, J.; Gluud, C. Estimating required information size by quantifying diversity in random-effects model meta-analyses. *BMC Med. Res. Methodol.* **2009**, *9*, 86. [CrossRef]
93. Zhang, W.; Zhang, S.; Deng, Y.; Wu, S.; Ren, J.; Sun, G.; Yang, J.; Jiang, Y.; Xu, X.; Wang, T.D.; et al. Trial of Intensive Blood-Pressure Control in Older Patients with Hypertension. *N. Engl. J. Med.* **2021**, *385*, 1268–1279. [CrossRef]
94. Zhang, Y.; Li, J.J.; Wang, A.J.; Wang, B.; Hu, S.L.; Zhang, H.; Li, T.; Tuo, Y.H. Effects of intensive blood pressure control on mortality and cardiorenal function in chronic kidney disease patients. *Ren. Fail* **2021**, *43*, 811–820. [CrossRef]
95. Blood Pressure Lowering Treatment Triallists' Collaboration. Age-stratified and blood-pressure-stratified effects of blood-pressure-lowering pharmacotherapy for the prevention of cardiovascular disease and death: An individual participant-level data meta-analysis. *Lancet* **2021**, *398*, 1053–1064. [CrossRef]
96. Volpe, M.; Patrono, C. Age-independent benefits of blood pressure lowering: Are they applicable to all patients? *Eur. Heart J.* **2021**, *43*, 448–449. [CrossRef]
97. Aronow, W.S. Blood Pressure Goals and Targets in the Elderly. *Curr. Treat. Options Cardiovasc. Med.* **2015**, *17*, 394. [CrossRef] [PubMed]
98. Weber, M.A.; Schiffrin, E.L.; White, W.B.; Mann, S.; Lindholm, L.H.; Kenerson, J.G.; Flack, J.M.; Carter, B.L.; Materson, B.J.; Ram, C.V.; et al. Clinical practice guidelines for the management of hypertension in the community a statement by the American Society of Hypertension and the International Society of Hypertension. *J. Hypertens.* **2014**, *32*, 3–15. [CrossRef] [PubMed]
99. Wang, K.M.; Stedman, M.R.; Chertow, G.M.; Chang, T.I. Factors Associated With Failure to Achieve the Intensive Blood Pressure Target in the Systolic Blood Pressure Intervention Trial (SPRINT). *Hypertension* **2020**, *76*, 1725–1733. [CrossRef] [PubMed]
100. Verdecchia, P.; Reboldi, G.; Angeli, F.; Trimarco, B.; Mancia, G.; Pogue, J.; Gao, P.; Sleight, P.; Teo, K.; Yusuf, S. Systolic and diastolic blood pressure changes in relation with myocardial infarction and stroke in patients with coronary artery disease. *Hypertension* **2015**, *65*, 108–114. [CrossRef] [PubMed]
101. Kjeldsen, S.E.; Berge, E.; Bangalore, S.; Messerli, F.H.; Mancia, G.; Holzhauer, B.; Hua, T.A.; Zappe, D.; Zanchetti, A.; Weber, M.A.; et al. No evidence for a J-shaped curve in treated hypertensive patients with increased cardiovascular risk: The VALUE trial. *Blood Press.* **2016**, *25*, 83–92. [CrossRef] [PubMed]
102. Maione, A.; Navaneethan, S.D.; Graziano, G.; Mitchell, R.; Johnson, D.; Mann, J.F.; Gao, P.; Craig, J.C.; Tognoni, G.; Perkovic, V.; et al. Angiotensin-converting enzyme inhibitors, angiotensin receptor blockers and combined therapy in patients with micro- and macroalbuminuria and other cardiovascular risk factors: A systematic review of randomized controlled trials. *Nephrol. Dial. Transpl.* **2011**, *26*, 2827–2847. [CrossRef] [PubMed]

103. Bjorck, S.; Mulec, H.; Johnsen, S.A.; Norden, G.; Aurell, M. Renal protective effect of enalapril in diabetic nephropathy. *BMJ* **1992**, *304*, 339–343. [CrossRef]
104. Lewis, E.J.; Hunsicker, L.G.; Bain, R.P.; Rohde, R.D. The effect of angiotensin-converting-enzyme inhibition on diabetic nephropathy. The Collaborative Study Group. *N. Engl. J. Med.* **1993**, *329*, 1456–1462. [CrossRef]
105. Brenner, B.M.; Cooper, M.E.; de Zeeuw, D.; Keane, W.F.; Mitch, W.E.; Parving, H.H.; Remuzzi, G.; Snapinn, S.M.; Zhang, Z.; Shahinfar, S. Effects of losartan on renal and cardiovascular outcomes in patients with type 2 diabetes and nephropathy. *N. Engl. J. Med.* **2001**, *345*, 861–869. [CrossRef]
106. Lewis, E.J.; Hunsicker, L.G.; Clarke, W.R.; Berl, T.; Pohl, M.A.; Lewis, J.B.; Ritz, E.; Atkins, R.C.; Rohde, R.; Raz, I. Renoprotective effect of the angiotensin-receptor antagonist irbesartan in patients with nephropathy due to type 2 diabetes. *N. Engl. J. Med.* **2001**, *345*, 851–860. [CrossRef]
107. Parving, H.H.; Lehnert, H.; Brochner-Mortensen, J.; Gomis, R.; Andersen, S.; Arner, P. The effect of irbesartan on the development of diabetic nephropathy in patients with type 2 diabetes. *N. Engl. J. Med.* **2001**, *345*, 870–878. [CrossRef] [PubMed]
108. Reboldi, G.; Gentile, G.; Angeli, F.; Verdecchia, P. Optimal therapy in hypertensive subjects with diabetes mellitus. *Curr. Atheroscler. Rep.* **2011**, *13*, 176–185. [CrossRef] [PubMed]
109. Reboldi, G.; Gentile, G.; Angeli, F.; Verdecchia, P. Exploring the optimal combination therapy in hypertensive patients with diabetes mellitus. *Expert Rev. Cardiovasc. Ther.* **2009**, *7*, 1349–1361. [CrossRef] [PubMed]
110. Schroeder, E.B.; Chonchol, M.B.; Shetterly, S.; Powers, J.D.; Adams, J.L.; Schmittdiel, J.A.; Nichols, G.A.; o Connor, P.J.; Steiner, J.F. Add-On Antihypertensive Medications to Angiotensin-Aldosterone System Blockers in Diabetes: A Comparative Effectiveness Study. *Clin. J. Am. Soc. Nephrol.* **2018**, *13*, 727–734. [CrossRef] [PubMed]
111. Tsika, E.P.; Poulimenos, L.E.; Boudoulas, K.D.; Manolis, A.J. The J-Curve in Arterial Hypertension: Fact or Fallacy? *Cardiology* **2014**, *129*, 126–135. [CrossRef] [PubMed]

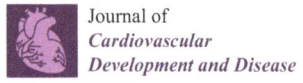

Article

Cardio-Ankle Vascular Index as an Arterial Stiffness Marker Improves the Prediction of Cardiovascular Events in Patients without Cardiovascular Diseases

Yuko Okamoto [1,2], Toru Miyoshi [1,*], Keishi Ichikawa [1], Yoichi Takaya [1], Kazufumi Nakamura [1] and Hiroshi Ito [1]

1. Department of Cardiovascular Medicine, Okayama University Graduate School of Medicine, Dentistry and Pharmaceutical Sciences, Okayama 700-8558, Japan
2. Department of Medical Technology, Kawasaki University of Medical Welfare, Kurashiki 701-0193, Japan
* Correspondence: miyoshit@cc.okayama-u.ac.jp

Abstract: Several studies have reported that the cardio-ankle vascular index (CAVI), a non-invasive measurement of arterial stiffness, is associated with the incidence of cardiovascular events. We investigated whether adding CAVI to a risk score improves the prediction of cardiovascular events in the setting of primary prevention. This retrospective observational study included consecutive 554 outpatients with cardiovascular disease risk factors but without known cardiovascular disease (68 ± 9 years, 64% men). The CAVI was measured using the VaSera vascular screening system. Major adverse cardiovascular events (MACE) included cardiovascular death, myocardial infarction, stroke, hospitalization for heart failure, and coronary revascularization. During a median follow-up of 4.3 years, cardiovascular events occurred in 65 patients (11.7%). Multivariate Cox analysis showed that abnormal CAVI (>9.0) was significantly associated with the incidence of MACE (hazard ratio 2.31, 95% confidence interval 1.27–4.18). The addition of CAVI to the Suita score, a conventional risk score for coronary heart disease in Japan, significantly improved the C statics from 0.642 to 0.713 ($p = 0.04$). In addition to a conventional risk score, CAVI improved the prediction of cardiovascular events in patients with cardiovascular disease risk factors but without known cardiovascular diseases.

Keywords: arterial stiffness; cardio-ankle vascular index; cardiovascular events; risk factors

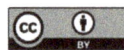

1. Introduction

Arterial stiffness is closely associated with the risk of cardiovascular disease (CVD) and mortality [1]. Carotid-femoral pulse wave velocity (PWV) has been reported to be associated with an increased risk of first cardiovascular events in the general population and improved risk prediction when added to standard risk factors [2]. Brachial-ankle PWV can be performed more easily than carotid-femoral PWV measurement, while both carotid-femoral PWV and brachial-ankle PWV are affected by blood pressure [1,3], which is an important confounding factor for CVD. To overcome this limitation, the cardio-ankle vascular index (CAVI), a marker of arterial stiffness based on stiffness parameter β, was developed in Japan in 2004 [4]. CAVI can be obtained automatically by wrapping pressure cuffs around the upper and lower legs and is less dependent on blood pressure. Previous studies have reported the association between a greater CAVI and a high incidence of cardiovascular events in patients with diabetes mellitus, obesity, and several CVD risk factors [5–16].

The measures of arterial stiffness benefit the prevention of cardiovascular disease, although they have not been widely incorporated into routine clinical practice. To facilitate the use of the CAVI, we proposed a criterion for CAVI based on the expert consensus from the Physiological Diagnosis Criteria for Vascular Failure Committee of the Japan Society for Vascular Failure [17]. We set three ranges in the document: normal range (CAVI ≤ 8.0), borderline range (8.0 < CAVI ≤ 9.0), and abnormal range (CAVI > 9.0). Abnormal CAVI was considered a cutoff value for discriminating the presence of cardiovascular disease or the risk of future cardiovascular events. However, the cutoff value for CAVI has not been adequately validated.

For the risk assessment of CVD, pooled cohort risk equations were introduced by the American College of Cardiology [18] and the European Society of Cardiology [19] to estimate the 10-year atherosclerotic cardiovascular disease. The Suita score was proposed and validated to estimate the 10-year risk of coronary heart disease in the Japanese population [20]. These risk scores are beneficial for assessing patient risk stratification in the setting of primary prevention. As CAVI has been reimbursed by insurance in Japan, its measurement has been included in routine clinical practice. However, the usefulness of CAVI, in addition to the Suita score, has not yet been evaluated.

This study aimed to investigate [1] whether abnormal CAVI (>9.0) is a good predictor of cardiovascular events in patients with CVD risk factors but without known CVD and [2] whether CAVI offers incremental value in addition to the Suita score for predicting cardiovascular events in a retrospective cohort.

2. Methods

2.1. Study Population

This retrospective, single-center cohort study evaluated the impact of CAVI on prognosis. We enrolled 554 outpatients between May 2012 and December 2016. They had no history of CVD but had at least one CVD risk factor and were referred to our hospital for examination of coronary artery disease. Patients were excluded for the following reasons: peripheral artery disease, defined as ankle–brachial pressure index < 0.9, left ventricular ejection fraction < 50%, a history of CVD, atrial fibrillation, and hemodialysis. Hypertension was defined as systolic blood pressure $\geq$ 140 mmHg, diastolic blood pressure $\geq$ 90 mmHg, and/or the use of antihypertensive medication. Diabetes mellitus was defined as a fasting blood glucose concentration of 126 mg/dL and/or the use of insulin or oral hypoglycemic medication. Dyslipidemia was defined as low-density lipoprotein cholesterol (LDL-C) $\geq$ 140 mg/dL, triglyceride $\geq$ 150 mg/dL, high-density lipoprotein cholesterol (HDL-C) < 40 mg/dL, and/or the use of antidyslipidemic medication. The estimated glomerular filtration rate (eGFR) was calculated using the Modification of Diet in Renal Disease equation with the Japanese coefficient [21].

This study was conducted in accordance with the principles of the Declaration of Helsinki and approved by the ethics committees of the Okayama University Graduate School of Medicine, Dentistry, and Pharmaceutical Sciences. The requirement for informed patient consent was waived owing to the low-risk nature of the study and the inability to obtain consent directly from all study subjects.

2.2. Measurement of CAVI

Arterial stiffness was evaluated using CAVI, as previously described [6]. After a 5-min rest and with the subject seated, extremity blood pressure was measured using the oscillometric method. CAVI was measured automatically using a VaSera vascular screening system (Fukuda Denshi, Tokyo, Japan) from the measurement of blood pressure and pulse wave velocity (PWV) while monitoring the electrocardiogram and heart sounds. PWV was calculated by dividing the distance from the aortic valve to the ankle artery by the sum of the time between the aortic valve closing sound and the notch of the brachial pulse wave and the time between the rise of the brachial pulse wave and the rise of the ankle pulse wave. CAVI was determined using the following equation: $CAVI = a[(2\rho/\Delta P) \times \ln(Ps/Pd) \times PWV^2] + b$, where Ps and Pd are the systolic and diastolic blood pressures, respectively, PWV is the pulse wave velocity between the heart and ankle, ΔP is $Ps - Pd$, ρ is blood density, and a and b are constants. The averages of the right and left CAVI were used for the analysis. Patients were classified into three groups based on CAVI levels, as previously described [17]: normal group (CAVI $\leq$ 8.0), borderline group (8.0 < CAVI $\leq$ 9.0), and abnormal group (CAVI > 9.0).

2.3. The Suita Score

The Suita score has been used to predict the risk of CVD development; hence we used the Suita score in this study [20]. The Suita score is an established CVD risk score based on risk factor categories for predicting coronary heart disease in the Japanese population. According to a previous report, the Suita score LDL-C version was calculated using age, sex, HDL-C and LDL-C levels, systolic blood pressure, diastolic blood pressure, smoking, diabetes mellitus, and eGFR [21]. High-, medium-, and low-risk were classified as Suita scores ≥ 56, 41–55, and <40, respectively. The estimated risks of developing coronary heart disease in 10 years in high, medium-, and low-risk groups were >9%, 2–9%, and <2%, respectively.

2.4. Outcome Data

Follow-up information was obtained from a review of medical records or telephone interviews blinded to the CAVI data. Major adverse cardiovascular events (MACE) included cardiovascular death, nonfatal myocardial infarction, nonfatal stroke, coronary revascularization, and heart failure requiring hospitalization. Strokes included ischemic and hemorrhagic strokes. The definitions of MACE have been previously described [6]. The time to the first primary endpoint was retrospectively evaluated.

2.5. Statistical Analysis

Data are expressed as mean ± standard deviation. Dichotomous variables are expressed as numbers and percentages. Categorical data were compared using the χ^2 analysis or Fisher's exact test. One-way analysis of variance was used to compare normally distributed continuous variables, and Bonferroni correction was used for post hoc testing. The relationship between continuous variables was investigated using Spearman's correlation coefficient. Cumulative survival estimates were calculated using the Kaplan–Meier method and compared using the log-rank test. To ascertain the association between CAVI and MACE, we performed univariate and multivariate Cox regression analyses, and the results were reported as hazard ratios (HRs) with 95% confidence intervals (CI). Multivariate Cox regression analysis included variables with $p < 0.05$ in the univariate analysis. The incremental prognostic value of CAVI was assessed using receiver operating characteristic (ROC) curve analysis, continuous net reclassification improvement, and integrated discrimination improvement. All reported *p*-values were two-sided, and statistical significance was set at $p < 0.05$. Statistical analyses were performed using SPSS statistical software (version 28; IBM Corp., Armonk, NY, USA) and the R statistical package (version 3.5.2; R Foundation for Statistical Computing, Vienna, Austria).

3. Results

3.1. Comparison of Baseline Characteristics

The mean age of the patients was 68 ± 9 years, and 64% were male. The average CAVI was 8.8 ± 1.3. The baseline characteristics of 554 patients according to CAVI (normal group, CAVI < 8; borderline group, CAVI 8.0–9.0; abnormal group, CAVI > 9.0) are shown in Table 1. Patients with higher CAVI levels were older and more likely to be male. The mean systolic blood pressure and the prevalence of hypertension increased significantly with higher CAVI. The mean diastolic pressure, HDL-C levels, triglyceride levels, hemoglobinA1c, the prevalence of diabetes mellitus, dyslipidemia, smoking habits, and use of statins did not differ among the groups.

Table 1. Baseline Characteristics According to the CAVI.

Variables	All (n = 554)	Normal CAVI (CAVI < 8) (n = 140)	Borderline CAVI (8 ≤ CAVI < 9) (n = 141)	Abnormal CAVI (9 ≤ CAVI) (n = 273)	p-Value for Trend
Age, year	66 ± 9	62 ± 10	67 ± 9	71 ± 7	<0.01
Male, n (%)	353 (64)	92 (66)	76 (54)	185 (68)	0.01
Body mass index, kg/m^2	23.4 ± 3.9	24.7 ± 4.6	23.9 ± 3.8	22.9 ± 3.5	<0.01
Hypertension, n (%)	418 (75)	84 (60)	110 (78)	224 (82)	<0.01
Diabetes mellitus, n (%)	283 (51)	69 (43)	76 (54)	138 (51)	0.72
Dyslipidemia, n (%)	343 (62)	82 (59)	92 (65)	169 (62)	0.52
Current smoking, n (%)	159 (29)	44 (31)	41 (29)	74 (27)	0.65
Systolic blood pressure, mmHg	129 ± 19	122 ± 19	128 ± 16	133 ± 18	<0.01
Diastolic blood pressure, mmHg	74 ± 11	72 ± 11	74 ± 10	75 ± 11	0.04
Laboratory data					
Triglyceride, mg/dL	140 ± 119	136 ± 126	137 ± 94	144 ± 126	0.78
HDL-C, mg/dL	55 ± 17	58 ± 19	54 ± 18	545 ± 16	0.08
LDL-C, mg/dL	109 ± 31	113 ± 33	110 ± 31	107 ± 32	0.17
HemoglobinA1c, %	6.4 ± 1.4	6.3 ± 1.5	6.5 ± 1.4	6.5 ± 1.4	0.69
eGFR, mL/min/1.73 m^2	66.1 ± 19.4	70.0 ± 17.3	68.0 ± 20.9	63.3 ± 18.2	0.02
Medications					
Antihypertensive agents, n (%)	406 (73)	85 (61)	107 (76)	214 (78)	<0.01
Antidiabetic agents, n (%)	178 (42)	34 (37)	52 (47)	92 (42)	0.31
Lipid-lowering agents, n (%)	310 (56)	64 (46)	86 (61)	160 (59)	0.01

HDL-C, high-density lipoprotein cholesterol; LDL-C, low-density lipoprotein cholesterol; eGFR, estimated glomerular filtration rate.

3.2. Association between Cumulative Incidence of Major Adverse Cardiovascular Events (MACE) and CAVI

During this follow-up period (median 4.3 years), 65 patients had MACE, including cardiac death (n = 2), myocardial infarction (n = 3), stroke (n = 13), heart failure with hospitalization (n = 14), or coronary revascularization (n = 34). The cumulative incidence rates of MACE according to CAVI levels are shown in Figure 1, and the rates were significantly higher in the abnormal group than in the other groups (p-value for trend < 0.001). Figure 2 shows the ROC curve analysis of CAVI for predicting MACE. The sensitivity and specificity of CAVI at a cutoff value of 9.0 were 75% and 54%, respectively (area under the curve, 0.688; $p < 0.001$). The multivariable-adjusted Cox proportional hazard model, CAVI (>9.0), was associated with an increased risk of MACE after adjusting for covariates (HR, 1.941 [95% CI, 1.092–3.448]; $p = 0.024$) (Table 2).

Table 2. Association Between the CAVI and Cardiovascular Events.

	Univariate		Multivariate	
	HR (95% CI)	p-Value	HR (95% CI)	p-Value
CAVI > 9	3.07 (1.78–5.41)	<0.01	2.31 (1.27–4.18)	<0.01
Age per year	1.05 (1.01–1.08)	<0.01	1.02 (0.98–1.06)	0.18
Male	1.97 (1.09–3.57)	0.02	1.86 (1.02–3.39)	0.04
Hypertension	2.56 (1.16–5.62)	0.01	0.86 (0.38–2.27)	0.86
Diabetes mellitus	1.44 (0.87–2.37)	0.14		
Dyslipidemia	1.68 (0.96–2.93)	0.06		
Current smoking	1.34 (0.80–2.25)	0.25		
Antihypertensive agents	5.36 (1.94–14.78)	<0.01	4.16 (1.29–13.40)	0.01
Antidiabetic agents	1.41 (0.32–2.40)	0.20		
Lipid-lowering agents	1.79 (1.05–3.07)	0.03	1.56 (0.91–2.68)	0.10

The multivariate analysis included CAVI > 9, age, male sex, hypertension, antihypertensive agents, and lipid-lowering agents. CAVI, cardio-ankle vascular index; HR, hazard ratio; CI, confidence interval.

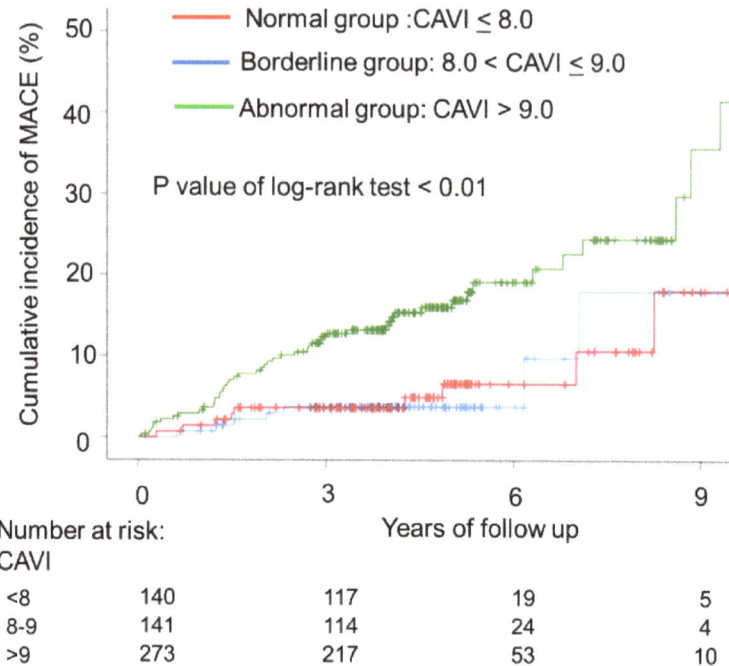

Figure 1. Kaplan–Meier plot of cumulative probability of cardiovascular events by cardio-ankle vascular index (CAVI) levels. Time to cardiovascular events, including cardiovascular death, nonfatal stroke, nonfatal myocardial infarction, heart failure requiring hospitalization, and coronary revascularization, according to baseline CAVI. The cumulative incidence rates of cardiovascular events according to CAVI levels were significantly higher in the abnormal group (CAVI > 9.0) than in the normal (CAVI < 8) and abnormal groups (8 < CAVI ≤ 9) (p-value for trend < 0.01).

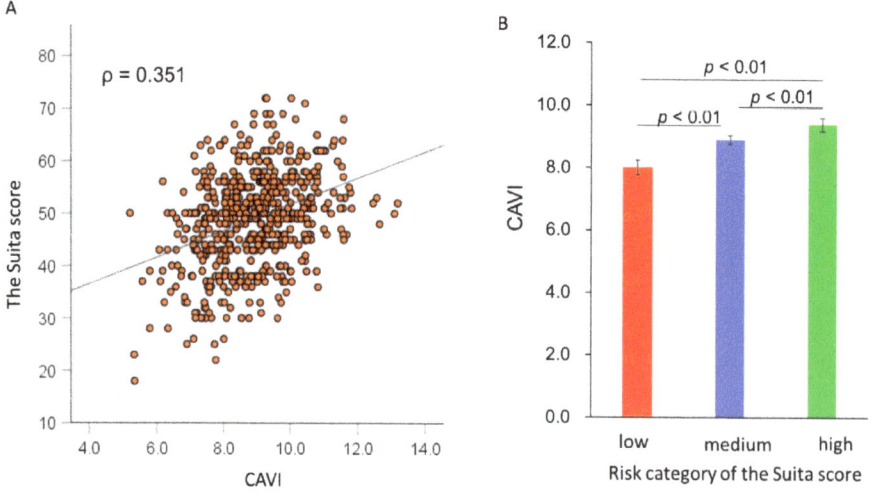

Figure 2. Correlation between CAVI and the Suita score. Scatter plot showing the correlation between CAVI and the Suita score (**A**) and CAVI according to the risk category of the Suita score (**B**).

3.3. Incremental Predictive Value of CAVI over the Suita Score

As shown in Figure 2A, the CAVI was weakly correlated with the Suita score ($\rho = 0.351$, $p < 0.01$). When patients were classified into three groups (low-risk, medium-risk, and high-risk groups) according to the Suita score, the CAVI value increased stepwise from the low-risk group to the high-risk group (8.1 ± 0.2, 8.9 ± 0.1, and 9.3 ± 0.2, respectively; p-value for trend < 0.01) (Figure 2B). An ROC curve analysis was performed to determine the incremental value of CAVI for predicting MACE (Figure 3). The addition of CAVI to the Suita score significantly improved the C statics from 0.642 to 0.713 ($p = 0.04$). The addition of the CAVI yielded a continuous net reclassification index of 0.293 (95% CI, 0.036–0.551; $p = 0.025$) and an integrated discrimination improvement of 0.0479 (95% CI, 0.0218–0.0740; $p < 0.001$).

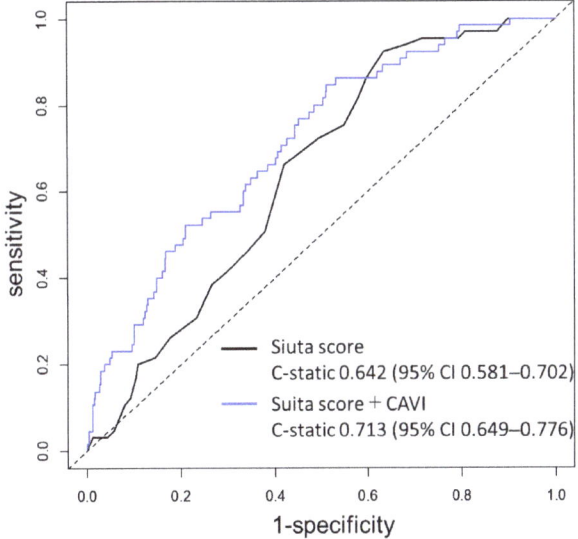

Figure 3. Comparison of the receiver-operating characteristic (ROC) curves. Black curve: predictive ability based on the Suita score. Blue curve: predictive ability based on the Suita score and CAVI. CI: confidence interval.

4. Discussion

This study demonstrated that abnormal CAVI (>9.0) was significantly associated with the incidence of MACE in patients with CVD risk factors but without known CVD. Furthermore, the CAVI and Suita scores improved the prediction of MACE in these patients. To our knowledge, this is the largest study showing the incremental value of CAVI in addition to a clinical risk score for predicting cardiovascular events in the setting of primary prevention.

Several studies have shown that CAVI is associated with the incidence of cardiovascular events in patients with known CVD [5–9] and without CVD [10–16]. However, evidence on the incremental value of CAVI over a clinical risk score for predicting cardiovascular events has been limited. Satoh-Asahara et al. showed that in 300 obese patients without CVD, CAVI, in addition to the atherosclerotic cardiovascular disease risk score, moderately improved the prediction of cardiovascular events [16]. We showed an incremental value of CAVI for predicting cardiovascular events in a large cohort study, where one-third of the participants had a history of CVD [6]. The present study is in line with these two previous studies and clearly demonstrates the usefulness of CAVI for predicting cardiovascular events in patients with CVD risk factors but without known CVD.

This study showed that the best cutoff value of CAVI for predicting cardiovascular events was 9.0, which was consistent with our proposal for abnormal CAVI (>9.0) [17].

However, Satoh-Asahara et al. showed that, including 300 obese patients, the threshold of CAVI for cardiovascular events was 7.8 [16]. Compared to the study by Satoh-Asahara et al., the patients in our study were heterogeneous with hypertension, diabetes, or dyslipidemia who visited the Department of Cardiovascular Medicine. In addition, the mean age in their study was 52 years, which was lower than that in our study (mean age = 66 years). Therefore, these differences may be the reason for the higher cutoff values in the present study. Although our study validated that a CAVI of 9.0 was a cutoff for predicting cardiovascular events in the setting of primary prevention, further research is needed to confirm the optimal threshold of CAVI to predict cardiovascular events in each population.

Several measures of arterial stiffness, such as carotid-femoral PWV and brachial-ankle PWV, have been introduced [1]. However, notable differences were observed among the arterial stiffness measurements. Carotid-femoral PWV is obtained by applanation tonometry, which is a complicated technique compared with CAVI and brachial-ankle PWV [3]. CAVI and brachial-ankle PWV are automatically derived from a plethysmography cuff [1]. CAVI has an advantage over PWV for measuring arterial stiffness because it is less dependent on blood pressure at the time of measurement [4]. A reproducible assessment of arterial properties may allow detailed monitoring of changes in arterial stiffness in clinical practice. CAVI can be easily obtained automatically with a device, leading to its widespread use in clinical situations if cost constraints are ignored. Further investigations are needed to elucidate this matter, with due consideration given to cost-effectiveness.

This study has several limitations. First, we acknowledge that an observational study cannot definitively prove that there is a causal link underlying the association between increased CAVI and increased CVD events. Second, the study population included only Asian individuals. Although several studies on non-Asian populations have recently been reported [12,14], the generalizability of our data to other races/ethnicities remains uncertain. Third, we failed to estimate the cutoff value of CAVI for each event because of the small number of events. Hence, further studies with larger sample sizes are required.

5. Conclusions

We demonstrated that abnormal CAVI (>9) was significantly associated with the incidence of cardiovascular events in patients with CVD risk factors but without known CVD. Furthermore, CAVI in addition to the Suita score improved the prediction of cardiovascular events in these patients. The data in this study suggest that the measurement of CAVI is a clinically useful means to predict the development of cardiovascular events in the setting of primary prevention.

Author Contributions: Conceptualization, Y.O. and T.M.; Methodology, T.M.; Formal Analysis, Y.O. and T.M.; Investigation, Y.O., T.M., K.I., Y.T. and K.N.; Writing—original draft preparation, Y.O. and T.M.; Writing—review and editing, H.I. All authors have read and agreed to the published version of the manuscript.

Funding: This study was supported by the Japan Society for the Promotion of Science KAKENHI (grant number JP 19K08558).

Institutional Review Board Statement: This study was conducted in accordance with the principles of the Declaration of Helsinki and approved by the ethics committees of the Okayama University Graduate School of Medicine, Dentistry, and Pharmaceutical Sciences (2203-024).

Informed Consent Statement: The requirement for informed patient consent was waived owing to the low-risk nature of the study and the inability to obtain consent directly from all study subjects.

Data Availability Statement: The data presented in this study are available upon request from the corresponding authors. The data were not publicly available because of privacy concerns.

Conflicts of Interest: T.M. revived the honorarium from Fukuda Denshi Inc. The authors declare no conflict of interest associated with this manuscript.

References

1. Miyoshi, T.; Ito, H. Arterial stiffness in health and disease: The role of cardio-ankle vascular index. *J. Cardiol.* 2021, 78, 493–501. [CrossRef] [PubMed]
2. Mitchell, G.F.; Hwang, S.J.; Vasan, R.S.; Larson, M.G.; Pencina, M.J.; Hamburg, N.M.; Vita, J.A.; Levy, D.; Benjamin, E.J. Arterial stiffness and cardiovascular events: The Framingham Heart Study. *Circulation* 2010, 121, 505–511. [CrossRef] [PubMed]
3. Chirinos, J.A.; Segers, P.; Hughes, T.; Townsend, R. Large-artery stiffness in health and disease: JACC state-of-the-art review. *J. Am. Coll. Cardiol.* 2019, 74, 1237–1263. [CrossRef] [PubMed]
4. Shirai, K.; Utino, J.; Otsuka, K.; Takata, M. A novel blood pressure-independent arterial wall stiffness parameter; cardio-ankle vascular index (CAVI). *J. Atheroscler. Thromb.* 2006, 13, 101–107. [CrossRef] [PubMed]
5. Kubota, Y.; Maebuchi, D.; Takei, M.; Inui, Y.; Sudo, Y.; Ikegami, Y.; Fuse, J.; Sakamoto, M.; Momiyama, Y. Cardio-Ankle Vascular Index is a predictor of cardiovascular events. *Artery Res.* 2011, 5, 91–96. [CrossRef]
6. Miyoshi, T.; Ito, H.; Shirai, K.; Horinaka, S.; Higaki, J.; Yamamura, S.; Saiki, A.; Takahashi, M.; Masaki, M.; Okura, T.; et al. Predictive value of the cardio-ankle vascular index for cardiovascular events in patients at cardiovascular risk. *J. Am. Heart Assoc.* 2021, 10, e020103. [CrossRef]
7. Gohbara, M.; Iwahashi, N.; Sano, Y.; Akiyama, E.; Maejima, N.; Tsukahara, K.; Hibi, K.; Kosuge, M.; Ebina, T.; Umemura, S.; et al. Clinical impact of the cardio-ankle vascular index for predicting cardiovascular events after acute coronary syndrome. *Circ. J.* 2016, 80, 1420–1426. [CrossRef]
8. Sumin, A.N.; Shcheglova, A.V.; Zhidkova, I.I.; Ivanov, S.V.; Barbarash, O.L. Assessment of arterial stiffness by cardio-ankle vascular index for prediction of five-year cardiovascular events after coronary artery bypass surgery. *Glob. Heart* 2021, 16, 90. [CrossRef]
9. Kirigaya, J.; Iwahashi, N.; Tahakashi, H.; Minamimoto, Y.; Gohbara, M.; Abe, T.; Akiyama, E.; Okada, K.; Matsuzawa, Y.; Maejima, N.; et al. Impact of cardio-ankle vascular index on long-term outcome in patients with acute coronary syndrome. *J. Atheroscler. Thromb.* 2020, 27, 657–668. [CrossRef]
10. Chung, S.L.; Yang, C.C.; Chen, C.C.; Hsu, Y.C.; Lei, M.H. Coronary artery calcium score compared with cardio-ankle vascular index in the prediction of cardiovascular events in asymptomatic patients with Type 2 diabetes. *J. Atheroscler. Thromb.* 2015, 22, 1255–1265. [CrossRef]
11. Kusunose, K.; Sato, M.; Yamada, H.; Saijo, Y.; Bando, M.; Hirata, Y.; Nishio, S.; Hayashi, S.; Sata, M. Prognostic implications of non-invasive vascular function tests in high-risk atherosclerosis patients. *Circ. J.* 2016, 80, 1034–1040. [CrossRef]
12. Laucevičius, A.; Ryliškytė, L.; Balsytė, J.; Badarienė, J.; Puronaitė, R.; Navickas, R.; Solovjova, S. Association of cardio-ankle vascular index with cardiovascular risk factors and cardiovascular events in metabolic syndrome patients. *Medicina* 2015, 51, 152–158. [CrossRef]
13. Sato, Y.; Nagayama, D.; Saiki, A.; Watanabe, R.; Watanabe, Y.; Imamura, H.; Yamaguchi, T.; Ban, N.; Kawana, H.; Nagumo, A.; et al. Cardio-ankle vascular index is independently associated with future cardiovascular events in outpatients with metabolic disorders. *J. Atheroscler. Thromb.* 2016, 23, 596–605. [CrossRef]
14. Limpijankit, T.; Vathesatogkit, P.; Matchariyakul, D.; Yingchoncharoen, T.; Siriyotha, S.; Thakkinstian, A.; Sritara, P. Cardio-ankle vascular index as a predictor of major adverse cardiovascular events in metabolic syndrome patients. *Clin. Cardiol.* 2021, 44, 1628–1635. [CrossRef]
15. Yasuharu, T.; Setoh, K.; Kawaguchi, T.; Nakayama, T.; Matsuda, F.; Nagahama study group. Brachial-ankle pulse wave velocity and cardio-ankle vascular index are associated with future cardiovascular events in a general population: The Nagahama Study. *J. Clin. Hypertens.* 2021, 23, 1390–1398. [CrossRef]
16. Satoh-Asahara, N.; Kotani, K.; Yamakage, H.; Yamada, T.; Araki, R.; Okajima, T.; Adachi, M.; Oishi, M.; Shimatsu, A.; Japan Obesity and Metabolic Syndrome Study (JOMS) Group. Cardio-ankle vascular index predicts for the incidence of cardiovascular events in obese patients: A multicenter prospective cohort study (Japan Obesity and Metabolic Syndrome Study: JOMS). *Atherosclerosis* 2015, 242, 461–468. [CrossRef]
17. Tanaka, A.; Tomiyama, H.; Maruhashi, T.; Matsuzawa, Y.; Miyoshi, T.; Kabutoya, T.; Kario, K.; Sugiyama, S.; Munakata, M.; Ito, H.; et al. Physiological diagnostic criteria for vascular failure. *Hypertension* 2018, 72, 1060–1071. [CrossRef]
18. Arnett, D.K.; Blumenthal, R.S.; Albert, M.A.; Buroker, A.B.; Goldberger, Z.D.; Hahn, E.J.; Himmelfarb, C.D.; Khera, A.; Lloyd-Jones, D.; McEvoy, J.W.; et al. 2019 ACC/AHA Guideline on the Primary Prevention of Cardiovascular Disease: Executive Summary: A Report of the American College of Cardiology/American Heart Association Task Force on Clinical Practice Guidelines. *J. Am. Coll. Cardiol.* 2019, 74, 1376–1414. [CrossRef]
19. SCORE2 working group and ESC Cardiovascular risk collaboration. SCORE2 risk prediction algorithms: New models to estimate 10-year risk of cardiovascular disease in Europe. *Eur. Heart J.* 2021, 42, 2439–2454. [CrossRef]
20. Nishimura, K.; Okamura, T.; Watanabe, M.; Nakai, M.; Takegami, M.; Higashiyama, A.; Kokubo, Y.; Okayama, A.; Miyamoto, Y. Predicting coronary heart disease using risk factor categories for a Japanese urban population, and comparison with the Framingham risk score: The suita study. *J. Atheroscler. Thromb.* 2014, 21, 784–798. [CrossRef]
21. Matsuo, S.; Imai, E.; Horio, M.; Yasuda, Y.; Tomita, K.; Nitta, K.; Yamagata, K.; Tomino, Y.; Yokoyama, H.; Hishida, A.; et al. Revised equations for estimated GFR from serum creatinine in Japan. *Am. J. Kidney Dis.* 2009, 53, 982–992. [CrossRef] [PubMed]

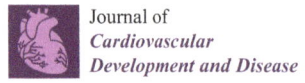

Journal of
Cardiovascular Development and Disease

Article

H-Type Hypertension among Black South Africans and the Relationship between Homocysteine, Its Genetic Determinants and Estimates of Vascular Function

Jacomina P. du Plessis [1], Leandi Lammertyn [2,3], Aletta E. Schutte [2,3,4] and Cornelie Nienaber-Rousseau [1,3,*]

1. Centre of Excellence for Nutrition, North-West University, Potchefstroom 2520, South Africa
2. Hypertension in Africa Research Team, North-West University, Potchefstroom 2520, South Africa
3. Medical Research Council Unit for Hypertension and Cardiovascular Disease, North-West University, Potchefstroom Campus, Potchefstroom 2520, South Africa
4. School of Population Health, University of New South Wales, The George Institute of Global Health, Sydney, NSW 2000, Australia
* Correspondence: cornelie.nienaber@nwu.ac.za

Abstract: Elevated homocysteine (Hcy) increases cardiovascular disease (CVD) risk. Our objective was to emphasize Hcy's contribution in hypertension and CVD management by determining H-type hypertension (hypertension with Hcy ≥ 10 µmol/L) and associations between Hcy, blood pressure (BP) and estimates of vascular function among Black South Africans. We included 1995 adults (63% female). Plasma Hcy and cardiovascular measures (systolic and diastolic BP (SBP, DBP), pulse pressure, heart rate (HR), carotid-radialis pulse wave velocity (cr-PWV), intercellular adhesion molecule-1 (ICAM-1) and vascular cell adhesion molecule-1) were quantified. Five Hcy-related polymorphisms (*cystathionine β-synthase* (*CBS* 844ins68, T833C, G9276A); *methylenetetrahydrofolate reductase* (*MTHFR* C677T) and *methionine synthase* (*MTR* A2756G)) were genotyped. Hcy was >10 µmol/L in 41% (n = 762), and of the 47% (n = 951) hypertensives, 45% (n = 425) presented with H-type. Hcy was higher in hypertensives vs. normotensives (9.86 vs. 8.78 µmol/L, $p < 0.0001$, effect size 0.56) and correlated positively with SBP, DBP, cr-PWV and ICAM-1 ($r > 0.19$, $p < 0.0001$). Over Hcy quartiles, SBP, DBP, HR, cr-PWV and ICAM-1 increased progressively (all p-trends ≤ 0.001). In multiple regression models, Hcy contributed to the variance of SBP, DBP, HR, cr-PWV and ICAM-1. H-type hypertensives also had the lowest *MTHFR* 677 CC frequency (p = 0.03). Hcy is positively and independently associated with markers of vascular function and raised BP.

Keywords: blood pressure management; endothelial function; endothelial structure; H-type hypertension; hyperhomocysteinemia; *MTHFR* C677T; sub-Saharan Africa; vascular inflammation

Citation: du Plessis, J.P.; Lammertyn, L.; Schutte, A.E.; Nienaber-Rousseau, C. H-Type Hypertension among Black South Africans and the Relationship between Homocysteine, Its Genetic Determinants and Estimates of Vascular Function. *J. Cardiovasc. Dev. Dis.* 2022, 9, 447. https://doi.org/10.3390/jcdd9120447

Academic Editor: Narayanaswamy Venketasubramanian

Received: 29 September 2022
Accepted: 7 December 2022
Published: 9 December 2022

Publisher's Note: MDPI stays neutral with regard to jurisdictional claims in published maps and institutional affiliations.

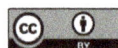

Copyright: © 2022 by the authors. Licensee MDPI, Basel, Switzerland. This article is an open access article distributed under the terms and conditions of the Creative Commons Attribution (CC BY) license (https://creativecommons.org/licenses/by/4.0/).

1. Introduction

Homocysteine (Hcy) is a nonproteinogenic, nonessential, sulfhydryl-containing amino acid. When Hcy is elevated, it conveys an independent risk toward hypertension [1], with Mendelian randomization evidence alluding to a causal relationship [2]. Observations made in the US National Health and Nutrition Examination Survey revealed that hypertensive men and women with Hcy concentrations below 10 µmol/L were 5.4 and 7.1 times more likely to suffer a stroke than normotensives, respectively. However, a combination of both hypertension and Hcy elevated above 10 µmol/L increased the risk substantially to 12.0 and 17.3 times for men and women, respectively [3]. Consequently, hypertension and hyperhomocysteinemia (HHcy) are independent risk factors of stroke, and the combination of both—that is, H-type hypertension—is a major risk factor of vascular diseases [3,4]. H-type hypertension is defined as essential hypertension combined with circulating Hcy greater than 10 µmol/L. Despite its risk to health, however, H-type hypertension has not been investigated in continental African populations [5], who currently demonstrate rapidly increasing hypertension prevalence rates [6,7]. The benefits of reducing Hcy concentrations are unjustifiably underestimated in treatment-resistant hypertension [8].

Because the etiology of essential hypertension has not been fully explained and understood, all factors that could contribute to the condition—including the influence of Hcy-related genes as well as environmental factors and their interactions—should be scrutinized further, some aspects of which we report here. Single genetic polymorphisms within the *methylenetetrahydrofolate reductase* (*MTHFR*) gene, such as the cytosine replacement at position 677 by a thymine (C677T), and other genes coding for proteins involved in Hcy's metabolism can alter the amino acid's concentrations [9]. A large-scale meta-analysis reported on the *MTHFR* C677T genotype's association with hypertension and the homozygote TT genotype conferring an increased risk [2]. However, a follow-up meta-analysis with false-positive report probability interrogations found that the *MTHFR* C677T polymorphism's relationship was not robust enough [5]. The results of genetic studies are equivocal; this might be because of the variations in the roles played by genotypes in the different ethnic studies reported [2]. If so, it makes it desirable to conduct research on a wider range of ethnic groups in order to establish to what extent Hcy and its genetic markers could influence the high prevalence of hypertension observed in, for example, sub-Saharan Africans [6]. We hope this study will help to re-emphasize Hcy's contribution in the integral multimodal approach of hypertension and related cardiovascular disease (CVD) management. Consequently, we determined, for the first time, the prevalence of H-type hypertension among Black South African adults and the relationship between plasma Hcy—and its genetic determinants—and blood pressure (BP), as well as estimates of vascular function.

2. Materials and Methods

2.1. Study Design and Participants

For this cross-sectional investigation, we analyzed the baseline data of 2010 randomly selected participants from the South African arm of the Prospective Urban and Rural Epidemiology (PURE–SA) study. The screening period involved visiting 6000 households in two urbanization strata (rural and urban) within the North West province of South Africa, from which eligible participants were identified as apparently healthy Black South African men and women over the age of 35 years without acute medical conditions. Interested individuals were well informed of all aspects of the study and invited to partake. Written, voluntary, informed consent was required before any measurements were taken, and participants could withdraw from the study at any stage without adverse consequences. The use of hypertension medication was not regarded as a basis for exclusion. For the analytic purposes of this study, volunteers who did not have blood pressure measurements were excluded from the investigation, and analyses proceeded with the remaining 1995 individuals (see Figure 1).

2.2. Questionnaires

Standardized questionnaires [10] obtained detailed information from respondents regarding their demographic and lifestyle characteristics by means of face-to-face interviews; these details included age, sex, education level, marital status, medication use, smoking and alcohol consumption.

2.3. Anthropometric Measurements

In accordance with the International Society for the Advancement of Kinanthropometry (ISAK), anthropometrical measurements were taken by ISAK-trained researchers using calibrated instruments. Measurements included height (IP 1465, Invicta, London, UK) and weight (Precision Health Scale, A&D Company, Tokyo, Japan). Hip and waist circumferences were recorded by means of a Lufkin steel tape (Cooper Tools, Apex, NC, USA), and the measurements were in turn used to calculate body mass index (BMI) (kg/m^2).

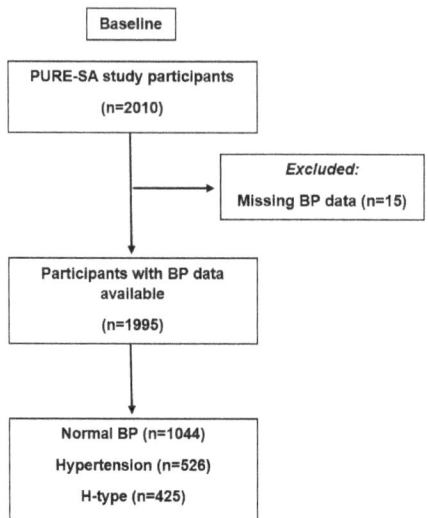

Figure 1. Study design flow chart.

2.4. Cardiovascular Marker Measurements

After a 5 min rest period, brachial systolic BP (SBP), diastolic BP (DBP) and heart rate (HR) were measured in duplicate using a validated Omron HEM-757 device (Omron Healthcare, Kyoto, Japan) while volunteers were in a seated position with the measuring (right) arm supported at the heart level. Pulse pressure (PP) was calculated by subtracting DBP from SBP. Carotid radialis pulse wave velocity (cr-PWV) was measured in the supine position and on the left side using the Complior SP device (Artech-Medical, Pantin, France). BP escalating behaviors such as caffeine use (participants were instructed to be fasting, with only water allowed), exercise and smoking were avoided at least 30 min prior to measurements, to ensure accuracy (standardized conditions set by the Joint National Committee on Prevention, Detection, Evaluation and Treatment of High Blood Pressure [11]). Normal BP was identified as BP values <140/90 mmHg. Hypertension was identified in those with a BP $\geq$ 140 and/or 90 mmHg or who reported anti-hypertensive medication use [12]. H-type hypertension was classified as hypertensive patients with concomitant [Hcy] $\geq$ 10 µmol/L [13]. Anti-hypertensive medications including thiazide diuretics, calcium channel blockers and renin-angiotensin system inhibitors were grouped together in a categorical variable created for antihypertensive medication use.

2.5. Laboratory Biochemical Measurements

A registered nurse sampled blood from the antecubital vein in the mornings between 7 a.m. and 11 a.m. after an overnight fast. Blood samples were centrifuged at 2000× g for at least 15 min to obtain serum, plasma and the buffy coat. After being transferred to tubes, the specimens were snap-frozen and then transported on dry ice to be stored at −80 °C.

A recognized pathology firm used an Abbott automated immunoassay analyzer (AxSYM) to quantify Hcy concentrations based on fluorescence polarization immunoassay technology (coefficient of variation (CV) = 4.52%). Both sequential multiple analyzers (Konelab 20i, Thermo Scientific (Vantaa, Finland) and Cobas Integra 400 Plus (Roche, Switzerland)) were used to analyze high-sensitivity C-reactive protein (CRP), gamma-glutamyl transferase (GGT) and blood lipids (triglycerides, total cholesterol (TC) and high-density lipoprotein cholesterol (HDL-C)). The remaining blood lipid, low-density lipoprotein cholesterol (LDL-C) concentration, was calculated using the Friedewald–Levy–Fredrickson formula [14]. Fasting glycated hemoglobin A1c (HbA1c) was measured with a D-10 hemoglobin testing system from Bio-Rad Laboratories (Hercules, CA, USA), and fasting plasma glucose was determined by the hexokinase method of the SynchronR System (Beckman Coulter Co., Fullerton, CA, USA). Serum intercellular adhesion molecule-1 (ICAM-1) and vascular cell adhesion molecule-1 (VCAM-1) levels were determined using sandwich ELISAs (Human sICAM-1 and human sVCAM-1 assay, IBL, Hamburg, Germany).

Genomic DNA was extracted from peripheral blood leukocytes using the commercially available QIAGEN®, Flexigene® DNA extraction kits (QIAGEN® Valencia, CA, USA; catalogue number 51 206). Concentrations were determined with the NanoDrop™ spectrophotometer (ND-1000, Wilmington, DE, USA), and polymerase chain reaction coupled with restriction fragment length polymorphism methods enabled the identification of individual genotypes, as described elsewhere [9]. The five Hcy-related single nucleotide polymorphisms (SNPs) genotyped were *cystathionine β-synthase* (*CBS* 844ins68, T833C, G9276A), *methylenetetrahydrofolate reductase* (*MTHFR* C677T) and *methionine synthase* (*MTR* A2756G).

2.6. Statistical Analysis

The data were statistically analyzed using the following software packages: Statistica version 14.0 (TIBCO Software Inc., Tulsa, OK, USA) and R statistical software version 4.2.0 (R Core Team; R: A language and environment for statistical computing. R Foundation for Statistical Computing, Vienna, Austria; 2020; URL https://www.r-project.org/; accessed 18 May 2022). Data were tested for normality. Because the data deviated from the normal distribution, as determined by the Shapiro–Wilk W-test and the Kolmogorov–Smirnov tests, descriptive statistics were expressed as medians with interquartile ranges. To determine statistically significant differences in continuous variables, the Kruskal–Wallis ANOVA among three independent sub-groups (normal BP, hypertension and H-type) and the Mann–Whitney U test between two independent groups (normal BP vs. hypertension, normal BP vs. H-type hypertension and hypertension vs. H-type hypertension) were used. Practical significance was determined for differences using Cohen's effect sizes. For categorical variables, the Pearson chi-squared test was used to detect statistically significant differences and Cramer's V effect sizes to observe practical significance. Both normal and partial Spearman rank correlations (adjusting for age, sex, BMI and GGT for all analyses and additionally for mean arterial pressure in cr-PWV) were computed to establish the relationship between Hcy and related variables.

Participants were divided into quartiles according to their [Hcy]: <7.44 µmol/L (quartile 1), between $\geq$7.45 and <9.17 µmol/L (quartile 2), between $\geq$9.18 and <12.04 µmol/L (quartile 3) and $\geq$12.05 µmol/L (quartile 4). Differences among the CVD variables and Hcy quartiles were determined using general linear models (GLMs), adjusting for age, sex, BMI and GGT. Where significant differences between groups were indicated, we followed this with a Tukey post hoc test.

Genotype counts and frequencies were determined for the whole group and sub-groups: normal BP, hypertension and H-type hypertension. The Phi correlation coefficient measured the strength of associations between variables, and the chi-squared test was used to determine the significance between groups.

The relationships between BP as well as related cardiovascular variables and Hcy were explored by regression analyses. For regression analyses, the parametric and logarithmically transformed data were used to determine the practical significance of one unit increase in Hcy. For all analyses, a *p* value < 0.05 was regarded as statistically significant.

3. Results

The demographic characteristics of the study population are shown in Table 1. The median Hcy and SBP/DBP values were as follows: for all (9.18 µmol/L, 130/87 mmHg), those with a normal BP (8.78 µmol/L, 117/78 mmHg), hypertensives (9.86 µmol/L, 148/97 mmHg), and H-type hypertensives (12.8 µmol/L, 135/89 mmHg). There were no cases of severe HHcy (>100 µmol/L). However, 759 (41%) individuals presented with Hcy >10 µmol/L, 469 (25%) presented with mild Hcy >12 µmol/L and 207 (11%) presented with moderate HHcy >15 µmol/L.

Table 1. Demographic characteristics of participants over blood pressure sub-groups.

		Median (25th–75th) or n (%)				Differences Among Groups # p Value
		Whole Group (n = 1995)	Normal BP (n = 1044)	Hypertension (n = 526)	H-Type Hypertension * (n = 425)	
Age (years)		48.0 (41.0–56.0) @	45.0 (40.0–53.0) @	49.0 (43.0–57.0) @	53.0 (46.0–61.0) @	<0.0001
Sex	Male	743	393 (52.9) @	160 (21.5) @	190 (25.6) @	<0.0001
	Female	1252	651 (52.0) @	366 (29.2) @	235 (18.8) @	
Urbanization level	Urban	996	456 (45.8) @	330 (33.1) @	210 (21.1) @	<0.0001
	Rural	999	588 (58.9) @	196 (19.6) @	215 (21.5) @	
Tobacco use	Current	1033	544 (52.7)	272 (26.3)	217 (21.0)	0.71
	Former	77	39 (50.6)	19 (24.7)	19 (24.7)	
	Never	875	455 (52.0)	231 (26.4)	189 (21.6)	
Anthro markers	BMI (kg/m^2)	23.0 (19.3–28.9)	22.1 (18.9–27.5) @,†	25.3 (20.2–31.7) @,$	23.1 (19.5–28.8) $,†	<0.0001
	Waist circumference (cm)	77.45 (70.2–87.7)	74.7 (68.8–84.3) @	81.9 (72.5–92.7) @	80.1 (72.2–89.1) @	<0.0001
	Hip circumference (cm)	93.13 (84.8–106)	91.4 (83.8–103) @	97.3 (87.4–111) @	92.2 (85.2–104) @	<0.0001
	Waist-to-hip ratio	0.83 (0.78–0.88)	0.82 (0.77–0.87) @	0.83 (0.78–0.88) @	0.85 (0.81–0.90) @	<0.0001
Biochemical markers	HIV sero-negative	1655	820 (49.5) @	448 (27.1) @	387 (23.4) @	<0.0001
	HIV sero-positive	324	215 (66.4) @	73 (22.5) @	36 (11.1) @	
	HIV status unknown	14	9 (64.3)	4 (28.6)	1 (7.10)	
	TC (mmol/L)	4.82 (4.01–5.87)	4.68 (3.87–5.67) @	5.02 (4.22–6.12) @	4.96 (4.15–6.06) @	<0.0001
	LDL-C (mmol/L)	2.77 (2.07–3.63)	2.73 (2.06–3.52) $	2.91 (2.20–3.82) $	2.77 (1.97–3.67)	0.01
	HDL-C (mmol/L)	1.42 (1.06–1.87)	1.35 (1.01–1.80) @	1.37 (1.05–1.85) @	1.60 (1.18–2.11) @	<0.0001
	Triglycerides (mmol/L)	1.08 (0.82–1.55)	1.01 (0.79–1.40) @	1.18 (0.86–1.70) @,$	1.12 (0.82–1.70) $	<0.0001
	Fasting glucose (mmol/L)	4.80 (4.30–5.30)	4.80 (4.30–5.20) †	4.80 (4.30–5.40)	4.90 (4.40–5.45) †	0.01
	HbA1c (%)	5.50 (5.30–5.80)	5.50 (5.30–5.80) †	5.60 (5.30–5.90) †	5.50 (5.20–5.85)	0.02
	GGT (µkat/L)	46.0 (29.7–88.0)	40.4 (28.0–69.0) @,$	49.5 (30.8–82.3) $	57.4 (33.8–139.8) @	<0.0001
	Hcy (µmol/L)	9.18 (7.50–12.1)	8.78 (7.16–11.0) @	8.00 (6.78–8.99) @	12.8 (11.4–15.9) @	<0.0001
	CRP (mg/L)	3.29 (0.96–9.34)	2.80 (0.73–9.29) @	3.77 (1.39–9.08) †	3.76 (1.16–9.67)	<0.0001

Table 1. Cont.

		Median (25th–75th) or n (%)				Differences Among Groups # p Value
		Whole Group (n = 1995)	Normal BP (n = 1044)	Hypertension (n = 526)	H-Type Hypertension * (n = 425)	
Cardiovascular markers	SBP (mmHg)	130 (116–147)	117 (109–126) @	146 (136–160) @	135 (120–152) @	<0.0001
	DBP (mmHg)	87.0 (78.0–97.0)	78.0 (72.0–84.0) @	97.0 (92.0–105) @	89.0 (80.0–99.0) @	<0.0001
	Pulse pressure (mmHg)	43.0 (35.0–53.0)	39.0 (33.0–45.0) @	50.0 (40.0–61.0) @	45.0 (36.0–56.0) @	<0.0001
	Heart rate (bpm)	72.0 (62.0–84.0)	71.0 (62.0–84.0) @	71.0 (61.0–81.0) @	74.0 (63.0–87.0) @	<0.0001
	cr-PWV (m/s)	10.9 (9.55–12.2)	10.5 (9.17–11.8) @	11.2 (9.98–12.3) @,†	11.2 (10.0–12.8) @,†	<0.0001
	ICAM-1 (ng/mL)	371 (234–507)	377 (247–510)	489 (327–805)	440 (286–548)	0.83
	VCAM-1 (ng/mL)	693 (390–1279)	679 (384–1295)	751 (357–1308)	662 (449–1139)	0.99
Anti-hypertensives use n (%)		283	82 (29.0) @	122 (43.1) @	79 (27.9) @	<0.0001

BMI, body mass index; CRP, C-reactive protein; cr-PWV, carotid-radialis pulse wave velocity; DBP, diastolic blood pressure; GGT, gamma glutamyl transferase; Hcy, homocysteine; HDL-C, high-density lipoprotein cholesterol; HbA1c, glycated hemoglobin; HIV, human immunodeficiency virus; HR, heart rate; ICAM-1, intercellular adhesion molecule 1; LDL-C, low-density lipoprotein cholesterol; PP, pulse pressure; SBP, systolic blood pressure; VCAM-1, vascular cell adhesion molecule 1. * H-type hypertension is a subset of those presenting with both hypertension and Hcy > 12.0 μmol/L and has thus been excluded from the hypertension group to form two independent groups. # Kruskal-Wallis ANOVA p values for continuous values and Pearson Chi-squared p value for categorical values. Post hoc analysis differences indicated with the same symbol; @ denotes p > 0.0001, $ denotes p < 0.001, † denotes p < 0.05.

Almost half of the participants (951 (48%)) were hypertensive, and 425 (45%) of those with hypertension presented with H-type hypertension. Of those with Hcy >10 μmol/L, 56% presented with hypertension compared with those with lower Hcy ($p < 0.0001$). Only 262 (13%) participants reported using anti-hypertension medication, of whom 180 (69%) were still hypertensive, including 79 (44%) participants with H-type hypertension.

Statistically significant differences were observed among the BP sub-groups (Tables 1 and 2). Noteworthy effect sizes were also observed for Hcy and triglycerides (moderate effect sizes) and HbA1c and PP (large effect sizes) in the normal BP vs. hypertension sub-groups. Between the normal BP and H-type hypertension sub-groups, age had a moderate effect size, whereas Hcy and PP had large effect sizes. Hcy attained a large effect size, and ICAM-1 attained a moderate effect size when BP groups of hypertension vs. H-type hypertension were compared. The categorical characteristics such as sex, urbanization and HIV status differed between BP sub-groups, although the effect sizes were small.

Table 2. Comparison of demographic, anthropometric and biochemical variables between hypertension status sub-groups.

	Variables	Normal vs. HTN		Normal vs. H-Type HTN		HTN vs. H-Type HTN *	
		p Value	Effect Size	p Value	Effect Size	p Value	Effect Size
	Continuous Variables						
	Age (years)	<0.0001	0.36	<0.0001	0.69	<0.0001	0.33
Anthro markers	BMI (kg/m^2)	<0.0001	0.40	0.58	0.17	0.001	0.21
	Waist circumference (cm)	<0.0001	0.45	<0.001	0.35	0.16	0.10
	Hip circumference (cm)	<0.0001	0.37	0.55	0.09	<0.0001	0.26
	Waist-to-hip ratio	<0.0001	0.16	<0.0001	0.45	<0.0001	0.27
Biochemical markers	TC (mmol/L)	<0.0001	0.24	<0.01	0.26	0.31	0.01
	LDL-C (mmol/L)	0.04	0.15	0.34	0.03	0.89	0.11
	HDL-C (mmol/L)	<0.0001	0.11	<0.0001	0.37	0.001	0.26
	Triglycerides (mmol/L)	<0.0001	0.79	0.03	0.23	0.23	0.08
	Fasting glucose (mmol/L)	0.001	0.23	0.05	0.13	0.32	0.10
	HbA1c (%)	0.04	0.88	0.41	0.07	0.11	0.15
	GGT (μkat/L)	<0.0001	0.11	<0.0001	0.33	0.03	0.15
	Hcy (μmol/L)	<0.0001	0.56	<0.0001	1.13	<0.0001	1.87
	CRP (mg/L)	<0.01	0.09	0.28	0.05	0.86	0.05
Cardiovascular markers	SBP (mmHg)	<0.0001	2.10	<0.0001	2.42	0.53	0.11
	DBP (mmHg)	<0.0001	2.35	<0.0001	2.38	0.57	0.09
	Pulse pressure (mmHg)	<0.0001	1.00	<0.0001	1.19	0.67	0.08
	Heart rate (bpm)	0.45	0.13	<0.0001	0.22	<0.0001	0.34
	cr-PWV (m/s)	<0.0001	0.33	<0.0001	0.49	0.04	0.17
	ICAM-1 (ng/mL)	0.14	0.02	0.03	0.03	0.21	0.51
	VCAM-1 (ng/mL)	0.30	0.06	0.01	0.14	0.86	0.17
	Categorical Variables						
Sex	Male/Female	0.01	0.07	0.01	0.07	<0.0001	0.15
Urbanization level	Urban/Rural	<0.0001	0.18	0.05	0.05	<0.0001	0.14
Tobacco use	Current/Former/Never	0.96	0.01	0.40	0.05	0.27	0.06
HIV status	Sero-negative/-positive/Unknown	0.01	0.08	<0.0001	0.16	0.02	0.09
Anti-hypertensives use	Yes/No	<0.0001	0.18	<0.0001	0.21	0.27	0.04

Continuous variables: Mann–Whitney U test for differences between groups and Cohen's effect sizes. Categorical variables: Pearson's chi-squared test for differences between groups and Cramer's V effect sizes. * H-type hypertension is a subset of those presenting with both hypertension and Hcy >12.0 μmol/L and has thus been excluded from the hypertension group to form two independent groups.

In Table 3, Hcy correlated with age, HDL-C, GGT, SBP, cr-PWV and ICAM-1 ($r \geq 0.19$), but after adjustment for age, sex, BMI and GGT (cr-PWV was additionally adjusted for mean arterial pressure), only correlations with age, HDL-C and GGT remained ($r \geq 0.19$). Hcy's relationship with HDL-C and GGT is discussed in detail elsewhere (Du Plessis JP et al. [15] and Nienaber-Rousseau C et al. [16], respectively).

Table 3. Spearman correlations between Hcy and characteristics of participants.

Variables	Unadjusted		Adjusted		Sensitivity Analysis	
	r	p	r	p	r	p
Age (year)	0.28	<0.0001	0.27	<0.0001	0.27	<0.0001
Anthropometrical Markers						
BMI (kg/m^2)	−0.13	<0.0001	−0.04	0.35	−0.16	<0.0001
Waist circumference (cm)	−0.03	0.24	0.02	0.69	−0.04	0.09
Hip circumference (cm)	−0.14	<0.0001	0.01	0.82	−0.16	<0.0001
Waist-to-hip ratio	0.17	<0.0001	−0.02	0.67	0.17	<0.0001
Biochemical Markers						
TC (mmol/L)	0.05	0.02	0.10	0.03	0.05	0.06
LDL-C (mmol/L)	−0.05	0.03	0.01	0.91	−0.07	<0.01
HDL-C (mmol/L)	0.19	<0.0001	0.20	<0.0001	0.20	<0.0001
Triglycerides (mmol/L)	0.001	0.96	−0.06	0.16	−0.02	0.54
Fasting glucose (mmol/L)	0.002	0.92	−0.07	0.10	−0.02	0.34
HbA1c (%)	−0.05	0.02	−0.02	0.64	−0.06	0.01
GGT (µkat/L)	0.24	<0.0001	0.24	<0.0001	0.23	<0.0001
CRP (mg/L)	0.03	0.15	0.01	0.86	0.01	0.60
Cardiovascular Markers						
Blood pressure (mmHg) SBP	0.19	<0.0001	0.07	0.14	0.19	<0.0001
Blood pressure (mmHg) DBP	0.16	<0.0001	0.08	0.09	0.15	<0.0001
Pulse pressure (mmHg)	0.14	<0.0001	0.01	0.76	0.14	<0.0001
Heart rate (bpm)	0.11	<0.0001	0.12	0.01	0.09	<0.001
cr-PWV (m/s)	0.19	<0.0001	0.04	0.32	0.21	<0.0001
ICAM-1 (ng/mL)	0.23	<0.0001	−0.02	0.68	0.21	<0.0001
VCAM-1 (ng/mL)	0.04	0.35	0.03	0.53	0.05	0.23

In the unadjusted model, the r values are for Spearman correlations; in the adjusted model, the r values are for Spearman partial correlations adjusted for age, sex, BMI and GGT. cr-PWV was additionally adjusted for mean arterial pressure. Anthropometrical markers were not adjusted for BMI, and the age and GGT variables were not adjusted for age and GGT, respectively. In the sensitivity analysis, individuals using anti-hypertensive medication were excluded from analyses. BMI, body mass index; CRP, C-reactive protein; cr-PWV, carotid-radialis pulse wave velocity; DBP, diastolic blood pressure; GGT, gamma glutamyl transferase; HDL-C, high-density lipoprotein cholesterol; HbA1c, glycated hemoglobin; HR, heart rate; ICAM-1, intercellular adhesion molecule 1; LDL-C, low-density lipoprotein cholesterol; PP, pulse pressure; SBP, systolic blood pressure; VCAM-1, vascular cell adhesion molecule 1.

In Table 4, post hoc tests exhibited differences over Hcy quartiles for most of the cardiovascular markers after adjusting for age, sex, BMI and GGT. With ascending Hcy quartiles, SBP, DBP, HR, cr-PWV, ICAM-1 and HDL-C levels increased, with the highest levels reported in the last Hcy quartile. Two blood lipids, TC and LDL-C, were higher in the second Hcy quartile than they were in the other quartiles. Because of the low reporting rate and the high resistance to anti-hypertensive treatment, participants reporting anti-hypertensive medication use were not excluded from analyses; however, additional sensitivity analyses were performed, adjusting for anti-hypertensive medication use (Tables 3 and 4).

Hcy contributed to the variance of SBP, DBP, HR, cr-PWV and ICAM-1, with the highest contribution in DBP and HR controlling for age, sex, BMI and GGT. With one higher unit of Hcy, DBP and HR increased with 0.12 and 0.16 units, respectively (Table 5).

Table 4. Cardiovascular markers across Hcy quartiles.

CVD Marker	Homocysteine (Adjusted Means with 95% CI Determined through GLM)				GLM p Value	Sensitivity p Value
	Quartile 1 (n = 464) <7.44 μmol/L	Quartile 2 (n = 467) ≥7.45 to <9.17 μmol/L	Quartile 3 (n = 469) ≥9.18 to <12.04 μmol/L	Quartile 4 (n = 467) >12.05 μmol/L		
CRP (mg/L)	8.12 (6.97–9.27)	8.17 (7.05–9.29)	8.16 (7.04–9.29)	8.94 (7.78–10.1)	0.73	0.88
Fasting glucose (μmol/L)	5.05 (4.90–5.21)	4.95 (4.81–5.10)	5.01 (4.86–5.15)	4.90 (4.75–5.06)	0.58	0.11
SBP (mmHg)	131 (129–133) c,d,f	133 (131–135) c,g	133 (130–135) d,h	137 (135–139) f,g,h	0.001	0.01
DBP (mmHg)	85.4 (84.1–86.7) c,f	85.9 (84.6–87.2) g	87.5 (86.2–88.8) c,d	90.9 (89.6–92.2) f,d,g	<0.0001	<0.0001
PP (mmHg)	45.6 (44.3–46.9)	46.9 (45.6–48.2)	45.0 (43.8–46.3)	46.1 (44.8–47.4)	0.21	0.37
HR (bpm)	71.9 (70.4–73.3) g	71.6 (70.3–73.0) f	73.3 (71.9–74.7) h	77.5 (76.1–79.0) f,g,h	<0.0001	<0.0001
cr-PWV (m/s)	10.7 (10.5–10.9) a,f,g	10.9 (10.7–11.2) a,h	11.1 (10.9–11.3) f,b	11.3 (11.1–11.5) g,h,b	<0.0001	0.001
ICAM-1 (ng/mL)	335 (310–360) a,g	351 (326–377) c	383 (356–409) a	420 (393–449) c,g	<0.0001	0.001
VCAM-1 (ng/mL)	1053 (853–1254)	1127 (914–1340)	1042 (814–1269)	909 (661–1157)	0.63	0.59
TC (mmol/L)	4.87 (4.74–5.00) c	5.14 (5.02–5.26) c	5.02 (4.89–5.14)	5.04 (4.91–5.17)	0.03	0.07
LDL-C (mmol/L)	2.90 (2.80–3.01)	3.03 (2.93–3.14) c	2.92 (2.82–3.03)	2.80 (2.69–2.91) c	0.001	0.04
HDL-C (mmol/L)	1.38 (1.32–1.44) c,d,g	1.52 (1.46–1.57) c,f	1.52 (1.47–1.58) d,e	1.66 (1.60–1.71) g,f,e	<0.0001	<0.0001
Triglicerides (mmol/L)	1.29 (1.22–1.36)	1.29 (1.23–1.36)	1.26 (1.19–1.33)	1.29 (1.22–1.36)	0.89	0.65

Post hoc test revealed significant differences between the quartiles indicated with letter(s); quartiles with the same symbol differ with the level of significance denoted as follows $p < 0.05$ a,b, ≤ 0.01 c, <0.001 d,e, <0.0001 f,g,h. GLMs were adjusted for age, sex, BMI and GGT. Additional analyses that excluded individuals using anti-hypertensive medication are reported as sensitivity p value. CRP, C-reactive protein; cr-PWV, carotid-radialis pulse wave velocity; DBP, diastolic blood pressure; HDL-C, high-density lipoprotein cholesterol; HR, heart rate; ICAM-1, intercellular adhesion molecule 1; LDL-C, low-density lipoprotein cholesterol; PP, pulse pressure; SBP, systolic blood pressure; TC, total cholesterol; VCAM-1, vascular cell adhesion molecule 1.

Table 5. Multivariable-adjusted relationships of cardiovascular measures with Hcy.

Variables	SBP ($R^2 = 0.18$)			
	B	SE	β	p
Age	0.71	0.05	0.30	<0.0001
Sex	5.34	1.21	0.11	<0.0001
BMI (kg/m^2)	0.41	0.09	0.12	<0.0001
GGT (μkat/L)	0.004	0.003	0.03	0.13
Hcy (μmol/L)	0.43	0.12	0.08	<0.0001
Anti-hypertensive use	8.92	1.51	0.14	<0.0001
	DBP ($R^2 = 0.10$)			
	B	SE	β	p
Age	0.17	0.03	0.12	<0.0001
Sex	0.21	0.75	0.01	0.79
BMI (kg/m^2)	0.33	0.05	0.16	<0.0001
GGT (μkat/L)	0.01	0.002	0.09	<0.0001
Hcy (μmol/L)	0.38	0.08	0.12	<0.0001
Anti-hypertensive use	5.13	0.94	0.13	<0.0001
	PP ($R^2 = 0.19$)			
	B	SE	β	p
Age	0.54	0.03	0.37	<0.0001
Sex	5.14	0.74	0.16	<0.0001
BMI (kg/m^2)	0.08	0.05	0.04	0.11
GGT (μkat/L)	−0.002	0.002	−0.03	0.19
Hcy (μmol/L)	0.04	0.07	0.01	0.57
Anti-hypertensive use	3.80	0.92	0.09	<0.0001
	HR ($R^2 = 0.10$)			
	B	SE	β	p
Age	−0.20	0.04	−0.13	<0.0001
Sex	−8.25	0.83	−0.25	<0.0001
BMI (kg/m^2)	−0.21	0.06	−0.09	<0.0001
GGT (μkat/L)	0.01	0.002	0.13	<0.0001
Hcy (μmol/L)	0.56	0.08	0.16	<0.0001
Anti-hypertensive use	2.40	1.04	0.06	0.02
	cr-PWV ($R^2 = 0.15$)			
	B	SE	β	p
Age	0.01	0.01	0.05	0.04
Sex	0.77	0.12	0.16	<0.0001
BMI (kg/m^2)	−0.08	0.01	−0.25	<0.0001
GGT (μkat/L)	0.001	<0.0001	0.05	0.02
Hcy (μmol/L)	0.04	0.01	0.09	<0.0001
Anti-hypertensive use	0.20	0.15	0.03	0.17
	ICAM-1 ($R^2 = 0.08$)			
	B	SE	β	p
Age	2.27	2.04	0.05	0.27
Sex	−5.73	45.9	−0.01	0.90
BMI (kg/m^2)	−3.34	3.20	−0.05	0.30
GGT (μkat/L)	0.71	0.11	0.28	<0.0001
Hcy (μmol/L)	−11.7	4.58	−0.11	0.01
Anti-hypertensive use	95.1	57.2	0.07	0.10
	VCAM ($R^2 = 0.01$)			
	B	SE	β	p
Age	4.51	5.61	0.04	0.42

Table 5. Cont.

Variables	SBP ($R^2 = 0.18$)			
	B	SE	β	p
Sex	59.11	126	0.02	0.64
BMI (kg/m^2)	−7.08	8.79	−0.04	0.42
GGT (μkat/L)	0.02	0.29	0.003	0.95
Hcy (μmol/L)	−15.0	12.6	−0.05	0.23
Anti-hypertensive use	−57.0	157	−0.02	0.71

β, standardized beta; B, unstandardized beta; BMI, body mass index; DBP, diastolic blood pressure; cr-PWV, carotid-radialis pulse wave velocity; GGT, gamma glutamyl transferase; Hcy, homocys-teine; HR, heart rate; ICAM-1, intercellular adhesion molecule 1; PP, pulse pressure; SBP, systolic blood pressure; SE, standard error; VCAM-1, vascular cell adhesion molecule 1.

Genotype distributions were as predicted without deviating from the Hardy–Weinberg equilibrium ($p > 0.05$) (Table 6). The lowest frequency of the *MTHFR* 677CC genotype and, in turn, the highest T allele prevalence were observed in those with H-type hypertension compared to the other BP sub-groups ($p = 0.03$).

Table 6. Hcy-related SNPs and their genotype frequencies in population subdivisions for blood pressure.

Gene; SNP ID (rs Number; Location)	Whole Group	Normotensive	Hypertension	H-Type Hypertension
	Genotype Counts (Frequencies %)			
MTHFR; C677T Ala222Val (rs1801133; 1:11796321)	CC 1561 (84.0) CT 282 (15.2) TT 15 (0.80)	821 (83.3) 156 (15.8) 9 (0.90)	404 (87.1) 58 (12.5) 2 (0.40) Phi = 0.08 Chi-square $p = 0.03$	336 (82.4) 68 (16.7) 4 (0.90)
MTR; A2756G Asp919Gly (rs1805087; 1:236885200)	AA 1181 (63.7) AG 583 (31.5) GG 89 (4.80)	621 (63.3) 315 (32.1) 45 (4.60)	284 (61.2) 154 (33.2) 26 (5.60) Phi = 0.06 Chi-square $p = 0.28$	276 (67.7) 114 (27.9) 18 (4.40)
CBS; T833C Ile278Thr (rs5742905; 21:43063074)	TT 984 (52.9) TC 740 (39.8) CC 137 (7.30)	520 (52.7) 396 (40.2) 70 (7.10)	246 (52.9) 187 (40.2) 32 (6.90) Phi = 0.05 Chi-square $p = 0.55$	218 (53.2) 157 (38.3) 35 (8.50)
CBS; 844ins68 indel (no rs#)	WT 985 (52.9) HT 742 (39.8) MT 135 (7.30)	521 (52.8) 396 (40.2) 69 (7.00)	245 (52.7) 188 (40.4) 32 (6.90) Phi = 0.04 Chi-square $p = 0.80$	219 (53.3) 158 (38.4) 34 (8.30)
CBS; G9276A (novel SNP no rs#; 21:43071860)	GG 966 (51.9) GA 750 (40.3) AA 144 (7.80)	517 (52.4) 391 (39.7) 78 (7.90)	232 (50.0) 199 (42.9) 33 (7.10) Phi = 0.04 Chi-square $p = 0.73$	217 (52.9) 160 (39.0) 33 (8.10)

844ins68, insertion of 68 base pairs at nucleotide position 844; A, adenine (nucleotide); Ala, alanine; Asp, aspartic acid; C, cytosine (nucleotide); *CBS*, *cystathionine β-synthase gene*; G, guanine (nucleotide); Gly, glycine; HT, heterozygous; ID, identity; Ile, isoleucine; indel, insertion/deletion; MT, homozygous insert; *MTHFR*, *methylenetetrahydrofolate reductase gene*; *MTR*, *methionine synthase gene*; rs, reference SNP; SNP, single nucleotide polymorphism; T, thymine (nucleotide); Thr, threonine; Val, valine; WT, homozygous non-insert. Genotype information expressed here is for individuals for whom we had genetic and BP data available. * Individuals with H-type hypertension are a subset of those presenting with hypertension for whom we had BP and Hcy data, with Hcy being >10 μmol/L.

4. Discussion

Here, we report, for the first time, an H-type hypertension prevalence of 23% among all participants and a 45% prevalence among those with hypertension in a relatively large sample of Black South Africans recruited from both rural and urban communities. We observed that BP related positively and independently to Hcy, which may be due to the adverse effects of Hcy on the measures of vascular structure and function reported here. To complement our investigation, we report on Hcy-related polymorphisms and conclude that, of those considered, the prevalence of the *MTHFR* 677 T allele was greater in those presenting with H-type hypertension.

4.1. Homocysteine and Blood Pressure—H-Type Hypertension

Approximately half of the participants (aged 51.0 ± 7 years) were hypertensive, with a positive relationship observed between Hcy and BP; however, these correlations diminished after adjustments. Nonetheless, both SBP and DBP values rose progressively over increasing Hcy quartiles, and DBP even exceeded the upper BP range (<90 mmHg) in the highest Hcy quartile, regardless of adjustments. These findings, together with the large effect sizes observed between BP sub-groups, confirm that Hcy plays a meaningful role in both SBP and DBP levels, irrespective of age, sex, BMI and GGT, in Black South African adults. Previous studies reported a similar association between Hcy and BP in adults [17,18] as well as in Black South African adolescents [19].

The participants in the hypertension sub-group also had higher Hcy concentrations, with a concomitant increase in the prevalence of H-type hypertension. The prevalence of H-type hypertension observed here reflects that reported by Towfighi et al. [3], who recorded a 48% prevalence among American adults, less than the 75% and higher prevalence reported in Chinese adults [20,21], reaffirming the importance of multi-ethnic investigations before evaluating intervention possibilities. The pathogenesis of H-type hypertension still needs further exploration. Because environmental and genetic factors as well as their interactions could contribute to the pathophysiology of H-type hypertension and resistant hypertension, investigations should incorporate both [2].

4.2. H-Type Hypertension and Genetic Determinants

Our findings provide an evidence-based reference for H-type hypertension in Black South Africans, with the possibility of the *MTHFR* C677T polymorphism becoming a new marker for the clinical evaluation of H-type hypertension in this population. Our results add to the body of evidence indicating that *MTHFR* C677T could be related to H-type hypertension susceptibility [22]. The frequency of the CC genotype of the *MTHFR* polymorphism, known to have protective qualities against hypertension [2,23], was the lowest in those with H-type hypertension, resulting in the T allele being the most prevalent in this BP sub-group. Those carrying genes predisposing them to hypertension and Hcy-related diseases could benefit from dietary interventions personalized according to their genetic make-up [15].

A recent study reported that patients treated with folic acid doses, individualized according to their *MTHFR* C677T genotype, exhibited reduced BP and Hcy and an improved prothrombotic status in those with H-type hypertension [24]. The *MTHFR* 677T allele causes a decrease in the essential cofactor flavin adenine dinucleotide's affinity, with riboflavin as a precursor, demonstrating higher BP values and increased hypertension risk. Genome-wide studies [25] and a randomized control trial [26] reported substantial reductions in BP after riboflavin (vitamin B_2) supplementation, more so than those with anti-hypertensive treatment alone. These studies emphasize an alternative and safe treatment opportunity for resistant hypertension through vitamin supplementation. Identifying genetic risk factors opens the possibility for risk stratification and personalized prevention as well as treatments such as genotype-guided dietary intake and even possible targeted gene therapy opportunities.

4.3. Hcy with Vascular Function and Inflammation Markers

As expected, we confirmed positive correlations between Hcy and some preclinical markers of vascular function and inflammation. However, after statistical adjustments, the associations diminished, with only HR remaining. When evaluating the cardiovascular markers over Hcy quartiles, peripheral arterial stiffness (cr-PWV) and vascular inflammation (ICAM-1) exceeded normal reference intervals (as provided by Bia and Zócalo [27] and Rothlein R et al. [28], respectively), corresponding to the greatest Hcy concentration quartile examined.

Elevated Hcy values have been indicated in both arterial stiffness and vascular inflammation, leading to endothelial dysfunction and hypertension development [29]. The postulated mechanisms involved include Hcy interfering with the production of vascular regulating nitric oxide and deregulating the signaling pathway associated with hydrogen sulfide (H_2S), resulting in endothelial imbalance [29]. A Chinese longitudinal community-based study reported Hcy to be positively associated with central arterial stiffness (carotid femoral-PWV) but not with peripheral arterial stiffness (cr-PWV), as observed in our study [30]. Further research is needed to evaluate the relationship between Hcy and different measures of arterial stiffness in multi-ethnic populations.

Hcy has been associated with vascular inflammation either directly or indirectly via the production of reactive oxygen species [31] and has also been indicated to initiate inflammatory responses within the vascular smooth muscle cells by stimulating CRP production [32]. Moreover, Barroso, Kao [30] reported that, in endothelial cells, the precursor of Hcy, S-adenosylhomocysteine, activates nuclear factor kappa B (NF-κB) and initiates the expression of pro-inflammatory molecules, including interleukin-1, ICAM-1, VCAM-1 and E-selectin. Durga, Van Tits [33], however, reported that a noticeable lowering of elevated Hcy concentrations did not influence inflammatory responses involving CRP, ICAM-1, oxidized LDL-C or autoantibodies against oxidized LDL-C. Further research is needed to clarify Hcy's role in vascular inflammation, because one of the enzymes in the Hcy transsulfuration pathway, CBS, is a major source of vascular H_2S, which inhibits vascular inflammation by inhibiting the NF-kB pathway [29].

4.4. Treatment and Recommendations

The least invasive and most cost-effective way of potentially manipulating Hcy is through diet and lifestyle changes. Consequently, the relationships between Hcy—and its genetic markers—and markers of vascular function should be further explored to confirm causality in trials where Hcy is lowered. Because African Americans and Asians have a 3–4 times higher risk of angioedema than Whites as a side effect of using anti-hypertensive medicine [11], alternative treatments are therefore necessary for those experiencing adverse pharmacological consequences. The Dietary Approaches to Stop Hypertension (DASH) lifestyle recommends a low-fat diet that is high in fruits, vegetables and low-fat dairy. The DASH lifestyle has been reported to reduce Hcy concentrations in addition to lowering BP [34,35]. Moreover, several other lifestyle factors are known to reduce BP, namely, weight loss, lowering sodium intake, regular physical activity and limiting alcohol consumption [11] and should also be investigated along with diet to lower Hcy and contingent CVD risk.

4.5. Limitations, Strengths and Future Studies

The large sample size reported here was critical, as it ensured the means to detect small changes in BP. This study could assess some associations, but, unfortunately, due to its cross-sectional nature, no inferences concerning the causal relationship of high Hcy and hypertension can be made. To examine any possible causal effect of Hcy lowering and BP, we suggest controlled intervention trials. Future research should investigate the interactions between dietary factors and Hcy-related genetic variations, especially the *MTHFR* C677T polymorphism, in relation to BP and markers of vascular structure and function or hard clinical outcomes. Thereafter, dietary supplementation trials stratified for genotypes should be conducted to evaluate their efficacy. Markers such as intima media thickness and carotid femoral-PWV, the "golden standard" measure for arterial stiffness, are not evaluated and should be included in future studies. H-type hypertension is an old concept with a new label, drawing attention to the relationship between Hcy and hypertension. By embracing the new single term, researchers will increase the searchabi-lity and visibility of articles still referring to HHcy and BP separately [36]. The use of the term "H-type hypertension" should be encouraged in future studies of this kind, which should include different ethnicities across their respective geographical regions to broaden the value and understanding of research on H-type hypertension.

5. Conclusions

This study has demonstrated a potentiating relationship between Hcy and raised BP, which could lead to safe, tailored prospects for CVD prevention. For example, Hcy can be lowered by lifestyle modifications including dietary supplementation with folate and B-vitamins. Such treatment can ultimately improve BP outcomes and subsequent stroke risk. Patients with elevated Hcy, hypertension or H-type hypertension should be consi-dered as candidates for screening and lifestyle changes. These modifications, together with appro-priate supplementation, can forestall hypertension in pre-hypertensives—especially using folic acid and riboflavin in addition to, or as alternatives to, expensive pharmacological medications when they are unavailable, ineffective or induce adverse side effects. More-over, this study indicates that specific genetic factors may dictate different prevention or treatment strategies. Future investigations should further explore the relationships between determinants of Hcy, especially gene–diet interactions, in relation to BP and markers of the vascular function of clinical outcomes such as stroke, to determine potential conflated associations informing intervention strategies.

Author Contributions: Conceptualization, investigation, data curation, writing—original draft prepa-ration, J.P.d.P. and C.N.-R.; methodology and formal analysis, J.P.d.P.; data interpretation, J.P.d.P., C.N.-R., L.L. and A.E.S.; writing—critical review and editing, L.L. and A.E.S.; supervision, C.N.-R.; funding acquisition, A.E.S., C.N.-R. and J.P.d.P. All authors have read and agreed to the published version of the manuscript.

Funding: This research was supported partially by grants from South Africa—Netherlands Research Programme on Alternatives in Development, the South African National Research Foundation, NWU, PHRI, the South African Medical Research Council (SAMRC) and the North West Province Health De-partment. The authors thank the SAMRC for the scholarship provided to J.P.d.P. through its Division of Research Capacity Development under the National Health Scholarship Program from funding received from the Public Health Enhancement Fund/South African National Department of Health. Disclosure Statement: The funders had no role in the study design, the data collection or analysis, the decision to publish or the preparation of the manuscript, whose content is the sole responsibility of the authors and does not necessarily represent the official views of the funding agencies.

Institutional Review Board Statement: The study protocol was approved by the Health Research Ethics Committee of North-West University (ethics number: 04M10 for the larger study and NWU-00142-18-A1 for this specific investigation, 27/112018) for studies involving humans and adhered to the principles of the Declaration of Helsinki laid down in 1975 and revised in 2013, with emphasis on voluntary participation, confidentiality and anonymity.

Informed Consent Statement: Informed consent was obtained from all subjects involved in the study.

Data Availability Statement: The data analyzed in this study are subject to the following licenses/restrictions: Raw data were generated at the North-West University. Obtained data supporting the findings of this study are available from the PI of the study after obtaining the necessary ethical approval. Due to ethical restrictions and the POPI act, data are not publicly available. Requests to access these datasets should be directed to lanthe.kruger@nwu.ac.za.

Acknowledgments: We sincerely thank the study participants of the PURE-SA study, all the supporting staff and the hardworking research team. We especially thank Annamarie Kruger (posthumous), the fieldworkers and the administrative personnel of the Africa Unit for Transdisciplinary Health Research (AUTHeR) from the Faculty of Health Sciences of NWU, the PURE-International research team, the office personnel and the PURE-study leader, Yusuf.

Conflicts of Interest: The authors declare no conflict of interest. The funders also had no role in the design of the study; in the collection, analyses or interpretation of the data; in the writing of the manuscript; or in the decision to publish the results.

References

1. Zhong, F.; Zhuang, L.; Wang, Y.; Ma, Y. Homocysteine levels and risk of essential hypertension: A meta-analysis of published epidemiological studies. *Clin. Exp. Hypertens.* **2017**, *39*, 160–167. [CrossRef] [PubMed]
2. Fu, L.; Li, Y.; Luo, D.; Deng, S.; Wu, B.; Hu, Y. Evidence on the causal link between homocysteine and hypertension from a meta-analysis of 40 173 individuals implementing Mendelian randomization. *J. Clin. Hypertens.* **2019**, *21*, 1879–1894. [CrossRef] [PubMed]
3. Towfighi, A.; Markovic, D.; Ovbiagele, B. Pronounced association of elevated serum homocysteine with stroke in subgroups of individuals: A nationwide study. *J. Neurol. Sci.* **2010**, *298*, 153–157. [CrossRef] [PubMed]
4. Li, J.; Jiang, S.; Zhang, Y.; Tang, G.; Wang, Y.; Mao, G.; Li, Z.; Xu, X.; Wang, B.; Huo, Y. H-type hypertension and risk of stroke in chinese adults: A prospective, nested case–control study. *J. Transl. Intern. Med.* **2015**, *3*, 171–178. [CrossRef]
5. Meng, H.; Huang, S.; Yang, Y.; He, X.; Fei, L.; Xing, Y. Association Between MTHFR Polymorphisms and the Risk of Essential Hypertension: An Updated Meta-analysis. *Front. Genet.* **2021**, *12*, 698590. [CrossRef]
6. E Schutte, A.; Botha, S.; Fourie, C.M.T.; Gafane-Matemane, L.F.; Kruger, R.; Lammertyn, L.; Malan, L.; Mels, C.M.C.; Schutte, R.; Smith, W.; et al. Recent advances in understanding hypertension development in sub-Saharan Africa. *J. Hum. Hypertens.* **2017**, *31*, 491–500. [CrossRef]
7. E Schutte, A.; Schutte, R.; Huisman, H.W.; van Rooyen, J.M.; Fourie, C.M.; Malan, N.T.; Malan, L.; MC Mels, C.; Smith, W.; Moss, S.J.; et al. Are behavioural risk factors to be blamed for the conversion from optimal blood pressure to hypertensive status in Black South Africans? A 5-year prospective study. *Int. J. Epidemiol.* **2012**, *41*, 1114–1123. [CrossRef]
8. Smith, A.D.; Refsum, H. Homocysteine—From disease biomarker to disease prevention. *J. Intern. Med.* **2021**, *290*, 826–854. [CrossRef]
9. Nienaber-Rousseau, C.; Ellis, S.M.; Moss, S.J.; Melse-Boonstra, A.; Towers, G.W. Gene–environment and gene–gene interactions of specific MTHFR, MTR and CBS gene variants in relation to homocysteine in black South Africans. *Gene* **2013**, *530*, 113–118. [CrossRef]
10. Teo, K.; Chow, C.K.; Vaz, M.; Rangarajan, S.; Yusuf, S. The Prospective Urban Rural Epidemiology (PURE) study: Examining the impact of societal influences on chronic noncommunicable diseases in low-, middle-, and high-income countries. *Am. Heart J.* **2009**, *158*, 1–7. [CrossRef]
11. Chobanian, A.V.; Bakris, G.L.; Black, H.R.; Cushman, W.C.; Green, L.A.; Izzo, J.L., Jr.; Jones, D.W.; Materson, B.J.; Oparil, S.; Wright, J.T., Jr.; et al. Seventh report of the joint national committee on prevention, detection, evaluation, and treatment of high blood pressure. *Hypertension* **2003**, *42*, 1206–1252. [CrossRef] [PubMed]
12. Unger, T.; Borghi, C.; Charchar, F.; Khan, N.A.; Poulter, N.R.; Prabhakaran, D.; Ramirez, A.; Schlaich, M.; Stergiou, G.S.; Tomaszewski, M.; et al. 2020 International Society of Hypertension Global Hypertension Practice Guidelines. *Hypertension* **2020**, *75*, 1334–1357. [CrossRef] [PubMed]
13. Tan, S.; Zhao, L.; Wang, H.; Song, B.; Li, Z.; Gao, Y.; Lu, J.; Chandra, A.; Xu, Y. H-type Hypertension and Recurrence of Ischemic Stroke. *Life Sci. J.* **2011**, *8*, 460–463.
14. Friedewald, W.T.; Levy, R.I.; Fredrickson, D.S. Estimation of the Concentration of Low-Density Lipoprotein Cholesterol in Plasma, Without Use of the Preparative Ultracentrifuge. *Clin. Chem.* **1972**, *18*, 499–502. [CrossRef]
15. du Plessis, J.P.; Melse-Boonstra, A.; Zandberg, L.; Nienaber-Rousseau, C. Gene interactions observed with the HDL-c blood lipid, intakes of protein, sugar and biotin in relation to circulating homocysteine concentrations in a group of black South Africans. *Mol. Genet. Metab. Rep.* **2019**, *22*, 100556. [CrossRef] [PubMed]
16. Nienaber-Rousseau, C.; Pisa, P.T.; Venter, C.S.; Ellis, S.M.; Kruger, A.; Moss, S.J.; Melse-Boonstra, A.; Towers, G.W. Nutritional Genetics: The Case of Alcohol and the MTHFR C677T Polymorphism in Relation to Homocysteine in a Black South African Population. *Lifestyle Genom.* **2013**, *6*, 61–72. [CrossRef] [PubMed]
17. Nygård, O.; Vollset, S.E.; Refsum, H.; Stensvold, I.; Tverdal, A.; Nordrehaug, J.E.; Ueland, P.M.; Kvåle, G. Total Plasma Homocysteine and Cardiovascular Risk Profile. *JAMA* **1995**, *274*, 1526–1533. [CrossRef] [PubMed]
18. Kahleová, R.; Palyzová, D.; Zvára, K.; Zvarova, J.; Hrach, K.; Nováková, I.; Hyánek, J.; Bendlová, B.; Kožich, V. Essential hypertension in adolescents: Association with insulin resistance and with metabolism of homocysteine and vitamins. *Am. J. Hypertens.* **2002**, *15*, 857–864. [CrossRef]

19. du Plessis, J.P.; Nienaber-Rousseau, C.; Lammertyn, L.; Schutte, A.E.; Pieters, M.; Kruger, H.S. The Relationship of Circulating Homocysteine with Fibrinogen, Blood Pressure, and Other Cardiovascular Measures in African Adolescents. *J. Pediatr.* **2021**, *234*, 158–163. [CrossRef]
20. Qian, X.-L.; Cao, H.; Zhang, J.; Gu, Z.-H.; Tang, W.-Q.; Shen, L.; Hu, J.-L.; Yao, Z.-F.; Zhang, L.; Tang, M.-N.; et al. The prevalence, relative risk factors and MTHFR C677T genotype of H type hypertension of the elderly hypertensives in Shanghai, China: A 'cross-section study. *BMC Cardiovasc. Disord.* **2021**, *21*, 1–10. [CrossRef]
21. Zhong, C.; Lv, L.; Liu, C.; Zhao, L.; Zhou, M.; Sun, W.; Xu, T.; Tong, W. High Homocysteine and Blood Pressure Related to Poor Outcome of Acute Ischemia Stroke in Chinese Population. *PLoS ONE* **2014**, *9*, e107498. [CrossRef] [PubMed]
22. Liao, S.; Guo, S.; Ma, R.; He, J.; Yan, Y.; Zhang, X.; Wang, X.; Cao, B.; Guo, H. Association between methylenetetrahydrofolate reductase (MTHFR) C677T polymorphism and H-type hypertension: A systematic review and meta-analysis. *Ann. Hum. Genet.* **2022**. *e-pub ahead of print*. [CrossRef]
23. Candrasatria, R.M.; Adiarto, S.; Sukmawan, R. Methylenetetrahydrofolate Reductase C677T Gene Polymorphism as a Risk Factor for Hypertension in a Rural Population. *Int. J. Hypertens.* **2020**, *2020*, 4267246. [CrossRef] [PubMed]
24. Zhang, S.; Wang, T.; Wang, H.; Tang, J.; Hou, A.; Yan, X.; Yu, B.; Ran, S.; Luo, M.; Tang, Y.; et al. Effects of individualized administration of folic acid on prothrombotic state and vascular endothelial function with H-type hypertension. *Medicine* **2022**, *101*, e28628. [CrossRef] [PubMed]
25. McNulty, H.; Strain, J.; Hughes, C.F.; Ward, M. Riboflavin, MTHFR genotype and blood pressure: A personalized approach to prevention and treatment of hypertension. *Mol. Asp. Med.* **2017**, *53*, 2–9. [CrossRef]
26. Wilson, C.P.; McNulty, H.; Ward, M.; Strain, J.; Trouton, T.G.; Hoeft, B.A.; Weber, P.; Roos, F.F.; Horigan, G.; McAnena, L.; et al. Blood Pressure in Treated Hypertensive Individuals with the *MTHFR* 677TT Genotype Is Responsive to Intervention with Riboflavin. *Hypertension* **2013**, *61*, 1302–1308. [CrossRef]
27. Bia, D.; Zócalo, Y. Physiological Age- and Sex-Related Profiles for Local (Aortic) and Regional (Carotid-Femoral, Carotid-Radial) Pulse Wave Velocity and Center-to-Periphery Stiffness Gradient, with and without Blood Pressure Adjustments: Reference Intervals and Agreement between Methods in Healthy Subjects (3–84 Years). *J. Cardiovasc. Dev. Dis.* **2021**, *8*, 3. [CrossRef]
28. Rothlein, R.; Mainolfi, E.A.; Czajkowski, M.; Marlin, S.D. A form of circulating ICAM-1 in human serum. *J. Immunol.* **1991**, *147*, 3788–3793.
29. Esse, R.; Barroso, M.; De Almeida, I.T.; Castro, R. The Contribution of Homocysteine Metabolism Disruption to Endothelial Dysfunction: State-of-the-Art. *Int. J. Mol. Sci.* **2019**, *20*, 867. [CrossRef]
30. Wang, X.-N.; Ye, P.; Cao, R.-H.; Yang, X.; Xiao, W.-K.; Zhang, Y.; Bai, Y.-Y.; Wu, H.-M. Plasma Homocysteine is a Predictive Factor for Arterial Stiffness: A Community-Based 4.8-Year Prospective Study. *J. Clin. Hypertens.* **2015**, *17*, 594–600. [CrossRef]
31. Barroso, M.; Kao, D.; Blom, H.J.; Tavares de Almeida, I.; Castro, R.; Loscalzo, J.; Handy, D.E. S-adenosylhomocysteine induces inflammation through NFkB: A possible role for EZH2 in endothelial cell activation. *Biochim. Biophys. Acta (BBA)-Mol. Basis Dis.* **2016**, *1862*, 82–92. [CrossRef] [PubMed]
32. Pang, X.; Liu, J.; Zhao, J.; Mao, J.; Zhang, X.; Feng, L.; Han, C.; Li, M.; Wang, S.; Wu, D. Homocysteine induces the expression of C-reactive protein via NMDAr-ROS-MAPK-NF-κB signal pathway in rat vascular smooth muscle cells. *Atherosclerosis* **2014**, *236*, 73–81. [CrossRef] [PubMed]
33. Durga, J.; Van Tits, L.J.H.; Schouten, E.G.; Kok, F.J.; Verhoef, P. Effect of Lowering of Homocysteine Levels on Inflammatory Markers. *Arch. Intern. Med.* **2005**, *165*, 1388–1394. [CrossRef] [PubMed]
34. Appel, L.J.; Moore, T.J.; Obarzanek, E.; Vollmer, W.M.; Svetkey, L.P.; Sacks, F.M.; Bray, G.A.; Vogt, T.M.; Cutler, J.A.; Windhauser, M.M.; et al. A clinical trial of the effects of dietary patterns on blood pressure. DASH Collaborative Research Group. *N. Engl. J. Med.* **1997**, *336*, 1117–1124. [CrossRef]
35. Seung-Hye, C.; Smi, C.-K.; Chung-Sil, K.; Haeyoung, L. The Effects of Korean DASH Diet Education Program on Oxidative Stress, Antioxidant Capacity, and Serum Homocysteine Level among Elderly Korean Women. *J. Korean Biol. Nurs. Sci.* **2017**, *19*, 141–150. [CrossRef]
36. Elias, M.F.; Brown, C.J. New Evidence for Homocysteine Lowering for Management of Treatment-Resistant Hypertension. *Am. J. Hypertens.* **2022**, *35*, 303–305. [CrossRef]

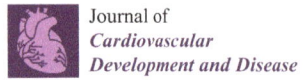

Article

Effectiveness of the Combination of Enalapril and Nifedipine for the Treatment of Hypertension versus Empirical Treatment in Primary Care Patients

Humberto Badillo-Alonso [1,2], Marisol Martínez-Alanis [3], Ramiro Sánchez-Huesca [4], Abel Lerma [5] and Claudia Lerma [1,4,*]

1. Centro de Investigación en Ciencias de la Salud (CICSA), FCS, Universidad Anáhuac México Campus Norte, Huixquilucan Edo. de Mexico 52786, Mexicoo; humbertobadilloalonso@gmail.com
2. Jalalpa el Grande Health Center, Mexico City Health Secreatariat, Mexico City 01377, Mexico
3. School of Engineering, Universidad Anahuac Mexico, Huixquilucan 52786, Mexico; marisol.martinez2@anahuac.mx
4. Instituto Nacional de Cardiologia Ignacio Chávez, Mexico City 04480, Mexico; farmacologia.medica@gmail.com
5. Institute of Health Sciences, Universidad Autónoma del Estado de Hidalgo, San Agustín Tlaxiaca 42160, Mexico; abel_lerma@uaeh.edu.mx
* Correspondence: claudia.lerma@anahuac.mx or dr.claudialerma@gmail.com; Tel.: +52-(55)-55732911 (ext. 26202)

Abstract: Hypertension in Mexico has a prevalence of 32% and is the second most widespread cause of consultation in primary care. Only 40% of patients in treatment have a blood pressure (BP) below 140/90 mmHg. This clinical trial aimed to compare the effectiveness of the combination of enalapril and nifedipine versus the empirical treatment for hypertension in patients with uncontrolled BP in a primary care center in Mexico City. Participants were randomized to treatment with enalapril and nifedipine (combination group) or to continue with the empirical treatment. Outcome variables were BP control, therapeutic adherence, and adverse effects at 6 months of follow-up. At the end of the follow-up period, BP control (64% versus 77%) and therapeutic adherence (53% versus 93%) showed an improvement from the baseline values in the group that received the combination treatment. BP control (51% versus 47%) and therapeutic adherence (64% versus 59%) in the group who received the empirical treatment did not show improvement from the baseline to follow-up. Combined treatment was 31% more efficacious than conventional empirical treatment (odds ratio = 3.9), which yielded an incremental clinical utility of 18% with high tolerability extent among patients in primary care in Mexico City. These results contribute to the control of arterial hypertension.

Keywords: hypertension control; primary care; clinical trial

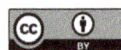

1. Introduction

Hypertension is a disease that contributes most to all-cause morbidity and mortality worldwide [1,2]. Hypertension can be detected in the community and in primary care settings, and several effective medications are available at low cost to treat patients with hypertension and reduce the risk of sequalae. Improving effective treatment coverage for patients with hypertension is a goal of many global, regional, and national initiatives and programs [3]. The care of hypertension, including detection, treatment, and management, varies substantially around the world and even within the same region of the world. In Mexico, the National Health and Nutrition Survey 2020 (ENSANUT 2020) reports that the prevalence of hypertension in Mexican adults was 49.4%, using the American Heart Association (AHA) classification as a reference. Among these adults, 70% were diagnosed with hypertension at the time of the survey. According to the JNC-7 classification (used in

ENSANUT 2020), only 30.2% of Mexican adults had hypertension and 51% of them were unaware of having this disease.

Hypertension can be detected at primary care and low-cost treatments can effectively control it. Although lifestyle modification (nonpharmacological treatment) is important, it has been very difficult to apply it at the individual and population level, and is often not sufficient by itself to control blood pressure. Therefore, effective pharmacological management is essential for controlling hypertension. However, with the increasing number and diversity of pharmacological agents available that encompasses several key and complementary drug classes, treatment options are now complex and need to be simplified [4]. Furthermore, other barriers to an effective antihypertensive treatment involve the healthcare providers, who may lack a complete understanding of the appropriate use of the different pharmacological classes and individual agents, be reluctant to use standardized treatment algorithms, and are driven by "clinical or therapeutic inertia" (the phenomenon of not initiating therapy immediately), which delays dose increases or the addition of other pharmacological agents when indicated. At the primary care level, factors, such as the lack of accessibility to health centers and clinics, the limited availability of affordable and reliable drugs, the inability to maintain follow-up and treatment programs once initiated, and budgetary constraints preventing the widespread use of antihypertensive drugs, all contribute to low rates of effective treatment [5]. In Mexico, the treatment of arterial hypertension is regulated by the Mexican Official Standard NOM_ 030-SSA2 for the prevention, treatment and control of arterial hypertension and clinical practice guidelines. However, in many cases, patients receive the empirical treatment, which is defined as "the treatment of diseases by means whose usefulness has been demonstrated by the experience of the primary care physician", without strictly following the current clinical practice guidelines, and includes four main classes of antihypertensive drugs: angiotensin-converting enzyme inhibitors, angiotensin receptor blockers, calcium channel blockers, and thiazide and thiazide-like diuretics. These drugs are generally prescribed in monotherapy. Any of these four classes of antihypertensive drugs can be used as initial treatment unless there are specific contraindications. However, to achieve blood pressure control (systolic blood pressure < 140 mmHg and diastolic blood pressure < 90 mmHg), effective hypertension treatment usually requires at least two antihypertensive medications from different complementary classes [6–10].

When combining antihypertensive drugs, the aim should be to maximize the effects with a decrease in adverse reactions. The combination chosen for this study is an angiotensin-converting enzyme inhibitor "enalapril" and a calcium channel blocker "nifedipine" which has an antihypertensive effect and the potential to mitigate side effects of the substances given separately. The combination based on enalapril and nifedipine is justified on several pharmacological, therapeutic, and clinical grounds [11]. This combination therapy is metabolically neutral and has been shown to offer consistent advantages in relation to new-onset diabetes mellitus when compared to other classical combination therapy, such as beta-blockers and thiazide diuretics [12]. This combination also presents an important clinical advantage in terms of tolerability, as it favors a significant reduction in the adverse effects of one component (ankle edema favored by calcium channel blockers) through the antagonistic peripheral vascular actions of angiotensin-converting enzyme inhibitors [13]. Moreover, the fixed-dose combination of angiotensin-converting enzyme inhibitors and calcium channel blockers may offer an important additional advantage in relation to patient compliance when compared to the separate administration of the two drugs, while maintaining blood pressure control and renal and cardiovascular protection efficacy [14]. Both enalapril and nifedipine are antihypertensive drugs that are included in the basic drug list at primary care and are in continuous supply due to their low cost in Mexico, representing an early antihypertensive response because it is made up of first-line drugs that simplify the treatment regimen with the benefit of contributing to therapeutic adherence.

The combination of enalapril and nifedipine has not been studied in relation to a treatment scheme, which is highly variable and is based on the experience of the primary care physician (empirical treatment). Although the effectiveness of drug combinations for the management of arterial hypertension has been demonstrated in several studies, the specific circumstances at primary care have not been evaluated. Prior to this clinical trial, no direct comparison studies between empirical treatment and this fixed-dose combination at primary care have been conducted that would demonstrate if the combination of enalapril and nifedipine is superior to non-fixed free combinations. The aim of this work was to compare the effectiveness of the combination of enalapril and nifedipine for the treatment of hypertension versus empirical treatment, with respect to blood pressure control, therapeutic adherence, and adverse effects, in patients with uncontrolled blood pressure at primary care.

2. Materials and Methods

2.1. Study Design and Patients

The study design was a randomized clinical trial. It was an experimental study comparing two groups with the aim to evaluate the antihypertensive effectivity of a combined treatment, while describing therapeutic adherence and any possible adverse effects. The combined treatment consisted of enalapril (one tablet of 10 mg every 12 h) and nifedipine (one tablet of 10 mg every 12 h).

The participants included in the study were selected from a group of patients with a hypertension diagnosis that attended "Dr. Manuel Escontria" Health Center in Mexico City. All participants agreed to take part in the study by signing an informed consent. Participants were selected in a non-probabilistic manner with consecutive cases and random assignment to the intervention groups. This was a prospective, randomized, open, blinded-endpoint study. Inclusion criteria considered patients, both male and female, over 40 years of age who had a systolic blood pressure between 140 and 180 mmHg and a diastolic blood pressure between 90 and 110 mmHg. All patients had to be recently diagnosed with hypertension or based on a medical opinion, must benefit from a change in treatment.

Exclusion criteria considered any patient who had suffered an acute myocardial infarction in prior months, who had arrhythmias, unstable angina, heart failure, diagnosis of a cerebrovascular accident or renal failure. For fertile women, anyone taking contraception or pregnant were excluded, because oral contraceptives can prevent an effective antihypertensive treatment in certain patients [15]. Additionally, any patient taking an immunosuppressive treatment, with known hypersensitivity to calcium channel blockers or angiotensin converting enzyme inhibitors, were excluded from our study.

Any patient who voluntarily decided to leave, abandoned the study, or presented adverse effects that could put their health at risk, was eliminated.

This study was approved by the Bioethics Committee of our institution (protocol number 201626). It was carried out in accordance with the provisions contained in the General Health Law of Mexico and the ethical principles contained in the Declaration of Helsinki.

2.2. Sample Size and Sampling Method

The sample size was calculated considering the proportion of patients who are expected to experience a reduction in their blood pressure after application of a combined antihypertensive therapy treatment (40%) and the proportion of patients whose blood pressure figures will be reduced by continuing with an empirical treatment (25%). The sample size was calculated using the 2-proportion comparison formula for experimental studies (Equation (1)).

$$n = \left[\frac{z_\alpha \sqrt{2p(1-p)} + z_\beta \sqrt{p_1(1-p_1) + p_2(1-p_2)}}{p_1 - p_2} \right]^2 \quad (1)$$

A confidence level of 95% and a power of 80% were considered. The calculated minimum sample size was 145.86, rounded to 146 subjects for both the experimental group and the non-experimental group. Though only 292 patients were required, a total of 328 participated in this study.

The sampling process was carried out by a group of 12 primary care physicians and each of them selected a minimum of 30 patients via consecutive sampling. Allocation of the patients to each intervention group was randomized.

2.3. Study Protocol

Participating patients signed an informed consent after one of the physicians explained the purpose of this study. They could be either newly diagnosed as hypertensive or those who, in the opinion of their doctor, could benefit from a change in treatment based on the proposed combined therapy.

Patient monitoring lasted 6 months, during which 5 control visits were carried out (Figure 1). In the initial visit (V1), training was conducted and recorded, the medical team was formed, and they were given instructions on the management of the medication. The data collection formats were tested, and patients were selected and randomly assigned to the two intervention groups. The following visits were carried out every two months. In the first bimester visit (V2), the pharmacological treatment was started in the intervention groups. The next two visits (V3 and V4) were the follow-up of the treatment, and the final visit (V5) conducted was the last follow-up and closure of our study.

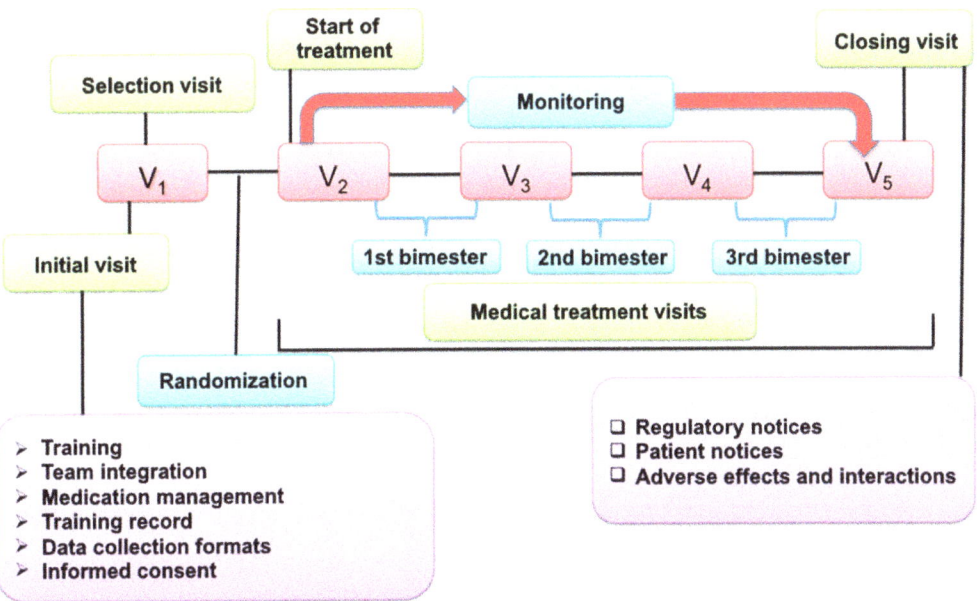

Figure 1. Flow chart of the study protocol.

During each visit, blood pressure, weight and height were recorded; and laboratory tests, including glycemia, glycated hemoglobin, total cholesterol, triglycerides, creatinine, and uric acid were conducted. At the start and the end of the study, systematic analytical controls were registered. The possibility of presenting adverse effects and their degree were recorded whenever they presented. Blood pressure was measured in the morning, before taking the medication, after resting for 5 min, and in the dominant arm. Two measurements were performed 2 min apart in a sitting position, and the average of both was recorded. In each consultation, the results of the Morisky–Green–Levine test for therapeutic adherence and notification of suspected adverse drug reactions were applied and recorded in the patient's medical record.

2.3.1. Assessment of Blood Pressure, Vital Signs, Anthropometric Variables, and Biochemical Variables

All blood pressure measurements were conducted using an automatic and validated electronic device (Omron M4). All anthropometric measurements were performed using a scale with a validated digital stadiometer (Seca 213). All laboratory samples were processed in the laboratory of the health center using automated equipment (Cobas c11).

2.3.2. Assessment of Therapeutic Adherence and Adverse Reactions

The Morisky–Green–Levine test consists of four questions where it is specified, according to the value of the answers obtained, if the patient has had therapeutic adherence to a pharmacological treatment or if the adherence is not adequate. In all cases, the questions must be answered with a "yes" or a "no". Adherents (ADT) are those who answer NO to the four questions and non-adherents (NADT) are those who answer YES to one or more questions. The test has shown a good correlation between adherence and blood pressure control [16].

In the event of any adverse reaction, the observation was conducted during the clinical interview using the Suspected Adverse Reactions Report format from the National Center for Pharmacovigilance in Mexico.

2.3.3. Study Variables

Systolic blood pressure and diastolic blood pressure were measured in mmHg as described above. The main outcome was controlled blood pressure (yes or no), defined as systolic blood pressure < 140 mmHg and diastolic blood pressure < 90 mmHg. Adherence to treatment and adverse reactions were the secondary outcomes. The intervention variable was the antihypertensive treatment (combined or empirical treatment).

Anthropometric variables were age (years), sex (female or male), body weight (kg), height (cm), and body mass index (kg/m^2). Clinical variables included comorbidities (diabetes, obesity, metabolic syndrome, and dyslipidemia). Blood chemistry laboratory variables included glucose (mg/dL), glycated hemoglobin (%), uric acid (mg/dL), creatinine (mg/dL), total cholesterol (mg/dL), and triglycerides (mg/dL).

2.4. Statistical Analysis

Most continuous variables did not have a normal distribution (Kolmogorov–Smirnov test with $p < 0.05$). Therefore, these variables were reported as median (25th percentile—75th percentile) and were compared between treatments using the Mann–Whitney U test. Within each treatment group, the medians evaluated at 2, 4, and 6 months were compared against the evaluation baseline using the Wilcoxon test. The study variables were compared with respect to uncontrolled hypertension (controlled vs. uncontrolled) using the Mann–Whitney U test (ordinal variables) or Chi-square test (nominal variables). To evaluate the efficacy of the combined treatment, we calculated several indices. For each treatment, we assessed the incidence of controlled blood pressure (number of patients with controlled blood pressure/total number of patients who received the treatment), expressed as percentage. Then, we calculated the clinical utility as the difference between incidence in the combined treatment—incidence in the empirical treatment (expressed as percentage), which corresponds to the absolute risk reduction (ARR), expressed as a proportion. The relative risk (RR) was calculated as incidence of combined treatment/incidence of empirical treatment. The number required to be treated (NRT) was calculated as 100%/clinical utility. Statistical analysis was performed using SPSS Statistics 21.0 (IBM Corp., Armonk, NY, USA) and Microsoft Excel 2017.

3. Results

3.1. Baseline Characteristics

The characteristics of the study participants are shown in Table 1. Both treatment groups were similar, except for a lower proportion of overweight or obese patients in the group with combined treatment compared to the group with empirical treatment.

Table 1. Sociodemographic and clinical characteristics of the study participants at baseline. Data are shown as median (percentile 25—percentile 75) or absolute value (percentage).

Variable	Empirical Treatment (N = 161)	Combined Treatment (Enalapril + Nifedipine) (N = 167)	p Value
Age (years)	61 (53–70)	62 (55–71)	0.501
BMI (kg/m^2)	29.2 (26.3–32.8)	28.6 (24.7–32.0)	0.092
Female sex	120 (75%)	123 (74%)	0.855
Overweight or obese	139 (86%)	122 (73%)	0.003
Diabetes mellitus	91 (56%)	94 (65%)	0.966
Dyslipidemia	58 (36%)	69 (41%)	0.325
Metabolic syndrome	72 (45%)	75 (45%)	0.972
Uncontrolled diabetes	43 (47%)	34 (36%)	0.126
Uncontrolled dyslipidemia	58 (36%)	69 (41%)	0.325
Uncontrolled metabolic syndrome	74 (45%)	75 (45%)	0.972

Table 2 shows a detailed description of the prescribed drugs in both the study groups. Compared to the group with empirical treatment, the group with combined treatment had more patients with prescribed oral hypoglycemic drugs (glibenclamide), less patients with other antihypertensive drugs (captopril, metoprolol, telmisartan and losartan), and less patients with diuretic prescription (hydrochlorothiazide, and chlorthalidone). There were no significant differences in other prescribed drugs.

Table 2. Prescribed drugs during the study. Data are shown as absolute value (percentage).

Variable	Empirical Treatment	Enalapril + Nifedipine	p Value
Acetylsalicylic acid	19 (12%)	16 (10%)	0.515
Metformin	74 (45%)	91 (54%)	0.098
Glibenclamide	20 (12%)	42 (25%)	0.003
Linagliptin	1 (1%)	1 (1%)	0.742
Acarbose	3 (2%)	3 (2%)	0.640
Fast insulin	2 (1%)	4 (2%)	0.360
Glargine insulin	39 (24%)	29 (17%)	0.126
NPH insulin	1 (1%)	2 (1%)	0.514
Captopril	49 (30%)	0 (0%)	<0.001
Hydrochlorothiazide	6 (4%)	0 (0%)	0.013
Chlorthalidone	4 (3%)	0 (0%)	0.057
Metoprolol	26 (16%)	0 (0%)	<0.001
Propranolol	2 (1%)	1 (1%)	0.486
Telmisartan	12 (7%)	0 (0%)	<0.001
Losartan	44 (27%)	0 (0%)	<0.001
Alopurinol	0 (0%)	2 (1%)	0.258
Pravastatin	33 (21%)	34 (20%)	0.542
Atorvastatin	5 (3%)	6 (4%)	0.525
Bezafibrate	17 (11%)	25 (15%)	0.232
Verapamil	1 (1%)	0 (0%)	0.491
Furosemide	1 (1%)	0 (0%)	0.491

3.2. Outcome Variables and Treatment Efficacy

Table 3 shows the results of the outcome variables. At baseline, compared to the empiric treatment group, the group with the combined treatment had a slightly larger proportion of patients with controlled blood pressure (51 vs. 64%), less treatment adherence (64 vs. 53%), and less adverse reaction (2 vs. 1%). However, after 6 months of treatment, compared to the empiric treatment group, the group with the combined treatment had a notably larger proportion of patients with controlled blood pressure (47 vs. 77%), more treatment adherence (59 vs. 93%), and less adverse reaction (2 vs. 1%).

Table 3. Outcome variables. Data are shown as absolute value (percentage).

Baseline	Empirical Treatment	Enalapril + Nifedipine	p Value
Controlled blood pressure			
Yes	82 (51%)	106 (64%)	0.022
No	79 (49%)	61 (36%)	
Treatment adherence			
Yes	103 (64%)	88 (53%)	0.038
No	58 (36%)	79 (74%)	
Adverse reactions			
Yes	3 (2%)	1 (1%)	0.298
No	158 (98%)	166 (99%)	
After 6 months of treatment	Empirical treatment	Enalapril + nifedipine	p value
Controlled blood pressure			
Yes	75 (47%)	129 (77%)	<0.001
No	86 (53%)	38 (23%)	
Treatment adherence			
Yes	95 (59%)	155 (93%)	<0.001
No	66 (41%)	12 (7%)	
Adverse reactions			
Yes	3 (2%)	1 (1%)	0.298
No	158 (98%)	166 (99%)	

Figure 2 shows the estimation procedure of treatment efficacy for hypertension control of the combined treatment (enalapril plus nifedipine) versus the empirical treatment group. At baseline, the combined treatment was 12.5% superior to the empirical treatment (63.5–50.9%), which corresponds to an absolute risk reduction ARR = 0.125, with a relative risk (63.5/50.9) = 1.246, and an odds ratio = $((106 \times 79)/(82 \times 61)) = 1.67$. After 6 months of treatment, the combined treatment was 30.7% superior (77.2–46.6%), which corresponds to an absolute risk reduction of 0.307, a relative risk = 77.2%/46.6% = 0.307, and an odds ratio = $((129 \times 86)/75 \times 38) = 3.89$). The relative risk (of controlling blood pressure) increased from 1.246 to 1.658 after 6 months of combined treatment, raising the clinical protective effect by 41.2% (24% to 64%), leading to a net increase in clinical utility of 18.1% (12.5% to 30.7%). This clinical utility indicates that the number of patients required to be treated (NRT) to control blood pressure decreased from eight to three patients.

3.3. Anthropometric, Blood Pressure and Laboratory Variables Follow-Up

Figure 3 shows that systolic blood pressure was higher in the empirical treatment group compared to the combined treatment group at all assessment times (including baseline). In both groups, the antihypertensive treatment decreased the systolic blood pressure at all times of follow-up compared to baseline.

Diastolic blood pressure was larger in the empirical treatment group compared to the combined treatment group at all assessment times (Figure 3). The combined treatment group had a significant decrease from the baseline at all the follow-up months. The combined treatment group had the largest decrease with respect to baseline after six months, while the empirical group remained unchanged compared at the same time.

Body weight was larger in the empirical treatment group compared to the combined treatment throughout the study (Figure 3). Compared to baseline, changes in body weight occurred in both groups after four months of follow-up, and the increase remained in the empirical treatment group.

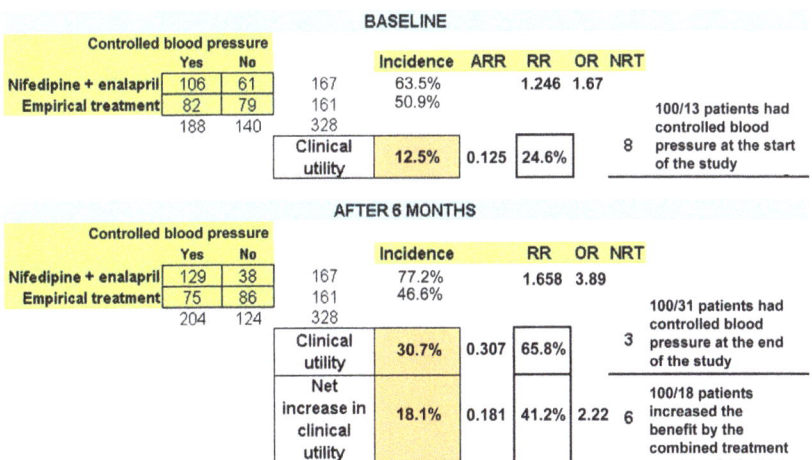

Figure 2. Assessment of treatment efficacy for blood pressure control with the combined treatment (nifedipine + enalapril) versus the empirical treatment. BP = blood pressure, ARR = absolute risk reduction, RR = relative risk, OR = odds ratio, NRT = number required to be treated.

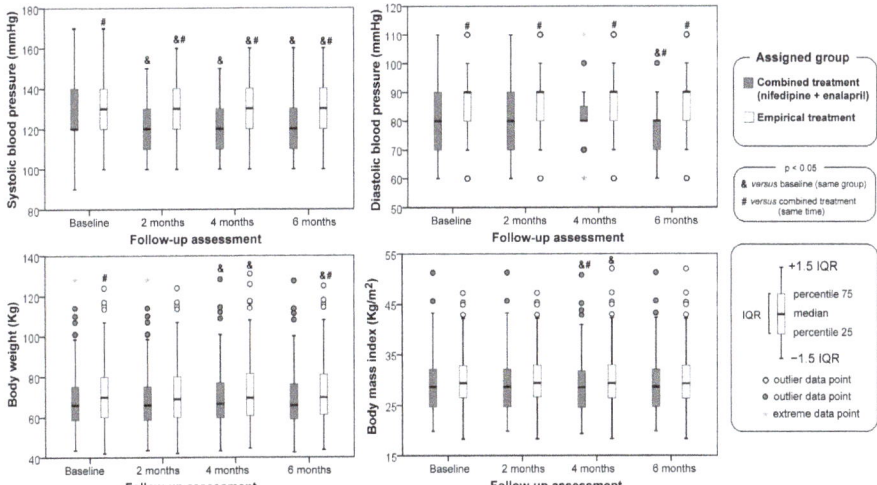

Figure 3. Baseline and follow-up assessment of blood pressure and anthropometry. IQR = interquartile range.

Regarding body mass index (Figure 3), compared to baseline, significant changes presented after four months of follow-up in both the groups; the empirical treatment group only presented changes at four months in relation to the combined treatment group at the same time.

Figure 4 shows the assessment of serum glucose, glycated hemoglobin, total cholesterol, triglycerides, uric acid, and creatinine. Glucose did not show significant changes in the combined treatment group during the study, but for the empirical treatment group, an increase was observed at 4 and 6 months of months of treatment. Glycosylated hemoglobin showed changes in the combined treatment group at 2, 4 and 6 months compared to the empirical treatment group. The combined treatment group presented changes at 2, 4 and 6 months in relation to the baseline of the same group, while the empirical treatment group showed changes at 4 and 6 months compared to baseline in the same group. Cholesterol was higher in the combined treatment group and showed no changes during the study. The empirical treatment group showed a slight decrease at 2, 4 and 6 months in relation to the combined treatment at the same time. Triglycerides showed a slight increase at 2, 4 and 6 months in the combined treatment group compared to baseline, while in the empirical treatment group changes were only recorded at 2 months with a slight decrease as compared to the combined treatment. At 6 months of evaluation, the combined treatment group had a slight decrease in uric acid levels in reference to the baseline of the same group, while the empirical treatment showed a decrease at 4 and 6 months with respect to the baseline of the same group. Serum creatinine in the empirical treatment group showed a decrease at 2 and 4 months with respect to the combined treatment group and a decrease at 6 months in the combined treatment group with respect to the beginning of the study.

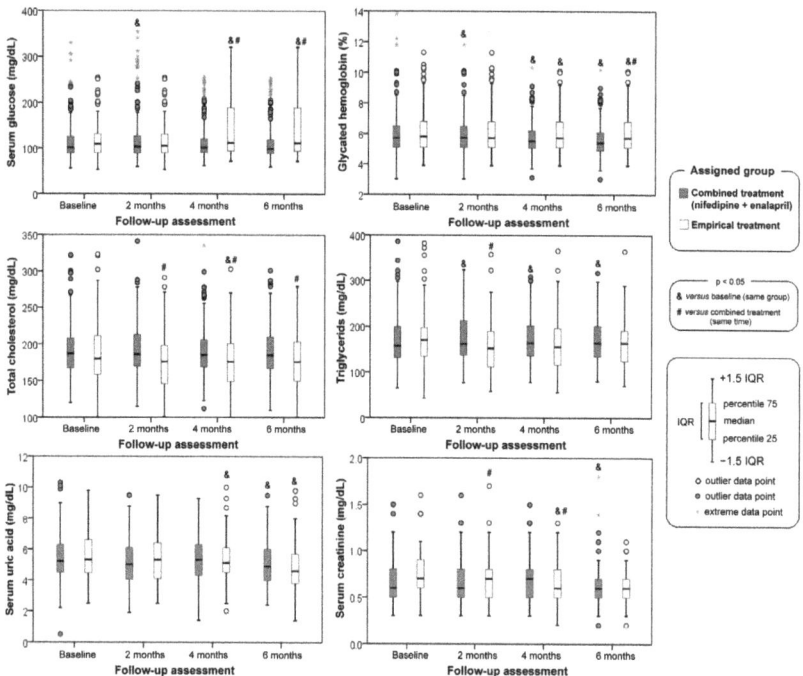

Figure 4. Baseline and follow-up assessment of serum glucose, glycated hemoglobin, total cholesterol, triglycerides, serum uric acid, and serum creatinine. IQR = inter-quartile range.

4. Discussion

The main aim of this work was to assess the efficacy of an intervention to improve the arterial blood pressure control in primary care patients diagnosed with systemic arterial hypertension by initiating (or changing) treatment to a fixed combination of enalapril and nifedipine and comparing it with the empirical treatment. The results show that after 6 months of treatment, the combination of enalapril and nifedipine improved the control of arterial blood pressure compared with the conventional empirical treatment. The combined therapy also improved the adherence without adverse effects. An important contribution is that this research was performed in the primary care setting, which is one of the largest settings that treats most of the population but has low rates of controlled blood pressure. In regions such as Latin America, low blood pressure control rates are a significant public health issue, considering the high hypertension prevalence, which is about 30 to 45% in the general population and this tend to increase rapidly with age [17].

For a long time, clinicians have been overconfident regarding monotherapy. Guidelines from the European Society for Hypertension (ESH), European Society of Cardiology (ESC) and the Joint National Committee 8 (JNC 8) from the United States of America indicate that most patients will need two or more medications to control arterial blood pressure and shed light on recommendations about possible combinations [18]. Moreover, it is recommended to reduce the number of pharmaceutical dosage forms throughout the combination of fixed doses [19]. A combined therapy is recommended to patients with high cardiovascular risk and subclinical organic damage, as well as those irresponsive to monotherapy [20]. Several clinical trials have documented that the physician's decision is one of the main reasons contributing to the lack of update in the antihypertensive treatment and thus in the control of blood pressure [21–23].

The combined therapy is aimed to provide a synergistic effect, more tolerability, higher patient's therapeutic adherence [24], simplify the treatment, improve the blood pressure control, and reduce the cardiovascular morbidity and mortality. Nowadays, double or triple drug combinations are available to hypertensive patients with good clinical results, that is, adequate therapeutic adherence and low profile of adverse effects [25]. The administration of an efficacious treatment is key to reducing the risk of other diseases related to systemic arterial hypertension, such as myocardial infarction and cerebrovascular event [26]. Despite these well-established concepts, systemic arterial hypertension is still treated inadequately around the world [27].

This study also contributes to a change in the way general practitioners prescribe medications, since it is common to find physicians who are reluctant to modify or increase the antihypertensive treatment in patients who present non-controlled blood pressure [28]. Therefore, to overcome this reluctance in upgrading medication, it is important for physicians and healthcare providers to become conscious about the elevated risk in those patients who do not reach the minimum goal of blood pressure within the first year of treatment. The use of educational programs also has an important role in enhancing the conduct of physicians during systemic arterial hypertension treatments [29].

The lack of adherence to antihypertensive therapy is probably the most important reason for non-controlled arterial blood pressure and it is influenced by multiple interrelated factors [30]. To understand the lack of therapeutic adherence and its associated factors, it is important to determine correct intervention strategies. There are several factors related to poor control of arterial blood pressure, for example, those related to patients or the role of the health system [29]. This study has shown that the combination of enalapril and nifedipine from the beginning of the treatment favors therapeutic adherence.

Follow-up laboratory tests were performed on all patients who participated in this study to describe the biochemical changes during the course of the combined therapy. Although the laboratory results were statistically significant for some analytes, these did not result in a change of the clinical state of the patients and the variations were minimal. Further studies are required to test if the combination of enalapril and nifedipine, as a treatment for systemic arterial hypertension, has any beneficial effects in other metabolic variables usually monitored by the blood biochemical tests in primary care.

It seems that drug combinations, not restricted to hypertensive drugs but also those with statins and antidiabetics, will be widely used in chronic and degenerative diseases in the near future [25]. Combined antihypertensive therapies are more effective, better tolerated, safer and has less economic impact than monotherapy [31], however, there is a lack of evidence to guide the selection of drugs under consideration of different populations, according to age, sex, ethnic group, and comorbidities. We hypothesize that the assessed drug combination may prevent complications in the long term.

A double-blind study was not performed, since no placebo was used and patients with arterial hypertension with different degrees of evolution and clinical complications were included, thereby making it necessary to test the intervention with groups with greater control and stratification to standardize the treatment. Furthermore, although the allocation of patients was randomized, the fact that the selection of patients could be decided based on medical opinion increased the risk of bias in the selection process. We do not know the impact of this intervention on other clinical aspects, such as biochemical parameters, adherence to treatment of diabetes and other comorbidities, survival or risk of hospitalization; these factors should be explored in future research.

5. Conclusions

The combination of enalapril and nifedipine for the treatment of hypertension is more effective in controlling blood pressure than the empirical treatment in patients with uncontrolled blood pressure in primary care. After six months of treatment, the combination showed an increase of 41.2% in the clinical protector effect and an increase of 18.1% in net clinical utility Treatment adherence also improved in the patients undergoing the combined treatment, without any difference in adverse reactions. These findings support the use of simple therapeutic schemes for an easier, more accessible, and effective treatment of hypertension in primary care patients.

Author Contributions: Conceptualization, H.B.-A., R.S.-H. and C.L.; methodology, H.B.-A., R.S.-H. and C.L.; validation, H.B.-A., A.L. and C.L.; formal analysis, A.L. and C.L.; investigation, H.B.-A., M.M.-A., R.S.-H. and C.L.; resources, H.B.-A. and C.L.; data curation, H.B.-A. and C.L.; writing—original draft preparation, H.B.-A., M.M.-A., R.S.-H. and C.L.; writing—review and editing, H.B.-A., M.M.-A., R.S.-H., A.L. and C.L.; visualization, H.B.-A., M.M.-A., A.L. and C.L.; supervision, H.B.-A. and C.L.; project administration, H.B.-A. and C.L.; funding acquisition, H.B.-A. and C.L. All authors have read and agreed to the published version of the manuscript.

Funding: This research received no external funding and the APC was funded by Universidad Anahuac Mexico.

Institutional Review Board Statement: The study was conducted in accordance with the Declaration of Helsinki and approved by the Institutional Review Board of Universidad Anahuac Mexico (protocol number 201626 and date of approval 11 August 2016).

Informed Consent Statement: Informed consent was obtained from all subjects involved in the study.

Data Availability Statement: The data presented in this study are available on request from the corresponding author.

Acknowledgments: The authors thank the valuable collaboration of the health staff and patients at the participant primary care center. The authors thank Victor Kawas-Bustamante for his helpful comments.

Conflicts of Interest: The authors declare no conflict of interest. The funders had no role in the design of the study; in the collection, analyses, or interpretation of data; in the writing of the manuscript; or in the decision to publish the results.

References

1. Oparil, S.; Acelajado, M.C.; Bakris, G.L.; Berlowitz, D.R.; Cífková, R.; Dominiczak, A.F.; Grassi, G.; Jordan, J.; Poulter, N.R.; Rodgers, A.; et al. Hypertension. *Nat. Rev. Dis. Prim.* **2018**, *4*, 18014. [CrossRef] [PubMed]
2. Roth, G.A.; Mensah, G.A.; Johnson, C.O.; Addolorato, G.; Ammirati, E.; Baddour, L.M.; Barengo, N.C.; Beaton, A.Z.; Benjamin, E.J.; Benziger, C.P.; et al. Global Burden of Cardiovascular Diseases and Risk Factors, 1990-2019: Update from the GBD 2019 Study. *J. Am. Coll. Cardiol.* **2020**, *76*, 2982–3021. [CrossRef]
3. NCD Risk Factor Collaboration (NCD-RisC). Worldwide trends in hypertension prevalence and progress in treatment and control from 1990 to 2019: A pooled analysis of 1201 population-representative studies with 104 million participants. *Lancet* **2021**, *398*, 957–980. [CrossRef] [PubMed]
4. Jaffe, M.G.; Frieden, T.R.; Campbell, N.R.C.; Matsushita, K.; Appel, L.J.; Lackland, D.T.; Zhang, X.H.; Muruganathan, A.; Whelton, P.K. Recommended treatment protocols to improve management of hypertension globally: A statement by Resolve to Save Lives and the World Hypertension League (WHL). *J. Clin. Hypertens.* **2018**, *20*, 829–836. [CrossRef]
5. Ordunez, P.; Martinez, R.; Niebylski, M.L.; Campbell, N.R. Hypertension Prevention and Control in Latin America and the Caribbean. *J. Clin. Hypertens.* **2015**, *17*, 499–502. [CrossRef]
6. Sica, D.A. Rationale for fixed-dose combinations in the treatment of hypertension: The cycle repeats. *Drugs* **2002**, *62*, 443–462. [CrossRef] [PubMed]

7. Bress, A.P.; Greene, T.; Derington, C.G.; Shen, J.; Xu, Y.; Zhang, Y.; Ying, J.; Bellows, B.K.; Cushman, W.C.; Whelton, P.K.; et al. Patient Selection for Intensive Blood Pressure Management Based on Benefit and Adverse Events. *J. Am. Coll. Cardiol.* **2021**, *77*, 1977–1990. [CrossRef]
8. Whelton, P.K.; Carey, R.M.; Aronow, W.S.; Casey, D.E., Jr.; Collins, K.J.; Dennison Him-melfarb, C.; DePalma, S.M.; Gidding, S.; Jamerson, K.A.; Jones, D.W.; et al. 2017 ACC/AHA/AAPA/ABC/ACPM/AGS/APhA/ASH/ASPC/NMA/PCNA Guideline for the Prevention, Detection, Evaluation, and Management of High Blood Pressure in Adults: A Report of the American College of Cardiology/American Heart Association Task Force on Clinical Practice Guidelines. *J. Am. Coll. Cardiol.* **2018**, *71*, e127–e248. [CrossRef]
9. Williams, B.; Mancia, G.; Spiering, W.; Agabiti Rosei, E.; Azizi, M.; Burnier, M.; Clement, D.L.; Coca, A.; de Simone, G.; Dominiczak, A.; et al. Authors/Task Force Members: 2018 ESC/ESH Guidelines for the management of arterial hypertension: The Task Force for the management of arterial hypertension of the European Society of Cardiology and the European Society of Hypertension: The Task Force for the management of arterial hypertension of the European Society of Cardiology and the European Society of Hypertension. *J. Hypertens.* **2018**, *36*, 1953–2041. [CrossRef]
10. Task Force of the Latin American Society of Hypertension. Guidelines on the management of arterial hypertension and related comorbidities in Latin America. *J. Hypertens.* **2017**, *35*, 1529–1545. [CrossRef]
11. de la Sierra, A. Mitigation of calcium channel blocker-related oedema in hypertension by antagonists of the renin-angiotensin system. *J. Hum. Hypertens.* **2009**, *23*, 503–511. [CrossRef] [PubMed]
12. Lam, S.K.; Owen, A. Incident diabetes in clinical trials of antihypertensive drugs. *Lancet* **2007**, *369*, 1513–1514. [CrossRef] [PubMed]
13. Karlberg, B.E.; Andrup, M.; Odén, A. Efficacy and safety of a new long-acting drug combination, trandolapril/verapamil as compared to monotherapy in primary hyper-tension. Swedish TARKA trialists. *Blood Press.* **2000**, *9*, 140–145. [CrossRef] [PubMed]
14. Mancia, G.; Asmar, R.; Amodeo, C.; Mourad, J.J.; Taddei, S.; Gamba, M.A.; Chazova, I.E.; Puig, J.G. Comparison of single-pill strategies first line in hypertension: Perin-dopril/amlodipine versus valsartan/amlodipine. *J. Hypertens.* **2015**, *33*, 401–411. [CrossRef] [PubMed]
15. Lubianca, J.N.; Moreira, L.B.; Gus, M.; Fuchs, F.D. Stopping oral contraceptives: An effective blood pressure-lowering intervention in women with hypertension. *J. Hum. Hypertens.* **2005**, *19*, 451–455. [CrossRef]
16. Val Jimenez, A.; Amoros Ballestero, G.; Martinez Visa, P.; Fernández Ferre, M.L.; León Sanroma, M. Estudio descriptivo del cumplimiento del tratamiento farmacológico antihipertensivo y validación del test de Morisky y Green [Descriptive study of patient compliance in pharmacologic antihypertensive treatment and validation of the Morisky and Green test]. *Aten Primaria.* **1992**, *10*, 767–770.
17. Ruilope, L.M.; Nunes Filho, A.C.B.; Nadruz, W., Jr.; Rodríguez Rosales, F.F.; Verdejo-Paris, J. Obesity and hypertension in Latin America: Current perspectives. *Hipertens. Riesgo Vasc.* **2018**, *3*, 70–76. [CrossRef]
18. Cohen, H.W.; Hailpern, S.M.; Fang, J.; Alderman, M.H. Sodium intake and mortality in the NHANES II follow-up study. *Am. J. Med.* **2006**, *119*, 275.e7–275.e14. [CrossRef]
19. Intersalt Cooperative Research Group. Intersalt: An international study of electrolyte excretion and blood pressure. Results for 24 hour urinary sodium and potassium excretion. *BMJ* **1988**, *297*, 319–328. [CrossRef]
20. Mancia, G.; Rea, F.; Corrao, G.; Grassi, G. Two-Drug Combinations as First-Step Antihypertensive Treatment. *Circ. Res.* **2019**, *124*, 1113–1123. [CrossRef] [PubMed]
21. Julius, S.; Kjeldsen, S.E.; Weber, M.; Brunner, H.R.; Ekman, S.; Hansson, L.; Hua, T.; Laragh, J.; McInnes, G.T.; Mitchell, L.; et al. Outcomes in hypertensive patients at high cardiovascular risk treated with regimens based on valsartan or amlodipine: The VALUE randomised trial. *Lancet* **2004**, *363*, 2022–2031. [CrossRef]
22. Liebson, P.R. ASCOT-Blood Pressure Trial (ASCOT-BPLA) and HOPE-TOO. *Prev. Cardiol.* **2006**, *9*, 60–63. [CrossRef] [PubMed]
23. Adrogué, H.J.; Madias, N.E. Sodium and potassium in the pathogenesis of hypertension. *N. Engl. J. Med.* **2007**, *356*, 1966–1978. [CrossRef] [PubMed]
24. Hyman, D.J.; Pavlik, V. Medication adherence and resistant hypertension. *J. Hum. Hypertens.* **2015**, *29*, 213–218. [CrossRef] [PubMed]
25. Lee, H.Y.; Kim, S.Y.; Choi, K.J.; Yoo, B.S.; Cha, D.H.; Jung, H.O.; Ryu, D.R.; Choi, J.H.; Lee, K.J.; Park, T.H.; et al. A Randomized, Multicenter, Double-blind, Placebo-controlled Study to Evaluate the Efficacy and the Tolerability of a Triple Combination of Amlodipine/Losartan/Rosuvastatin in Patients with Comorbid Essential Hypertension and Hyperlipidemia. *Clin. Ther.* **2017**, *39*, 2366–2379. [CrossRef]
26. Rosas-Peralta, M.; Jiménez-Genchi, G.M. New Challenges for Hypertension Treatment. *Arch. Med. Res.* **2018**, *49*, 548–557. [CrossRef]
27. Jarraya, F. Treatment of Hypertension: Which Goal for Which Patient? *Adv. Exp. Med. Biol.* **2017**, *956*, 117–127. [CrossRef]
28. De Backer, T.; Van Nieuwenhuyse, B.; De Bacquer, D. Antihypertensive treatment in a general uncontrolled hypertensive population in Belgium and Luxembourg in primary care: Therapeutic inertia and treatment simplification. The SIMPLIFY study. *PLoS ONE* **2021**, *16*, e0248471. [CrossRef]
29. Carey, R.M.; Muntner, P.; Bosworth, H.B.; Whelton, P.K. Prevention and Control of Hypertension: JACC Health Promotion Series. *J. Am. Coll. Cardiol.* **2018**, *72*, 1278–1293. [CrossRef]

30. Choi, H.Y.; Oh, I.J.; Lee, J.A.; Lim, J.; Kim, Y.S.; Jeon, T.H.; Cheong, Y.S.; Kim, D.H.; Kim, M.C.; Lee, S.Y. Factors Affecting Adherence to Antihypertensive Medication. *Korean J. Fam. Med.* **2018**, *39*, 325–332. [CrossRef]
31. Williams, B.; Mancia, G.; Spiering, W.; Agabiti Rosei, E.; Azizi, M.; Burnier, M.; Clement, D.; Coca, A.; De Simone, G.; Dominiczak, A.; et al. 2018 Practice Guidelines for the management of arterial hypertension of the European Society of Hypertension and the European Society of Cardiology: ESH/ESC Task Force for the Management of Arterial Hypertension. *J. Hypertens.* **2018**, *36*, 2284–2309. [CrossRef] [PubMed]

Disclaimer/Publisher's Note: The statements, opinions and data contained in all publications are solely those of the individual author(s) and contributor(s) and not of MDPI and/or the editor(s). MDPI and/or the editor(s) disclaim responsibility for any injury to people or property resulting from any ideas, methods, instructions or products referred to in the content.

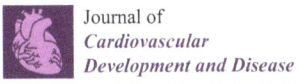

Journal of
Cardiovascular Development and Disease

Review

Mechanisms and Clinical Implications of Endothelial Dysfunction in Arterial Hypertension

Pasquale Ambrosino [1,*,†], Tiziana Bachetti [2,†], Silvestro Ennio D'Anna [3], Brurya Galloway [4], Andrea Bianco [4], Vito D'Agnano [4], Antimo Papa [1], Andrea Motta [5], Fabio Perrotta [4,‡] and Mauro Maniscalco [3,6,*,‡]

1. Istituti Clinici Scientifici Maugeri IRCCS, Cardiac Rehabilitation Unit of Telese Terme Institute, 82037 Telese Terme, Italy; antimo.papa@icsmaugeri.it
2. Istituti Clinici Scientifici Maugeri IRCCS, Scientific Direction, 27100 Pavia, Italy; tiziana.bachetti@icsmaugeri.it
3. Istituti Clinici Scientifici Maugeri IRCCS, Pulmonary Rehabilitation Unit of Telese Terme Institute, 82037 Telese Terme, Italy; silvestro.danna@icsmaugeri.it
4. Department of Translational Medical Sciences, University of Campania "Luigi Vanvitelli", 80131 Naples, Italy; brurya29@gmail.com (B.G.); andrea.bianco@unicampania.it (A.B.); vito.dagnano94@gmail.com (V.D.); fabio.perrotta@unicampania.it (F.P.)
5. Institute of Biomolecular Chemistry, National Research Council, 80078 Pozzuoli, Italy; andrea.motta@icb.cnr.it
6. Department of Clinical Medicine and Surgery, "Federico II" University, 80131 Naples, Italy
* Correspondence: pasquale.ambrosino@icsmaugeri.it (P.A.); mauro.maniscalco@icsmaugeri.it (M.M.)
† These authors contributed equally to this work.
‡ These authors contributed equally to this work.

Abstract: The endothelium is composed of a monolayer of endothelial cells, lining the interior surface of blood and lymphatic vessels. Endothelial cells display important homeostatic functions, since they are able to respond to humoral and hemodynamic stimuli. Thus, endothelial dysfunction has been proposed as a key and early pathogenic mechanism in many clinical conditions. Given the relevant repercussions on cardiovascular risk, the complex interplay between endothelial dysfunction and systemic arterial hypertension has been a matter of study in recent years. Numerous articles have been published on this issue, all of which contribute to providing an interesting insight into the molecular mechanisms of endothelial dysfunction in arterial hypertension and its role as a biomarker of inflammation, oxidative stress, and vascular disease. The prognostic and therapeutic implications of endothelial dysfunction have also been analyzed in this clinical setting, with interesting new findings and potential applications in clinical practice and future research. The aim of this review is to summarize the pathophysiology of the relationship between endothelial dysfunction and systemic arterial hypertension, with a focus on the personalized pharmacological and rehabilitation strategies targeting endothelial dysfunction while treating hypertension and cardiovascular comorbidities.

Keywords: arterial hypertension; endothelial dysfunction; occupational medicine; heart failure; chronic disease; arginine; rehabilitation; exercise; outcome; cardiovascular disease

1. Introduction

Systemic arterial hypertension (SAH) is the substrate of many cardiovascular and systemic disorders, leading to structural or functional impairment of the arterial vasculature and/or the organs it supplies [1]. Main end organ damage due to uncontrolled hypertension may affect the brain, heart, kidneys, central and peripheral arteries, and the eyes [2]. SAH has emerged as a major health problem because of the progressive growth in the ageing population coupled with the increased prevalence of predisposing risk factors, such as obesity, salt consumption, physical deconditioning, and inactivity [3]. The pathophysiology of hypertension is particularly complex and multifactorial and may be associated in a bidirectional relationship with endothelial dysfunction [4].

The endothelium is a thin layer of flat polygonal cells strategically located between the bloodstream and the vascular smooth muscle wall, exerting essential functions for the maintenance of vascular homeostasis [5]. Endothelial dysfunction is a phenotypic modification in the endothelium, leading to exalted prothrombotic and proinflammatory status [6]. The interaction between SAH and endothelial dysfunction may act at different levels: firstly, the compromised endothelial cells promote an altered reactivity of the vascular smooth muscle tone; secondly, the prothrombotic and proinflammatory phenotype induced by endothelial cell dysfunction amplifies the systemic effects of arterial hypertension, thus leading to end organ damage [7]. Currently, it is commonly believed that the relationship between endothelial dysfunction and hypertension is not linear, as each factor could influence the other, giving rise to a pathogenetic vicious circle [4]. Original research has documented that the integrity of endothelial cell function may control vascular smooth muscle tone in response to various agents, including acetylcholine, calcium ionophore, adenosine triphosphate (ATP), adenosine diphosphate (ADP), substance P, bradykinin, histamine, and thrombin [8]. Additionally, endothelial cells dynamically secern a plethora of mediators, including endothelins, cyclooxygenase-dependent vasoconstrictors, and endothelium-derived hyperpolarizing factors, that are involved in the pathophysiology of hypertension [5]. However, the prognostic significance of assessing endothelial dysfunction in hypertension is yet to be established [4].

In this review, we aimed to describe the molecular mechanisms involved in this complex interplay and define possible therapeutic targets modulating endothelial dysfunction in hypertensive patients.

2. Endothelial Cell Mediators in the Pathogenesis of Arterial Hypertension

A healthy endothelium releases a variety of factors in order to guarantee the appropriate vascular tone, the maintenance of a non-adhesive and unabridged surface, to prevent vascular remodeling, and to regulate the formation of new vessels [5]. Particularly, the vascular tone is balanced by endothelial-derived vasodilators and vasoconstrictors [9].

2.1. Endothelial-Derived Vasoactive Mediators

Among the vasodilator factors, a key player is undoubtedly nitric oxide (NO). NO is synthesized by the endothelial enzyme nitric oxide synthase (eNOS) starting from L-arginine and oxygen in the presence of several cofactors [6]. NO is a gas, freely diffusible and highly reactive. It induces vasodilation in the underlying smooth muscle cells by interacting with soluble guanylate cyclase, which activates a cascade of molecular pathways that ultimately lead to reduced intracellular calcium and increased intracellular potassium, favoring cell membrane hyperpolarization and muscle relaxation [10]. NO also has an antiproliferative effect on vascular smooth muscle cells [11]. When NO diffuses to the luminal side of the endothelial monolayer, it exerts an antithrombotic action by inhibiting platelet adhesion and aggregation [10]. Moreover, NO also prevents leukocyte adhesion to vascular endothelium and leukocyte migration into the vascular wall, thus exerting a physiological anti-atherosclerotic action [12].

Endothelial dysfunction is characterized by reduced release or availability of NO, which results in impaired endothelium-dependent vascular relaxation [10]. Therefore, endothelial dysfunction has been largely documented in hypertension [13,14]. The Framingham study was one of the first population-based studies showing that systolic blood pressure was inversely correlated with flow-mediated dilation (FMD) [15], which is largely accepted as an accurate, cost-effective, and noninvasive method to assess endothelial function in humans [16]. Although the study design could not allow the determination of a cause–effect relationship, the Framingham study demonstrated the presence of a link between these two conditions. Several factors may affect the production and bioavailability of NO. Oxidative stress can cause eNOS uncoupling due to reduced availability of the enzyme cofactor tetrahydrobiopterin (BH4) and deficiency of the substrate L-arginine, with the consequent production of superoxide radicals instead of NO [17]. Superoxide radicals scavenge NO, producing the toxic radical peroxynitrite. Thus, reactive oxygen species (ROS), which include also peroxides and hydroxyl radicals, have an important role in the homeostasis of vascular wall and they are likely factors promoting hypertension [18]. ROS are mainly produced in the cardiovascular and renal systems by a family of nicotinamide adenine dinucleotide phosphate (NADPH) oxidases (NOX) [19,20]. Several NOX isoforms have been shown to be involved in progression of hypertension in animal models [20]. Additionally, endoplasmic reticulum stress and mitochondrial oxidative stress also contribute to endothelial dysfunction and vascular remodeling in hypertension [21,22]. Although a causative link between ROS and increased blood pressure has not been demonstrated in hypertensive patients, positive associations between systemic biomarkers of oxidative stress and blood pressure values have been observed, as well as a reduced antioxidant capacity [23,24].

In addition to NO, the endothelium-derived hyperpolarizing factor (EDHF) can induce vascular relaxation [25]. Its chemical nature is unknown but is presumed to be either a chemical mediator or an electrical transducer, depending on the species and vascular beds considered. EDHF induces opening of Ca^{2+}-activated K^+ channels, thus hyperpolarizing the membrane potential of vascular smooth muscle cells, especially in resistance microvessels [26]. EDHF's potential role in the development of either human or animal hypertension is currently unknown.

Among endothelium-derived vasoconstrictors, the peptide endothelin-1 (ET-1) and angiotensin converting enzyme (ACE) play key roles. Endothelial cells generate ET-1 in response to several stimuli, such as ROS, inflammatory molecules, and hypoxia [27]. ET-1 can prompt vascular constriction by activating ET_A and ET_{B2} receptors on smooth muscle cells [28]. The vasoconstriction effect is mediated by increased intracellular calcium concentration and phosphorylation, resulting in myosin light chain activation [29]. ET-1 is also a potent mitogen able to stimulate the growth, proliferation, and migration of smooth muscle cells, with important implications in vascular remodeling [30]. However, ET-1 also has counter-regulatory properties, as it is able to interact with ET_{B1} receptors on the endothelial membrane and activate a signaling cascade, resulting in NO and prostacyclin (PGI_2) production, with consequent vascular relaxation [31]. ET-1 is constantly released by the endothelium but its concentrations are important in determining vascular function. In fact, low levels of ET-1 promote vasodilation, while high levels of ET-1 increase blood pressure and peripheral vascular resistance [32,33]. When the endothelium is dysfunctional, the balance between ET-1 vasodilator/vasoconstrictor effects is disrupted in favor of the latter [34]. Both experimental and clinical studies have shown high levels of ET-1 in hypertension, suggesting the presence of a link between ET-1 levels and development of systemic hypertension [35]. In addition, ET-1 is directly involved in the process of arterial remodeling causing hypertrophic thickening of small arteries [36]. The increased vascular wall thickness combined with the increased tone bring about increased peripheral vascular resistance, a typical hallmark of hypertension [37]. Moreover, ET-1 is also able to induce vascular inflammation, stimulating the expression of NOX in vascular cells with subsequent increased production of ROS, which, in turn, promotes the synthesis and release of inflammatory molecules, such as cytokines and adhesion molecules [38]. The inflammatory process is further amplified by the recruitment and activation of circulating immune cells by ET-1 [28].

ACE is constitutively expressed by the vascular endothelium and is particularly abundant in the lungs [39]. ACE is of paramount importance in the development of hypertension, since ACE is able to convert angiotensin I into angiotensin II (Ang II), a polypeptide with several biological effects in vascular smooth muscle cells [40]. Ang II interacts with the Ang II type I (AT1) receptor and activates a cascade of intracellular pathways that results in increased production of ROS, release of growth factors, release of ET-1 and adhesion molecules, triggering endothelial impairment, vasoconstriction, and remodeling of resistance arteries [41,42], ultimately leading to hypertension [43]. A physiological counter-regulatory pathway is activated when Ang II interacts with Ang II type II (AT2) receptor [44]. In this case, the biological effects elicited are opposite to the ones just described, eventuating in vasodilation and other homeostatic effects [45].

However, the affinity of Ang II for AT2 receptor is lower than that for AT1 receptor, making the first pathway prevalent over the second one, with consequent detrimental effects on blood pressure [45]. Another escape pathway for Ang II, which has recently come into prominence due to severe acute respiratory syndrome coronavirus-2 (SARS-CoV-2), is given by ACE2, an enzyme (and receptor for the coronavirus spike protein) able to transform Ang II into angiotensin 1-7 [46,47]. This very short peptide interacts with the proto-oncogene G-protein-coupled MAS receptor on endothelial cells, leading to higher NO availability and reduced ROS, with consequent beneficial effects on blood pressure [13,48] (Figure 1).

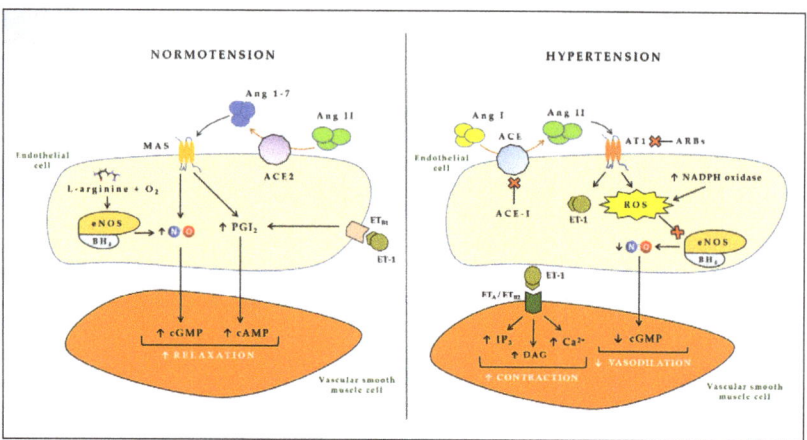

Figure 1. Effects of endothelial-derived vasoactive mediators in the cross-talk between endothelial and vascular smooth muscle cells. ACE: Angiotensin converting enzyme; ACE2: Angiotensin converting enzyme 2; Ang I: Angiotensin I; Ang II: Angiotensin II; Ang 1-7: Angiotensin 1-7; AT1: Angiotensin II type 1 receptor; MAS: Proto-oncogene G-protein-coupled receptor; eNOS: Endothelial nitric oxide synthase; BH4: Tetrahydrobiopterin; ET-1: Endothelin 1; ET_{B1}: Endothelin receptor B1; ET_{B2}: Endothelin receptor B2; ET_A: Endothelin receptor A; NO: Nitric oxide; PGI_2: Prostacyclin; NADPH: Nicotinamide adenine dinucleotide phosphate; ROS: Reactive oxygen species; cGMP: Cyclic guanosine monophosphate; cAMP: Cyclic adenosine monophosphate; IP_3: Inositol triphosphate; DAG: Diacylglycerol; ACE-I: Angiotensin-converting enzyme inhibitors; ARBs: Angiotensin II receptor blockers.

2.2. Extracellular Vesicles in the Cross-Talk between Endothelial and Smooth Muscle Cells

Besides traditional molecular effectors, other players able to modulate endothelial and vascular function have come to the arena in the last years. Among these, are the extracellular vesicles (EV).

EV are particles naturally released from various cell types that are unable to replicate [26]. They may contain a heterogeneous cargo of material ranging from microRNAs, long noncoding RNAs, DNA fragments, transcription factors, ROS, proteins, metabolites, and lipids [49]. EV can be divided into three subcategories: exosomes, microvesicles, and apoptotic bodies [50,51]. Exosomes are small EV (diameter: 40–160 nm), while microvesicles are large EV (diameter: 0.1–1 μm). Only the microvesicles are encased by a characteristic plasma membrane, while exosomes are delimited by endosomal membranes and are directly released by the cells to the extracellular space [50]. Apoptotic bodies are composed of discard material, such as intracellular fragments and damaged organelles, enveloped by plasma membranes [52]. Following binding to cells, circulating exosomes and microvesicles fuse with extracellular plasma membranes or internalize and release their content to the recipient cells [51].

The endothelium is both a recipient and a generator of EV [53], exerting multiple effects in the progression of hypertension, ranging from reduced NO release and increased

ROS production to stimulation of proliferation and migration of vascular smooth muscle cells [54]. EV may act in a paracrine or endocrine fashion and affect endothelial function at sites distant from their production, thus potentially representing a promising biomarker in endothelial dysfunction assessment [54]. Experimental studies have shown that infusion of concentrated EV is able to impair vasodilation in resistance arteries of normotensive animals [55] and that infusion of exosomes from spontaneously hypertensive rats increased systolic pressure of normotensive animals [56]. Results from clinical studies are in line with animal studies and show high circulating levels of endothelial- and platelet-derived EV in hypertensive patients [57,58], suggesting the involvement of EV in the pathogenesis of hypertension [54].

EV levels undoubtedly directly correlate with systolic blood pressure, arterial diameter, and pulse wave velocity [57]. In addition to EV levels, it is also important to take into account the composition of EV. A recent study showed in hypertensive patients with albuminuria that the profile of 29 plasma exosomal microRNAs is different from that of control subjects [59]. Animal studies have further provided mechanistic insights into the arterial remodeling induced by differently expressed microRNAs in EV of hypertensive versus normotensive animals [60].

3. Endothelial Dysfunction, Hypertension, and Cardiovascular Risk

The close inter-relationship between endothelial dysfunction and hypertension may represent the main pathogenic mechanism of small vessel disease in vital organs (e.g., heart, brain, kidney) [13]. Animal models of hypertension and cell culture studies have shown that, although endothelial and microvascular dysfunction are not exactly the same, an injured endothelium represents the earliest stage of an impaired functioning of the other vascular components (e.g., smooth muscle cells) [61]. The current tendency is to interpret small vessel disease as a systemic disorder with a common pathogenic background that differentially affects isolated organs [62]. Thus, cerebral small vessel disease is seen as the leading cause of cognitive decline and ischemic complications, being frequently observed also in Alzheimer's disease [61]. Similarly, hypertensive coronary microvascular dysfunction has been identified as a subclinical marker of end organ damage and heart failure [63]. The evidence that peripheral microvascular endothelial dysfunction is associated to cerebral small vessel disease, thus potentially predicting the risk of future stroke [64], supports the hypothesis that endothelial dysfunction reflects a systemic process of vascular remodeling initiated by hypertension and other cardiovascular risk factors [65]. This is further confirmed by the observation that peripheral endothelial dysfunction is able to predict the severity of cerebral small vessel disease even when evaluated in conduit arteries [66]. Conversely, the fact that microvascular dysfunction may be able to affect blood pressure and flow patterns is in line with the less traditional hypothesis that endothelial damage and subsequent microvascular dysfunction are causes rather than consequences of hypertension [67].

Overall, it is evident that peripheral endothelial function and arterial pressure are responsible for blood supply to the periphery and, therefore, for protection from cardiovascular events [68]. In a landmark study [69], endothelium-dependent and endothelium-independent coronary vasoreactivity were tested through intracoronary instillation of acetylcholine in 147 patients with a median follow-up period of 7.7 years. The authors demonstrated that the incidence of cardiovascular events (cardiovascular death, unstable angina, myocardial infarction, coronary revascularization, ischemic stroke, and peripheral artery revascularization) was lower in subjects with preserved endothelial responsiveness. Therefore, endothelial dysfunction emerged as a phenotype with high risk for cardiovascular events. In keeping with this, Yeboah et al. [70] examined 3026 subjects without cardiovascular disease from the Multi-Ethnic Study of Atherosclerosis (MESA) cohort, showing that each standard deviation increase in FMD corresponded to a hazard ratio of 0.84 for incident cardiovascular events after 5 years. These data were corroborated from another clinical research from Gokce et al. [71] in patients undergoing peripheral or coronary bypass surgery. Authors demonstrated a higher risk of postoperative cardiac events in subjects with impaired endothelial function, expressed by a low FMD (i.e., FMD < 8.1%). Using the MESA cohort, Shimbo et al. [72] were among the first demonstrating an association between FMD and hypertension. Moreover, when specifically considering participants without hypertension, the authors also documented a significant association between baseline FMD and incident hypertension at 4.8-year follow-up. However, the latter finding was not confirmed in multivariate analyses. In another study [73], the coexistence of left ventricular hypertrophy and endothelial dysfunction in hypertensive patients emerged as risk for subsequent major cardiovascular events. In particular, hypertensives with left ventricular hypertrophy showed attenuated brachial and coronary artery endothelium-dependent vasodilation, suggesting that both the endothelium and left ventricle may be damaged by hypertension. This study supports the hypothesis that hypertension may have a causal role in endothelial dysfunction, which is the earliest stage of atherosclerosis, thereby representing one of the main traditional cardiovascular risk factors [74]. This is in line with the evidence that, when NO synthase antagonists are administered to normotensive subjects, a significant increase in systemic blood pressure can be documented [75]. Accordingly, the Cardiovascular Risk in Young Finns Study found that hypertension in youth may predict future impaired endothelial function [76]. The widely accepted viewpoint that hypertension is a cause rather than a consequence of endothelial dysfunction is in contrast with the evidence on 957 postmenopausal women in which the incidence of hypertension at 3.6-year follow-up was nearly sixfold higher in those in the lowest FMD quartile, with a 16% increase in cardiovascular risk per unit of FMD [77]. The relatively healthy cohort of postmenopausal women is a strength of this study, supporting the hypothesis that monitoring endothelial function may be used to predict the risk of incident hypertension along with that of cardiovascular events.

4. Endothelial Function Evaluation

Given its systemic nature and potential reversibility in early stages, a number of laboratory and clinical methods have been proposed for endothelial function assessment and monitoring.

4.1. Laboratory Methods

In normal conditions, the endothelium has an anticoagulant, anti-inflammatory, and vasodilatory phenotype, which is reflected in the constitutive expression of NO, von Willebrand factor (vWF), plasminogen activator inhibitor-1 (PAI-1), and tissue factor (TF), as well as endothelium-derived adhesion molecules or chemokines, including intercellular adhesion molecule-1 (ICAM-1), vascular cell adhesion molecule-1 (VCAM-1), E-selectin, P-selectin, vascular endothelial-cadherin (VE-cadherin), and monocyte chemotactic protein-1 (MCP-1) [5]. The soluble forms of these endothelium-derived biomarkers can be measured in peripheral blood with different laboratory techniques.

More recently, the levels of some components of the glycocalyx (e.g., heparan sulfate, endocan, and syndecan-1) have been proposed as markers of endothelial function [78]. Finally, endothelial progenitor cells (EPCs) and circulating endothelial cells (CECs) have been used to test vascular repair capacity and the presence of endothelial injury [79].

4.2. Clinical Methods

Several clinical methods have been tested to assess endothelial function. If venous occlusion plethysmography (VOP) is substantially underutilized because of its invasiveness, laser doppler flowmetry (LDF) in cutaneous microcirculation has been increasingly employed in recent years [80]. Moreover, peripheral artery tonometry (PAT) has become a Food and Drug Administration (FDA)-approved test for an automated assessment of microvascular endothelial function [81]. Overall, although validated and highly reproducible, these methods may deal with the disadvantages of invasiveness and/or high cost, which may limit their use in routine clinical practice and sometimes in research [82].

About 20 years ago, the guidelines for FMD assessment in conduit arteries were first reported by Corretti et al. [83]. Since then, the procedure has been increasingly used in clinical research, given its noninvasiveness and cost-effectiveness [5]. In brief, FMD is the percentage change in brachial artery diameter as a response to the shear stress induced by a pneumatic cuff placed on the forearm inflated to a suprasystolic pressure for 5 min. After cuff deflation, the increased blood flow enhances the shear stress on endothelium, which stimulates NO synthesis and, therefore, vasodilatation [83]. The fact that FMD has been widely recognized as a reliable surrogate marker of cardiovascular risk and an independent predictor of cardiovascular events [16], together with the recent identification of age- and sex-specific reference values [84], makes this method as one of the most used in clinical research studies. More recently, the use of a dedicated software for real-time edge detection, shear-rate monitoring, and wall tracking has proven to further increase reproducibility of FMD assessment [85] (Figure 2).

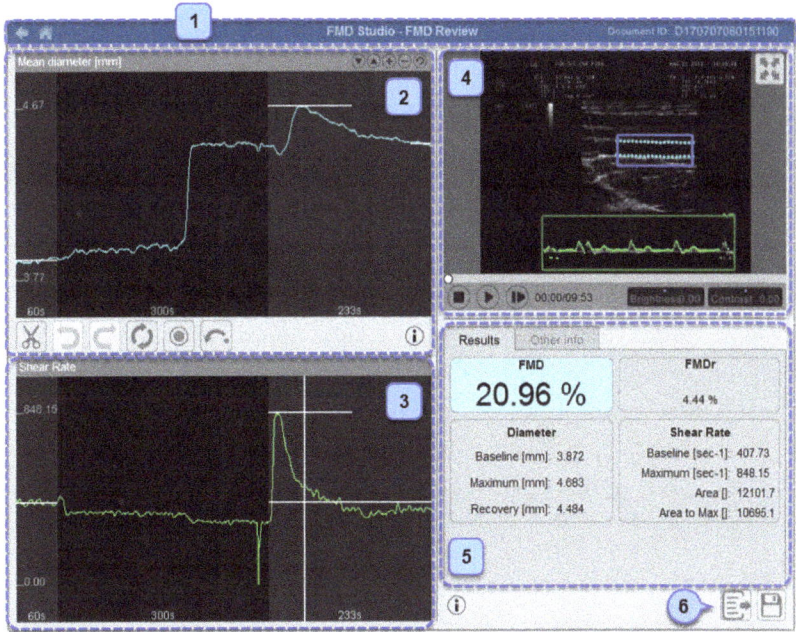

Figure 2. Automatic measurement of flow-mediated dilation (FMD) using a Food and Drug Administration (FDA)-cleared software. 1: Document identifier; 2: mean diameter; 3: shear rate; 4: video window; 5: results and info panel; 6: data exportation. Reproduced with permission from Quipu SRL, Pisa, Italy.

5. Therapeutic Targets for Endothelial Dysfunction in Hypertension

Whether endothelial and microvascular dysfunction may be causes or consequences of hypertension is still a matter of discussion [68]. However, the strict inter-relationship between the two conditions suggests that improving endothelial function may represent an attractive therapeutic target in the near future [86].

To date, renin–angiotensin system (RAS) inhibitors and statins are the main classes of drugs that have proven real effectiveness in reducing endothelial dysfunction in hypertension, thus restoring a vasodilatory and anticoagulant phenotype [87] while fighting microvascular dysfunction [88]. A number of other pharmacological and exercise-based strategies may positively impact endothelial homeostasis, microvascular function, and blood pressure. However, it is important to highlight that no routinely applied therapeutic approach can be considered specific to the endothelium, nor does any guideline currently recommend specific treatment in the presence of isolated endothelial dysfunction. Moreover, most of the novel promising candidates are still far from being translated into clinical practice [86]. Therefore, the impact on endothelium may be rather considered a welcome pleiotropic effect of many cardiovascular drugs and antihypertensive agents, including RAS inhibitors, calcium-channel blockers (CCBs), and β-blockers.

Here, we examined the main pharmacological, nutraceutical, and exercise-based approaches that a patient typically undergoes due to hypertension and cardiovascular comorbidities, focusing on the impact that these strategies may have on endothelial function as well.

5.1. ACE Inhibitors and Angiotensin II Receptor Blockers

ACE inhibitors and angiotensin II receptor blockers (ARBs) are key drugs in the treatment of hypertension, particularly in patients with multiple cardiovascular risk factors, heart failure, diabetes mellitus, and kidney impairment [89]. Therefore, given their capacity to reduce cardiovascular morbidity and mortality with an overall good tolerability [90,91], RAS inhibitors are widely prescribed as first-line drugs in essential hypertension [89] and coronary microvascular disease [88].

By reducing the synthesis of Ang II or blocking its AT1 receptor, these compounds are able to increase NO bioavailability, thus improving endothelial function [92] while also reducing the thrombotic risk due to their capacity to reduce TF and PAI-1 expression [93]. Overall, the lower stimulation of AT1 receptor results in a number of counter-regulatory actions on Ang II, also reducing inflammation and oxidative stress [13,48]. RAS inhibitors have been shown to increase the stability of eNOS mRNA while improving eNOS phosphorylation, reducing its uncoupling, reducing NOX expression, and increasing vascular levels of BH4 [94]. These drugs also lead to bradykinin accumulation in proximity of endothelial bradykinin receptors 1 and 2, which indirectly results in enhanced NO production [95]. Some studies also reported that, due to their antioxidant properties, RAS inhibitors have also an indirect effect on dimethylarginine dimethylaminohydrolase (DDAH), thus inducing the catabolism of asymmetric dimethylarginine (ADMA), which is an endogenous competitive inhibitor of eNOS [94].

Accordingly, using different outcome measures, including FMD, numerous clinical studies have demonstrated the ability of ACE inhibitors and ARBs to improve endothelial function [96,97], even in patients with concomitant coronary artery disease [98] and either type of diabetes mellitus [99,100].

Recently, the use of RAS inhibitors in COVID-19 has been put into question, given their capacity to upregulate ACE2 expression, thus hypothetically increasing the risk of infection. The evidence from randomized controlled trials of no difference in the risk of death between COVID-19 patients who use and those who do not use RAS inhibitors may be in line with the key pathogenic role of endothelial dysfunction in COVID-19 and with the capacity of these drugs to restore endothelial cells' homeostasis.

5.2. Calcium-Channel Blockers

CCBs are another category of first-line drugs for arterial hypertension. The protective effect of CCBs on cardiovascular risk in hypertensive patients has been established [101], and the beneficial effect on endothelial function has also been documented [102], particularly in the coronary microvasculature [103]. The protective mechanism of CCBs on endothelial integrity is still unclear but it has been demonstrated that CCBs are able to counteract ROS-induced endothelial cell death due to lipid peroxidation [104]. In fact, although they may vary in their chemical structure and antihypertensive effect, dihydropyridine CCBs contain aromatic rings that stabilize oxygen radicals and possess a hydrogen-donating reaction, which may also account for their antioxidant activity [104]. A study from Napoli et al. [105] in hypertensive patients documented that CCBs reduced low-density lipoprotein (LDL) oxidation and formation of oxidation-specific epitopes, thus resulting in exalted antioxidant activity. CCBs also reduce calcium inflow in the voltage-dependent channels of subendothelial vascular smooth muscle cells, thereby resulting in vasodilation of large conduit and resistance arteries [106]. Moreover, dihydropyridine CCBs are able to inhibit the effects of endothelin-1 in the vascular smooth muscle, thus facilitating the vasodilatory activity of NO [106]. Another mechanism by which CCBs have shown a beneficial effect on vascular endothelium is their capacity to reduce tissue plasminogen activator (t-PA) activity [107].

5.3. β-Blockers

Similar to other antihypertensive drugs, β-blockers also exhibit a cardioprotective effect [108], particularly in patients with high resting heart rate or increased sympathetic tone and in those with coronary microvascular disease [109]. Using FMD as an outcome measure, nebivolol has shown a positive impact on endothelial function [110] and superiority as compared to atenolol, a selective β1-receptor blocker without vasodilatory properties [111]. β-blockers are able to inhibit fibrinogen, homocysteine, and PAI-1 while increasing NO levels via stimulation of eNOS [112]. Furthermore, some agents (i.e., carvedilol) may add an antioxidant effect, given their scavenging activity on ROS [110,113].

5.4. Other Cardiovascular Therapies

SAH is a traditional cardiovascular risk factor, which is frequently associated to a number of additional risk factors in the context of a dysmetabolic phenotype [114]. Therefore, given the presence of comorbidities (e.g., obesity, diabetes mellitus, dyslipidemia), the use of antihypertensive drugs is often associated to the use of hypoglycemic, hypolipidemic, and antithrombotic agents [114].

Statins may represent another promising approach targeting endothelial function, given a multitude of potential mechanisms, including the activation of eNOS via phosphatidylinositol-3 (PI3)-kinase/Akt pathway, the inhibition of nuclear factor-κB (NF-κB) and other inflammatory pathways, and the reduction in TF expression with subsequent anticoagulant effect [87]. In particular, it has been shown that statins are able to reduce the mRNA levels of AT1 receptor, thus reducing its expression [94]. Moreover, by improving vascular BH4 bioavailability, statins are able to improve eNOS coupling, thus resulting in increased NO bioavailability [115]. Another potential mechanism, in common with other hypolipidemic agents, may be the reduction in LDL cholesterol, thus contrasting the LDL-induced endothelial dysfunction and oxidative stress [116,117]. Therefore, different statins coupled with hypolipidemic diet have been tested in experimental murine and clinical models, documenting positive effects on endothelial function [118]. This is in line with the meta-analytical evidence that statin administration is able to improve FMD [119] while lowering blood concentrations of P-selectin, E-selectin, and ADMA [120,121].

Similarly, hypoglycemic agents targeting peroxisome proliferator-activated receptor-γ (PPAR-γ) have been shown to restore endothelial function in subjects with early phases of insulin resistance through prompting PI3-kinase/Akt/eNOS pathway and increasing NO production [122]. Thiazolidinediones exhibited the capacity to reduce NOX expression in animal models, thus lowering the production of ROS. Moreover, by reducing the expression of VCAM-1 and ICAM-1, they have been shown to limit the chemotaxis of macrophages and monocytes to the endothelium [94]. Given the above mechanisms, randomized clinical studies demonstrated that thiazolidinediones administration is able to significantly improve FMD in both diabetic and nondiabetic patients [123]. Similar beneficial effects on endothelial function have been documented with metformin and sodium-glucose cotransporter-2 (SGLT2) inhibitors [124,125], likely due to similar mechanisms [122].

Considering that platelets play a key role in atherogenesis, antiplatelets with different mechanisms of action are widely used for primary and secondary prevention of cardiac, cerebral, and peripheral ischemic complications. Although the possibility that their effectiveness may also depend on a beneficial effect on endothelium is still debated [126], cilostazol administration has already shown to improve FMD in conduit arteries [127] while suppressing Ang II-induced apoptosis in endothelial cells [128] and mobilizing EPCs [129].

Animal models demonstrated that the adenosine monophosphate-activated protein kinase (AMPK) activation may contribute to the beneficial effects of cilostazol on endothelial function [130].

5.5. Antioxidants and Nutraceutical Strategies

Given the inter-relationship between endothelial dysfunction and oxidative stress, antioxidant therapies may also be useful in restoring a normal endothelial function [131]. In this regard, glutathione and its precursor, namely N-acetyl cysteine (NAC), are potent antioxidants involved in the removal of H_2O_2 and other ROS [132]. Furthermore, NAC has anticoagulant properties and inhibits ACE2, thus reducing the deleterious effects of Ang II [133]. Accordingly, although traditionally used for its mucolytic properties, NAC may also have antihypertensive effect [134]. While NAC has been shown to inhibit atherosclerosis and improve endothelial function in animal models [135], the evidence in clinical trials is scarce and somehow conflicting [136,137].

A number of nutraceutical strategies, including vitamin supplementation, have shown beneficial effects on oxidative stress and endothelial dysfunction [138], while potentially reducing blood pressure [139]. In this regard, there is recent meta-analytical evidence of hypertensive patients having relatively low levels of vitamin C [140], with its supplementation significantly reducing blood pressure in SAH [141]. Vitamin C and vitamin E are free radical scavengers and are able to reduce lipid peroxidation, thus improving eNOS coupling and stabilizing BH4 [94]. However, contrasting results have been reported in large epidemiological studies regarding the impact that oral supplementation of vitamins may have on vascular health [94], considering that it may even reduce the lipid-lowering properties of statins and their beneficial effect on endothelial function [142]. Therefore, pending further high-quality evidence, the fact that vitamin supplementation may not have significant effects on blood pressure [143] is another reason not to impose the routine and indiscriminate use of vitamin supplements to improve vascular health and reduce cardiovascular risk.

Conflicting results have also been reported for the NO precursor L-arginine, which is able to antagonize the effect of ADMA on eNOS function. The fact that its favorable impact on endothelial function depends on the basal levels of ADMA may account for the lack of effect in healthy subjects [144]. However, while the positive impact of L-arginine supplementation on endothelial homeostasis seems to depend on the baseline status, it may conversely have a dose-dependent effect on both systolic and diastolic blood pressure regardless of the baseline blood pressure category (normotensive or hypertensive) [145].

Most of the future perspectives on the treatment of endothelial dysfunction in hypertension and cardiovascular disease relate to the possibility of targeting oxidative stress through epigenetic approaches (e.g., regulation of microRNAs levels, histone acetylation/methylation, DNA methylation), the implementation of new pharmacological strategies targeting the oxidatively impaired eNOS or soluble guanylate cyclase, or the delivery of antioxidants directly to the endothelium through specific ligands or using vectors (e.g., liposomes) [86]. Although promising results have been obtained in vitro or in animal models, these strategies are still far from being translated into clinical practice.

5.6. Exercise and Rehabilitation

Rehabilitation has already proven its effectiveness in improving functional capacity, exercise performance, symptoms, and health-related quality of life in different clinical settings [146–148], while reducing the risk of exacerbations in chronic obstructive pulmonary disease (COPD) [149,150] and cardiovascular mortality in coronary artery disease [151,152]. Moreover, exercise-based approaches have been proposed also as promising interventions to modify the course of cerebral small vessel diseases and improve microvascular responsiveness [153,154]. Although not representing the primary outcome of multidisciplinary rehabilitation, the positive impact on blood pressure has been reported as a welcome pleiotropic effect of exercise-based approaches [155].

In the 1980s, the beneficial effect of exercise on endothelial function was first documented [156], being later confirmed in several reports focusing on specific clinical settings, including cardiovascular conditions [151,152]. Cardiac rehabilitation has a Class I recommendation in most guidelines [157], and the impact on endothelial function has been mainly tested in acute myocardial infarction, stable coronary artery disease, and heart failure [158–161]. Although with variable results, these studies agree on the beneficial effect of cardiac rehabilitation on endothelial function, particularly when it is significantly impaired. Similar findings have been recently reported when testing FMD in COPD patients undergoing pulmonary rehabilitation [162]. Some mechanisms have been proposed in this regard, including reduced uncoupling and increased eNOS phosphorylation, upregulation of superoxide dismutase, NOX downregulation, and EPCs mobilization [163]. It is reasonable to assume that the positive impact of exercise-based approaches on endothelial function may somehow account for the positive impact that these strategies may have also on blood pressure control [155]. This should be taken into consideration, given the evidence that hypertension is a frequent comorbid condition of the diseases that usually require rehabilitation programs [164,165]. More recently, the positive impact of in-hospital rehabilitation on both endothelial function and arterial blood pressure has been demonstrated also in the new coronavirus disease 2019 (COVID-19), with a potential reduction in the residual cardiovascular risk of COVID-19 survivors [166].

6. Conclusions

The relationship between systemic arterial hypertension and endothelial dysfunction comprises a bidirectional connection, which amplifies the magnitude of each factor. Endothelial cells, through canonical mediators and other paracrin systems, influence the pathogenesis of systemic hypertension. Similarly, systemic hypertension promotes endothelial dysfunction and contributes to the prothrombotic and proinflammatory status, increasing the cardiovascular risk. Endothelial dysfunction assessment among hypertensive patients may offer a new paradigm to define a specific cardiovascular phenotype with higher risk and should be carefully taken into consideration in clinical practice. Current agents, targeting systemic hypertension and metabolic disorders, may improve endothelial dysfunction by both favoring NO availability and restoring antioxidant properties. The fine modulation of these complex pathways is of primary importance based on the above reported data.

Author Contributions: Concept and design: P.A., T.B. Acquisition, analysis, or interpretation of data: S.E.D., B.G., A.B., V.D., A.P., A.M. Drafting of the manuscript: P.A., T.B., F.P. Critical revision of the manuscript for important intellectual content: A.B., A.P., A.M., F.P., M.M. English language revision from native speaker: B.G. Administrative, technical, or material support: V.D., S.E.D. Supervision: F.P., M.M. All authors have read and agreed to the published version of the manuscript.

Funding: This work was supported by the "Ricerca Corrente" funding scheme of the Ministry of Health, Italy.

Institutional Review Board Statement: Not applicable.

Informed Consent Statement: Not applicable.

Data Availability Statement: No new data were analyzed in this study.

Acknowledgments: Figure 2 has been reproduced after acquiring written permission from Quipu SRL, Pisa, Italy. We thank the copyright holder for this relevant contribution.

Conflicts of Interest: The authors declare no conflict of interest.

References

1. Oparil, S.; Acelajado, M.C.; Bakris, G.L.; Berlowitz, D.R.; Cifkova, R.; Dominiczak, A.F.; Grassi, G.; Jordan, J.; Poulter, N.R.; Rodgers, A.; et al. Hypertension. *Nat. Rev. Dis Prim.* **2018**, *4*, 18014. [CrossRef] [PubMed]
2. Unger, T.; Borghi, C.; Charchar, F.; Khan, N.A.; Poulter, N.R.; Prabhakaran, D.; Ramirez, A.; Schlaich, M.; Stergiou, G.S.; Tomaszewski, M.; et al. 2020 International Society of Hypertension global hypertension practice guidelines. *J. Hypertens* **2020**, *38*, 982–1004. [CrossRef]
3. Roth, G.A.; Mensah, G.A.; Johnson, C.O.; Addolorato, G.; Ammirati, E.; Baddour, L.M.; Barengo, N.C.; Beaton, A.Z.; Benjamin, E.J.; Benziger, C.P.; et al. Global burden of cardiovascular diseases and risk factors, 1990–2019: Update from the GBD 2019 study. *J. Am. Coll. Cardiol.* **2020**, *76*, 2982–3021. [CrossRef] [PubMed]
4. Konukoglu, D.; Uzun, H. Endothelial dysfunction and hypertension. *Adv. Exp. Med. Biol.* **2017**, *956*, 511–540. [CrossRef] [PubMed]
5. Ambrosino, P.; Grassi, G.; Maniscalco, M. Endothelial dysfunction: From a pathophysiological mechanism to a potential therapeutic target. *Biomedicines* **2021**, *10*, 78. [CrossRef]
6. Gokce, N.; Holbrook, M.; Duffy, S.J.; Demissie, S.; Cupples, L.A.; Biegelsen, E.; Keaney, J.F., Jr.; Loscalzo, J.; Vita, J.A. Effects of race and hypertension on flow-mediated and nitroglycerin-mediated dilation of the brachial artery. *Hypertension* **2001**, *38*, 1349–1354. [CrossRef]
7. Gonzalez, M.A.; Selwyn, A.P. Endothelial function, inflammation, and prognosis in cardiovascular disease. *Am. J. Med.* **2003**, *115* (Suppl. 8A), 99S–106S. [CrossRef]
8. Furchgott, R.F. Role of endothelium in responses of vascular smooth muscle. *Circ. Res.* **1983**, *53*, 557–573. [CrossRef]
9. Harrison, D.G.; Cai, H. Endothelial control of vasomotion and nitric oxide production. *Cardiol. Clin.* **2003**, *21*, 289–302. [CrossRef]
10. Arnold, W.P.; Mittal, C.K.; Katsuki, S.; Murad, F. Nitric oxide activates guanylate cyclase and increases guanosine 3′:5′-cyclic monophosphate levels in various tissue preparations. *Proc. Natl. Acad. Sci. USA* **1977**, *74*, 3203–3207. [CrossRef]
11. Forstermann, U.; Munzel, T. Endothelial nitric oxide synthase in vascular disease: From marvel to menace. *Circulation* **2006**, *113*, 1708–1714. [CrossRef] [PubMed]
12. da Silva, G.M.; da Silva, M.C.; Nascimento, D.V.G.; Lima Silva, E.M.; Gouvea, F.F.F.; de Franca Lopes, L.G.; Araujo, A.V.; Ferraz Pereira, K.N.; de Queiroz, T.M. Nitric oxide as a central molecule in hypertension: Focus on the vasorelaxant activity of new nitric oxide donors. *Biology* **2021**, *10*, 1041. [CrossRef] [PubMed]
13. Gallo, G.; Volpe, M.; Savoia, C. Endothelial dysfunction in hypertension: Current concepts and clinical implications. *Front. Med. (Lausanne)* **2021**, *8*, 798958. [CrossRef]
14. Brandes, R.P. Endothelial dysfunction and hypertension. *Hypertension* **2014**, *64*, 924–928. [CrossRef]
15. Benjamin, E.J.; Larson, M.G.; Keyes, M.J.; Mitchell, G.F.; Vasan, R.S.; Keaney, J.F., Jr.; Lehman, B.T.; Fan, S.; Osypiuk, E.; Vita, J.A. Clinical correlates and heritability of flow-mediated dilation in the community: The Framingham heart study. *Circulation* **2004**, *109*, 613–619. [CrossRef]
16. Ambrosino, P.; Lupoli, R.; Iervolino, S.; De Felice, A.; Pappone, N.; Storino, A.; Di Minno, M.N.D. Clinical assessment of endothelial function in patients with chronic obstructive pulmonary disease: A systematic review with meta-analysis. *Intern. Emerg. Med.* **2017**, *12*, 877–885. [CrossRef]
17. Karbach, S.; Wenzel, P.; Waisman, A.; Munzel, T.; Daiber, A. eNOS uncoupling in cardiovascular diseases—The role of oxidative stress and inflammation. *Curr. Pharm. Des.* **2014**, *20*, 3579–3594. [CrossRef]
18. Korsager Larsen, M.; Matchkov, V.V. Hypertension and physical exercise: The role of oxidative stress. *Medicina (Kaunas)* **2016**, *52*, 19–27. [CrossRef]
19. Sedeek, M.; Hebert, R.L.; Kennedy, C.R.; Burns, K.D.; Touyz, R.M. Molecular mechanisms of hypertension: Role of Nox family NADPH oxidases. *Curr. Opin. Nephrol. Hypertens.* **2009**, *18*, 122–127. [CrossRef]
20. Griendling, K.K.; Camargo, L.L.; Rios, F.J.; Alves-Lopes, R.; Montezano, A.C.; Touyz, R.M. Oxidative Stress and Hypertension. *Circ. Res.* **2021**, *128*, 993–1020. [CrossRef]
21. Shanahan, C.M.; Furmanik, M. Endoplasmic reticulum stress in arterial smooth muscle cells: A novel regulator of vascular disease. *Curr. Cardiol. Rev.* **2017**, *13*, 94–105. [CrossRef] [PubMed]
22. Ochoa, C.D.; Wu, R.F.; Terada, L.S. ROS signaling and ER stress in cardiovascular disease. *Mol. Asp. Med.* **2018**, *63*, 18–29. [CrossRef] [PubMed]
23. Yang, H.Y.; Lee, T.H. Antioxidant enzymes as redox-based biomarkers: A brief review. *BMB Rep.* **2015**, *48*, 200–208. [CrossRef]
24. Montezano, A.C.; Dulak-Lis, M.; Tsiropoulou, S.; Harvey, A.; Briones, A.M.; Touyz, R.M. Oxidative stress and human hypertension: Vascular mechanisms, biomarkers, and novel therapies. *Can. J. Cardiol.* **2015**, *31*, 631–641. [CrossRef]
25. Suzuki, H.; Chen, G.; Yamamoto, Y. Endothelium-derived hyperpolarizing factor (EDHF). *Jpn. Circ. J.* **1992**, *56*, 170–174. [CrossRef]
26. Oyama, J.; Node, K. Endothelium-derived hyperpolarizing factor and hypertension. *Hypertens. Res.* **2013**, *36*, 852–853. [CrossRef]
27. Kelly, J.J.; Whitworth, J.A. Endothelin-1 as a mediator in cardiovascular disease. *Clin. Exp. Pharmacol. Physiol.* **1999**, *26*, 158–161. [CrossRef]
28. Kostov, K. The causal relationship between endothelin-1 and hypertension: Focusing on endothelial dysfunction, arterial stiffness, vascular remodeling, and blood pressure regulation. *Life* **2021**, *11*, 986. [CrossRef]
29. Adam, L.P.; Milio, L.; Brengle, B.; Hathaway, D.R. Myosin light chain and caldesmon phosphorylation in arterial muscle stimulated with endothelin-1. *J. Mol. Cell. Cardiol.* **1990**, *22*, 1017–1023. [CrossRef]

30. Chen, M.; Lin, Y.Q.; Xie, S.L.; Wang, J.F. Mitogen-activated protein kinase in endothelin-1-induced cardiac differentiation of mouse embryonic stem cells. *J. Cell. Biochem.* **2010**, *111*, 1619–1628. [CrossRef]
31. Rafnsson, A.; Matic, L.P.; Lengquist, M.; Mahdi, A.; Shemyakin, A.; Paulsson-Berne, G.; Hansson, G.K.; Gabrielsen, A.; Hedin, U.; Yang, J.; et al. Endothelin-1 increases expression and activity of arginase 2 via ETB receptors and is co-expressed with arginase 2 in human atherosclerotic plaques. *Atherosclerosis* **2020**, *292*, 215–223. [CrossRef]
32. Davenport, A.P.; Hyndman, K.A.; Dhaun, N.; Southan, C.; Kohan, D.E.; Pollock, J.S.; Pollock, D.M.; Webb, D.J.; Maguire, J.J. Endothelin. *Pharmacol. Rev.* **2016**, *68*, 357–418. [CrossRef]
33. Kiowski, W.; Luscher, T.F.; Linder, L.; Buhler, F.R. Endothelin-1-induced vasoconstriction in humans. Reversal by calcium channel blockade but not by nitrovasodilators or endothelium-derived relaxing factor. *Circulation* **1991**, *83*, 469–475. [CrossRef]
34. Shreenivas, S.; Oparil, S. The role of endothelin-1 in human hypertension. *Clin. Hemorheol. Microcirc.* **2007**, *37*, 157–178.
35. Schiffrin, E.L. Role of endothelin-1 in hypertension and vascular disease. *Am. J. Hypertens.* **2001**, *14*, 83S–89S. [CrossRef]
36. Schiffrin, E.L. Vascular remodeling in hypertension: Mechanisms and treatment. *Hypertension* **2012**, *59*, 367–374. [CrossRef]
37. Mulvany, M.J. Vascular remodelling in hypertension. *Eur. Hear. J.* **1993**, *14* (Suppl. C), 2–4. [CrossRef]
38. Idris-Khodja, N.; Ouerd, S.; Trindade, M.; Gornitsky, J.; Rehman, A.; Barhoumi, T.; Offermanns, S.; Gonzalez, F.J.; Neves, M.F.; Paradis, P.; et al. Vascular smooth muscle cell peroxisome proliferator-activated receptor gamma protects against endothelin-1-induced oxidative stress and inflammation. *J. Hypertens.* **2017**, *35*, 1390–1401. [CrossRef]
39. Wallace, K.B.; Bailie, M.D.; Hook, J.B. Development of angiotensin-converting enzyme in fetal rat lungs. *Am. J. Physiol.* **1979**, *236*, R57–R60. [CrossRef]
40. Khurana, V.; Goswami, B. Angiotensin converting enzyme (ACE). *Clin. Chim. Acta* **2022**, *524*, 113–122. [CrossRef]
41. Navar, L.G.; Harrison-Bernard, L.M.; Imig, J.D.; Cervenka, L.; Mitchell, K.D. Renal responses to AT1 receptor blockade. *Am. J. Hypertens.* **2000**, *13*, 45S–54S. [CrossRef]
42. Thomas, W.G. Regulation of angiotensin II type 1 (AT1) receptor function. *Regul. Pept.* **1999**, *79*, 9–23. [CrossRef]
43. Nickenig, G.; Bohm, M. Interaction between insulin and AT1 receptor. Relevance for hypertension and arteriosclerosis. *Basic Res. Cardiol.* **1998**, *93* (Suppl. 2), 135–139. [CrossRef]
44. Carey, R.M. Update on the role of the AT2 receptor. *Curr. Opin. Nephrol. Hypertens.* **2005**, *14*, 67–71. [CrossRef]
45. Siragy, H.M. The role of the AT2 receptor in hypertension. *Am. J. Hypertens.* **2000**, *13*, 62S–67S. [CrossRef]
46. Scialo, F.; Vitale, M.; Daniele, A.; Nigro, E.; Perrotta, F.; Gelzo, M.; Iadevaia, C.; Cerqua, F.S.; Costigliola, A.; Allocca, V.; et al. SARS-CoV-2: One year in the pandemic. What have we learned, the new vaccine era and the threat of SARS-CoV-2 variants. *Biomedicines* **2021**, *9*, 611. [CrossRef]
47. Scialo, F.; Daniele, A.; Amato, F.; Pastore, L.; Matera, M.G.; Cazzola, M.; Castaldo, G.; Bianco, A. ACE2: The major cell entry receptor for SARS-CoV-2. *Lung* **2020**, *198*, 867–877. [CrossRef]
48. Perrotta, F.; Matera, M.G.; Cazzola, M.; Bianco, A. Severe respiratory SARS-CoV2 infection: Does ACE2 receptor matter? *Respir. Med.* **2020**, *168*, 105996. [CrossRef]
49. van Niel, G.; D'Angelo, G.; Raposo, G. Shedding light on the cell biology of extracellular vesicles. *Nat. Rev. Mol. Cell Biol* **2018**, *19*, 213–228. [CrossRef]
50. Raposo, G.; Stoorvogel, W. Extracellular vesicles: Exosomes, microvesicles, and friends. *J. Cell Biol.* **2013**, *200*, 373–383. [CrossRef]
51. Jeppesen, D.K.; Fenix, A.M.; Franklin, J.L.; Higginbotham, J.N.; Zhang, Q.; Zimmerman, L.J.; Liebler, D.C.; Ping, J.; Liu, Q.; Evans, R.; et al. Reassessment of exosome composition. *Cell* **2019**, *177*, 428–445.e18. [CrossRef]
52. Santavanond, J.P.; Rutter, S.F.; Atkin-Smith, G.K.; Poon, I.K.H. Apoptotic bodies: Mechanism of formation, isolation and functional relevance. *Subcell. Biochem.* **2021**, *97*, 61–88. [CrossRef]
53. Mathiesen, A.; Hamilton, T.; Carter, N.; Brown, M.; McPheat, W.; Dobrian, A. Endothelial extracellular vesicles: From keepers of health to messengers of disease. *Int. J. Mol. Sci.* **2021**, *22*, 4640. [CrossRef]
54. Liu, Z.Z.; Jose, P.A.; Yang, J.; Zeng, C. Importance of extracellular vesicles in hypertension. *Exp. Biol. Med. (Maywood)* **2021**, *246*, 342–353. [CrossRef]
55. Good, M.E.; Musante, L.; La Salvia, S.; Howell, N.L.; Carey, R.M.; Le, T.H.; Isakson, B.E.; Erdbrugger, U. Circulating extracellular vesicles in normotension restrain vasodilation in resistance arteries. *Hypertension* **2020**, *75*, 218–228. [CrossRef]
56. Otani, K.; Yokoya, M.; Kodama, T.; Hori, K.; Matsumoto, K.; Okada, M.; Yamawaki, H. Plasma exosomes regulate systemic blood pressure in rats. *Biochem. Biophys. Res. Commun.* **2018**, *503*, 776–783. [CrossRef]
57. Sansone, R.; Baaken, M.; Horn, P.; Schuler, D.; Westenfeld, R.; Amabile, N.; Kelm, M.; Heiss, C. Endothelial microparticles and vascular parameters in subjects with and without arterial hypertension and coronary artery disease. *Data Br.* **2018**, *19*, 495–500. [CrossRef]
58. Sun, Y.; Wang, Q.; Yang, G.; Lin, C.; Zhang, Y.; Yang, P. Weight and prognosis for influenza A(H1N1)pdm09 infection during the pandemic period between 2009 and 2011: A systematic review of observational studies with meta-analysis. *Infect. Dis. (Lond)* **2016**, *48*, 813–822. [CrossRef]
59. Perez-Hernandez, J.; Riffo-Campos, A.L.; Ortega, A.; Martinez-Arroyo, O.; Perez-Gil, D.; Olivares, D.; Solaz, E.; Martinez, F.; Martinez-Hervas, S.; Chaves, F.J.; et al. Urinary- and plasma-derived exosomes reveal a distinct MicroRNA signature associated with albuminuria in hypertension. *Hypertension* **2021**, *77*, 960–971. [CrossRef]
60. Wang, C.; Xing, C.; Li, Z.; Liu, Y.; Li, Q.; Wang, Y.; Hu, J.; Yuan, L.; Yang, G. Bioinspired therapeutic platform based on extracellular vesicles for prevention of arterial wall remodeling in hypertension. *Bioact. Mater.* **2022**, *8*, 494–504. [CrossRef]

61. Quick, S.; Moss, J.; Rajani, R.M.; Williams, A. A vessel for change: Endothelial dysfunction in cerebral small vessel disease. *Trends Neurosci.* **2021**, *44*, 289–305. [CrossRef] [PubMed]
62. Berry, C.; Sidik, N.; Pereira, A.C.; Ford, T.J.; Touyz, R.M.; Kaski, J.C.; Hainsworth, A.H. Small-Vessel disease in the heart and brain: Current knowledge, unmet therapeutic need, and future directions. *J. Am. Hear. Assoc.* **2019**, *8*, e011104. [CrossRef] [PubMed]
63. Zhou, W.; Brown, J.M.; Bajaj, N.S.; Chandra, A.; Divakaran, S.; Weber, B.; Bibbo, C.F.; Hainer, J.; Taqueti, V.R.; Dorbala, S.; et al. Hypertensive coronary microvascular dysfunction: A subclinical marker of end organ damage and heart failure. *Eur Hear. J.* **2020**, *41*, 2366–2375. [CrossRef] [PubMed]
64. Toya, T.; Sara, J.D.; Scharf, E.L.; Ahmad, A.; Nardi, V.; Ozcan, I.; Lerman, L.O.; Lerman, A. Impact of peripheral microvascular endothelial dysfunction on white matter hyperintensity. *J. Am. Hear. Assoc.* **2021**, *10*, e021066. [CrossRef] [PubMed]
65. Toya, T.; Sara, J.D.; Ahmad, A.; Nardi, V.; Taher, R.; Lerman, L.O.; Lerman, A. Incremental prognostic impact of peripheral microvascular endothelial dysfunction on the development of ischemic stroke. *J. Am. Hear. Assoc.* **2020**, *9*, e015703. [CrossRef]
66. Nezu, T.; Hosomi, N.; Aoki, S.; Kubo, S.; Araki, M.; Mukai, T.; Takahashi, T.; Maruyama, H.; Higashi, Y.; Matsumoto, M. Endothelial dysfunction is associated with the severity of cerebral small vessel disease. *Hypertens. Res.* **2015**, *38*, 291–297. [CrossRef]
67. Serne, E.H.; de Jongh, R.T.; Eringa, E.C.; RG, I.J.; Stehouwer, C.D. Microvascular dysfunction: A potential pathophysiological role in the metabolic syndrome. *Hypertension* **2007**, *50*, 204–211. [CrossRef]
68. Quyyumi, A.A.; Patel, R.S. Endothelial dysfunction and hypertension: Cause or effect? *Hypertension* **2010**, *55*, 1092–1094. [CrossRef]
69. Schachinger, V.; Britten, M.B.; Zeiher, A.M. Prognostic impact of coronary vasodilator dysfunction on adverse long-term outcome of coronary heart disease. *Circulation* **2000**, *101*, 1899–1906. [CrossRef]
70. Yeboah, J.; Folsom, A.R.; Burke, G.L.; Johnson, C.; Polak, J.F.; Post, W.; Lima, J.A.; Crouse, J.R.; Herrington, D.M. Predictive value of brachial flow-mediated dilation for incident cardiovascular events in a population-based study: The multi-ethnic study of atherosclerosis. *Circulation* **2009**, *120*, 502–509. [CrossRef]
71. Gokce, N.; Keaney, J.F., Jr.; Hunter, L.M.; Watkins, M.T.; Menzoian, J.O.; Vita, J.A. Risk stratification for postoperative cardiovascular events via noninvasive assessment of endothelial function: A prospective study. *Circulation* **2002**, *105*, 1567–1572. [CrossRef] [PubMed]
72. Shimbo, D.; Muntner, P.; Mann, D.; Viera, A.J.; Homma, S.; Polak, J.F.; Barr, R.G.; Herrington, D.; Shea, S. Endothelial dysfunction and the risk of hypertension: The multi-ethnic study of atherosclerosis. *Hypertension* **2010**, *55*, 1210–1216. [CrossRef] [PubMed]
73. Sciacqua, A.; Scozzafava, A.; Pujia, A.; Maio, R.; Borrello, F.; Andreozzi, F.; Vatrano, M.; Cassano, S.; Perticone, M.; Sesti, G.; et al. Interaction between vascular dysfunction and cardiac mass increases the risk of cardiovascular outcomes in essential hypertension. *Eur. Hear. J.* **2005**, *26*, 921–927. [CrossRef] [PubMed]
74. van Oort, S.; Beulens, J.W.J.; van Ballegooijen, A.J.; Grobbee, D.E.; Larsson, S.C. Association of cardiovascular risk factors and lifestyle behaviors with hypertension: A mendelian randomization study. *Hypertension* **2020**, *76*, 1971–1979. [CrossRef]
75. Sander, M.; Chavoshan, B.; Victor, R.G. A large blood pressure-raising effect of nitric oxide synthase inhibition in humans. *Hypertension* **1999**, *33*, 937–942. [CrossRef]
76. Juonala, M.; Viikari, J.S.; Ronnemaa, T.; Helenius, H.; Taittonen, L.; Raitakari, O.T. Elevated blood pressure in adolescent boys predicts endothelial dysfunction: The cardiovascular risk in young Finns study. *Hypertension* **2006**, *48*, 424–430. [CrossRef]
77. Rossi, R.; Chiurlia, E.; Nuzzo, A.; Cioni, E.; Origliani, G.; Modena, M.G. Flow-mediated vasodilation and the risk of developing hypertension in healthy postmenopausal women. *J. Am. Coll. Cardiol* **2004**, *44*, 1636–1640. [CrossRef]
78. Salmito, F.T.; de Oliveira Neves, F.M.; Meneses, G.C.; de Almeida Leitao, R.; Martins, A.M.; Liborio, A.B. Glycocalyx injury in adults with nephrotic syndrome: Association with endothelial function. *Clin. Chim. Acta* **2015**, *447*, 55–58. [CrossRef]
79. Sabatier, F.; Camoin-Jau, L.; Anfosso, F.; Sampol, J.; Dignat-George, F. Circulating endothelial cells, microparticles and progenitors: Key players towards the definition of vascular competence. *J. Cell Mol. Med.* **2009**, *13*, 454–471. [CrossRef]
80. Klonizakis, M.; Manning, G.; Donnelly, R. Assessment of lower limb microcirculation: Exploring the reproducibility and clinical application of laser Doppler techniques. *Ski. Pharm. Physiol* **2011**, *24*, 136–143. [CrossRef]
81. Rubinshtein, R.; Kuvin, J.T.; Soffler, M.; Lennon, R.J.; Lavi, S.; Nelson, R.E.; Pumper, G.M.; Lerman, L.O.; Lerman, A. Assessment of endothelial function by non-invasive peripheral arterial tonometry predicts late cardiovascular adverse events. *Eur. Hear. J.* **2010**, *31*, 1142–1148. [CrossRef]
82. Flammer, A.J.; Anderson, T.; Celermajer, D.S.; Creager, M.A.; Deanfield, J.; Ganz, P.; Hamburg, N.M.; Luscher, T.F.; Shechter, M.; Taddei, S.; et al. The assessment of endothelial function: From research into clinical practice. *Circulation* **2012**, *126*, 753–767. [CrossRef]
83. Corretti, M.C.; Anderson, T.J.; Benjamin, E.J.; Celermajer, D.; Charbonneau, F.; Creager, M.A.; Deanfield, J.; Drexler, H.; Gerhard-Herman, M.; Herrington, D.; et al. Guidelines for the ultrasound assessment of endothelial-dependent flow-mediated vasodilation of the brachial artery: A report of the International Brachial Artery Reactivity Task Force. *J. Am. Coll. Cardiol.* **2002**, *39*, 257–265. [CrossRef]
84. Holder, S.M.; Bruno, R.M.; Shkredova, D.A.; Dawson, E.A.; Jones, H.; Hopkins, N.D.; Hopman, M.T.E.; Bailey, T.G.; Coombes, J.S.; Askew, C.D.; et al. Reference intervals for brachial artery flow-mediated dilation and the relation with cardiovascular risk factors. *Hypertension* **2021**, *77*, 1469–1480. [CrossRef]

85. Greyling, A.; van Mil, A.C.; Zock, P.L.; Green, D.J.; Ghiadoni, L.; Thijssen, D.H.; TIFN International Working Group on Flow Mediated Dilation. Adherence to guidelines strongly improves reproducibility of brachial artery flow-mediated dilation. *Atherosclerosis* **2016**, *248*, 196–202. [CrossRef]
86. Daiber, A.; Steven, S.; Weber, A.; Shuvaev, V.V.; Muzykantov, V.R.; Laher, I.; Li, H.; Lamas, S.; Munzel, T. Targeting vascular (endothelial) dysfunction. *Br. J. Pharmacol.* **2017**, *174*, 1591–1619. [CrossRef]
87. Nagele, M.P.; Haubner, B.; Tanner, F.C.; Ruschitzka, F.; Flammer, A.J. Endothelial dysfunction in COVID-19: Current findings and therapeutic implications. *Atherosclerosis* **2020**, *314*, 58–62. [CrossRef]
88. Yong, J.; Tian, J.; Yang, X.; Xing, H.; He, Y.; Song, X. Effects of oral drugs on coronary microvascular function in patients without significant stenosis of epicardial coronary arteries: A systematic review and meta-analysis of coronary flow reserve. *Front. Cardiovasc. Med.* **2020**, *7*, 580419. [CrossRef]
89. Bakris, G.; Ali, W.; Parati, G. ACC/AHA versus ESC/ESH on hypertension guidelines: JACC guideline comparison. *J. Am. Coll. Cardiol.* **2019**, *73*, 3018–3026. [CrossRef]
90. Juggi, J.S.; Koenig-Berard, E.; Van Gilst, W.H. Cardioprotection by angiotensin-converting enzyme (ACE) inhibitors. *Can. J. Cardiol.* **1993**, *9*, 336–352.
91. Matoba, S.; Tatsumi, T.; Keira, N.; Kawahara, A.; Akashi, K.; Kobara, M.; Asayama, J.; Nakagawa, M. Cardioprotective effect of angiotensin-converting enzyme inhibition against hypoxia/reoxygenation injury in cultured rat cardiac myocytes. *Circulation* **1999**, *99*, 817–822. [CrossRef]
92. Shahin, Y.; Khan, J.A.; Samuel, N.; Chetter, I. Angiotensin converting enzyme inhibitors effect on endothelial dysfunction: A meta-analysis of randomised controlled trials. *Atherosclerosis* **2011**, *216*, 7–16. [CrossRef] [PubMed]
93. Napoleone, E.; Di Santo, A.; Camera, M.; Tremoli, E.; Lorenzet, R. Angiotensin-converting enzyme inhibitors downregulate tissue factor synthesis in monocytes. *Circ. Res.* **2000**, *86*, 139–143. [CrossRef] [PubMed]
94. Lee, R.; Channon, K.M.; Antoniades, C. Therapeutic strategies targeting endothelial function in humans: Clinical implications. *Curr. Vasc. Pharmacol.* **2012**, *10*, 77–93. [CrossRef] [PubMed]
95. Erdos, E.G.; Tan, F.; Skidgel, R.A. Angiotensin I-converting enzyme inhibitors are allosteric enhancers of kinin B1 and B2 receptor function. *Hypertension* **2010**, *55*, 214–220. [CrossRef]
96. Li, K.; Zemmrich, C.; Bramlage, P.; Persson, A.B.; Sacirovic, M.; Ritter, O.; Buschmann, E.; Buschmann, I.; Hillmeister, P. Effect of ACEI and ARB treatment on nitric oxide-dependent endothelial function. *Vasa* **2021**, *50*, 413–422. [CrossRef]
97. Radenkovic, M.; Stojanovic, M.; Prostran, M. Calcium channel blockers in restoration of endothelial function: Systematic review and meta-analysis of randomized controlled trials. *Curr. Med. Chem.* **2019**, *26*, 5579–5595. [CrossRef]
98. Mancini, G.B.; Henry, G.C.; Macaya, C.; O'Neill, B.J.; Pucillo, A.L.; Carere, R.G.; Wargovich, T.J.; Mudra, H.; Luscher, T.F.; Klibaner, M.I.; et al. Angiotensin-converting enzyme inhibition with quinapril improves endothelial vasomotor dysfunction in patients with coronary artery disease. The TREND (trial on reversing endothelial dysfunction) study. *Circulation* **1996**, *94*, 258–265. [CrossRef]
99. Chiesa, S.T.; Marcovecchio, M.L.; Benitez-Aguirre, P.; Cameron, F.J.; Craig, M.E.; Couper, J.J.; Davis, E.A.; Dalton, R.N.; Daneman, D.; Donaghue, K.C.; et al. Vascular effects of ACE (angiotensin-converting enzyme) inhibitors and statins in adolescents with type 1 diabetes. *Hypertension* **2020**, *76*, 1734–1743. [CrossRef]
100. Schmieder, R.E.; Delles, C.; Mimran, A.; Fauvel, J.P.; Ruilope, L.M. Impact of telmisartan versus ramipril on renal endothelial function in patients with hypertension and type 2 diabetes. *Diabetes Care* **2007**, *30*, 1351–1356. [CrossRef]
101. Chobanian, A.V.; Bakris, G.L.; Black, H.R.; Cushman, W.C.; Green, L.A.; Izzo, J.L., Jr.; Jones, D.W.; Materson, B.J.; Oparil, S.; Wright, J.T., Jr.; et al. The seventh report of the joint national committee on prevention, detection, evaluation, and treatment of high blood pressure: The JNC 7 report. *JAMA* **2003**, *289*, 2560–2572. [CrossRef] [PubMed]
102. Mohler, E.R., 3rd; Herrington, D.; Ouyang, P.; Mangano, C.; Ritter, S.; Davis, P.; Purkayastha, D.; Gatlin, M.; Vogel, R.A.; Investigators, E. A randomized, double-blind trial comparing the effects of amlodipine besylate/benazepril HCl vs amlodipine on endothelial function and blood pressure. *J. Clin. Hypertens. (Greenwich)* **2006**, *8*, 692–698. [CrossRef] [PubMed]
103. Frielingsdorf, J.; Seiler, C.; Kaufmann, P.; Vassalli, G.; Suter, T.; Hess, O.M. Normalization of abnormal coronary vasomotion by calcium antagonists in patients with hypertension. *Circulation* **1996**, *93*, 1380–1387. [CrossRef] [PubMed]
104. Yasu, T.; Kobayashi, M.; Mutoh, A.; Yamakawa, K.; Momomura, S.; Ueda, S. Dihydropyridine calcium channel blockers inhibit non-esterified-fatty-acid-induced endothelial and rheological dysfunction. *Clin. Sci.* **2013**, *125*, 247–255. [CrossRef]
105. Napoli, C.; Salomone, S.; Godfraind, T.; Palinski, W.; Capuzzi, D.M.; Palumbo, G.; D'Armiento, F.P.; Donzelli, R.; de Nigris, F.; Capizzi, R.L.; et al. 1,4-Dihydropyridine calcium channel blockers inhibit plasma and LDL oxidation and formation of oxidation-specific epitopes in the arterial wall and prolong survival in stroke-prone spontaneously hypertensive rats. *Stroke* **1999**, *30*, 1907–1915. [CrossRef]
106. Ruschitzka, F.T.; Noll, G.; Luscher, T.F. Combination of ACE inhibitors and calcium antagonists: A logical approach. *J. Cardiovasc. Pharmacol.* **1998**, *31* (Suppl. 2), S5–S16. [CrossRef]
107. Tiryaki, O.; Usalan, C.; Buyukhatipoglu, H.; Sayiner, Z.A.; Kilisli, H. Effects of lisinopril, irbesartan, and amlodipine on the thrombogenic variables in the early and late stages of the treatment in hypertensive patients. *Clin. Exp. Hypertens.* **2012**, *34*, 145–152. [CrossRef]
108. Wiysonge, C.S.; Bradley, H.A.; Volmink, J.; Mayosi, B.M.; Opie, L.H. Beta-blockers for hypertension. *Cochrane Database Syst. Rev.* **2017**, *2017*, CD002003. [CrossRef]

109. Ong, P.; Athanasiadis, A.; Sechtem, U. Pharmacotherapy for coronary microvascular dysfunction. *Eur. Hear. J.-Cardiovasc. Pharm.* **2015**, *1*, 65–71. [CrossRef]
110. Gomes, A.; Costa, D.; Lima, J.L.; Fernandes, E. Antioxidant activity of beta-blockers: An effect mediated by scavenging reactive oxygen and nitrogen species? *Bioorganic Med. Chem.* **2006**, *14*, 4568–4577. [CrossRef]
111. Pedersen, M.E.; Cockcroft, J.R. The vasodilatory beta-blockers. *Curr. Hypertens. Rep.* **2007**, *9*, 269–277. [CrossRef] [PubMed]
112. Kalinowski, L.; Dobrucki, L.W.; Szczepanska-Konkel, M.; Jankowski, M.; Martyniec, L.; Angielski, S.; Malinski, T. Third-generation beta-blockers stimulate nitric oxide release from endothelial cells through ATP efflux: A novel mechanism for antihypertensive action. *Circulation* **2003**, *107*, 2747–2752. [CrossRef]
113. Zepeda, R.J.; Castillo, R.; Rodrigo, R.; Prieto, J.C.; Aramburu, I.; Brugere, S.; Galdames, K.; Noriega, V.; Miranda, H.F. Effect of carvedilol and nebivolol on oxidative stress-related parameters and endothelial function in patients with essential hypertension. *Basic Clin. Pharmacol. Toxicol.* **2012**, *111*, 309–316. [CrossRef] [PubMed]
114. Eckel, R.H.; Grundy, S.M.; Zimmet, P.Z. The metabolic syndrome. *Lancet* **2005**, *365*, 1415–1428. [CrossRef]
115. Antoniades, C.; Bakogiannis, C.; Leeson, P.; Guzik, T.J.; Zhang, M.H.; Tousoulis, D.; Antonopoulos, A.S.; Demosthenous, M.; Marinou, K.; Hale, A.; et al. Rapid, direct effects of statin treatment on arterial redox state and nitric oxide bioavailability in human atherosclerosis via tetrahydrobiopterin-mediated endothelial nitric oxide synthase coupling. *Circulation* **2011**, *124*, 335–345. [CrossRef]
116. Liu, A.; Wu, Q.; Guo, J.; Ares, I.; Rodriguez, J.L.; Martinez-Larranaga, M.R.; Yuan, Z.; Anadon, A.; Wang, X.; Martinez, M.A. Statins: Adverse reactions, oxidative stress and metabolic interactions. *Pharmacol. Ther.* **2019**, *195*, 54–84. [CrossRef] [PubMed]
117. Di Minno, M.N.; Ambrosino, P.; Peluso, R.; Di Minno, A.; Lupoli, R.; Dentali, F.; Ca, R.S.G. Lipid profile changes in patients with rheumatic diseases receiving a treatment with TNF-alpha blockers: A meta-analysis of prospective studies. *Ann. Med.* **2014**, *46*, 73–83. [CrossRef]
118. Martinez-Gonzalez, J.; Badimon, L. Influence of statin use on endothelial function: From bench to clinics. *Curr. Pharm. Des.* **2007**, *13*, 1771–1786. [CrossRef]
119. Takagi, H.; Yamamoto, H.; Iwata, K.; Goto, S.N.; Umemoto, T. Low-density lipoprotein-independent improvement of flow-mediated dilatation with atorvastatin: A meta-analysis and meta-regression of randomized controlled trials. *Int. J. Cardiol.* **2012**, *158*, 285–289. [CrossRef]
120. Zinellu, A.; Mangoni, A.A. Systematic review and meta-analysis of the effect of statins on circulating E-selectin, L-selectin, and P-selectin. *Biomedicines* **2021**, *9*, 1707. [CrossRef]
121. Zinellu, A.; Mangoni, A.A. An updated systematic review and meta-analysis of the effect of statins on asymmetric dimethylarginine. *Nitric Oxide* **2022**, *120*, 26–37. [CrossRef]
122. Maruhashi, T.; Higashi, Y. Pathophysiological association between diabetes mellitus and endothelial dysfunction. *Antioxidants* **2021**, *10*, 1306. [CrossRef] [PubMed]
123. Stojanovic, M.; Prostran, M.; Radenkovic, M. Thiazolidinediones improve flow-mediated dilation: A meta-analysis of randomized clinical trials. *Eur. J. Clin. Pharmacol.* **2016**, *72*, 385–398. [CrossRef] [PubMed]
124. Sugiyama, S.; Jinnouchi, H.; Kurinami, N.; Hieshima, K.; Yoshida, A.; Jinnouchi, K.; Nishimura, H.; Suzuki, T.; Miyamoto, F.; Kajiwara, K.; et al. The SGLT2 inhibitor dapagliflozin significantly improves the peripheral microvascular endothelial function in patients with uncontrolled type 2 diabetes mellitus. *Intern. Med.* **2018**, *57*, 2147–2156. [CrossRef] [PubMed]
125. Nafisa, A.; Gray, S.G.; Cao, Y.; Wang, T.; Xu, S.; Wattoo, F.H.; Barras, M.; Cohen, N.; Kamato, D.; Little, P.J. Endothelial function and dysfunction: Impact of metformin. *Pharmacol. Ther.* **2018**, *192*, 150–162. [CrossRef]
126. Androulakis, E.; Norrington, K.; Bakogiannis, C.; Lioudaki, E.; Siasos, G.; Tousoulis, D. The impact of antiplatelet treatment on endothelial function. *Curr. Pharm. Des.* **2016**, *22*, 4512–4518. [CrossRef]
127. Lee, S.J.; Lee, J.S.; Choi, M.H.; Lee, S.E.; Shin, D.H.; Hong, J.M. Cilostazol improves endothelial function in acute cerebral ischemia patients: A double-blind placebo controlled trial with flow-mediated dilation technique. *BMC Neurol.* **2017**, *17*, 169. [CrossRef]
128. Shi, M.Q.; Su, F.F.; Xu, X.; Liu, X.T.; Wang, H.T.; Zhang, W.; Li, X.; Lian, C.; Zheng, Q.S.; Feng, Z.C. Cilostazol suppresses angiotensin II-induced apoptosis in endothelial cells. *Mol. Med. Rep.* **2016**, *13*, 2597–2605. [CrossRef]
129. Chao, T.H.; Chen, I.C.; Lee, C.H.; Chen, J.Y.; Tsai, W.C.; Li, Y.H.; Tseng, S.Y.; Tsai, L.M.; Tseng, W.K. Cilostazol enhances mobilization of circulating endothelial progenitor cells and improves endothelium-dependent function in patients at high risk of cardiovascular disease. *Angiology* **2016**, *67*, 638–646. [CrossRef]
130. Suzuki, K.; Uchida, K.; Nakanishi, N.; Hattori, Y. Cilostazol activates AMP-activated protein kinase and restores endothelial function in diabetes. *Am. J. Hypertens.* **2008**, *21*, 451–457. [CrossRef]
131. Warnholtz, A.; Mollnau, H.; Oelze, M.; Wendt, M.; Munzel, T. Antioxidants and endothelial dysfunction in hyperlipidemia. *Curr. Hypertens. Rep.* **2001**, *3*, 53–60. [CrossRef] [PubMed]
132. Dodd, S.; Dean, O.; Copolov, D.L.; Malhi, G.S.; Berk, M. N-acetylcysteine for antioxidant therapy: Pharmacology and clinical utility. *Expert Opin. Biol. Ther.* **2008**, *8*, 1955–1962. [CrossRef] [PubMed]
133. Shen, Y.; Miao, N.J.; Xu, J.L.; Gan, X.X.; Xu, D.; Zhou, L.; Xue, H.; Zhang, W.; Lu, L.M. N-acetylcysteine alleviates angiotensin II-mediated renal fibrosis in mouse obstructed kidneys. *Acta Pharmacol. Sin.* **2016**, *37*, 637–644. [CrossRef]
134. Ruiz, F.J.; Salom, M.G.; Ingles, A.C.; Quesada, T.; Vicente, E.; Carbonell, L.F. N-acetyl-L-cysteine potentiates depressor response to captopril and enalaprilat in SHRs. *Am. J. Physiol.* **1994**, *267*, R767–R772. [CrossRef] [PubMed]

135. Fang, X.; Liu, L.; Zhou, S.; Zhu, M.; Wang, B. Nacetylcysteine inhibits atherosclerosis by correcting glutathionedependent methylglyoxal elimination and dicarbonyl/oxidative stress in the aorta of diabetic mice. *Mol. Med. Rep.* **2021**, *23*, 291. [CrossRef]
136. Sahin, G.; Yalcin, A.U.; Akcar, N. Effect of N-acetylcysteine on endothelial dysfunction in dialysis patients. *Blood Purif.* **2007**, *25*, 309–315. [CrossRef]
137. Miner, S.E.; Cole, D.E.; Evrovski, J.; Forrest, Q.; Hutchison, S.J.; Holmes, K.; Ross, H.J. N-acetylcysteine neither lowers plasma homocysteine concentrations nor improves brachial artery endothelial function in cardiac transplant recipients. *Can. J. Cardiol.* **2002**, *18*, 503–507.
138. Kim, D.H.; Meza, C.A.; Clarke, H.; Kim, J.S.; Hickner, R.C. Vitamin D and endothelial function. *Nutrients* **2020**, *12*, 575. [CrossRef]
139. Chiu, H.F.; Venkatakrishnan, K.; Golovinskaia, O.; Wang, C.K. Impact of micronutrients on hypertension: Evidence from clinical trials with a special focus on meta-analysis. *Nutrients* **2021**, *13*, 588. [CrossRef]
140. Ran, L.; Zhao, W.; Tan, X.; Wang, H.; Mizuno, K.; Takagi, K.; Zhao, Y.; Bu, H. Association between serum vitamin C and the blood pressure: A systematic review and meta-analysis of observational studies. *Cardiovasc. Ther.* **2020**, *2020*, 4940673. [CrossRef]
141. Guan, Y.; Dai, P.; Wang, H. Effects of vitamin C supplementation on essential hypertension: A systematic review and meta-analysis. *Medicine (Baltimore)* **2020**, *99*, e19274. [CrossRef] [PubMed]
142. Tousoulis, D.; Antoniades, C.; Vassiliadou, C.; Toutouza, M.; Pitsavos, C.; Tentolouris, C.; Trikas, A.; Stefanadis, C. Effects of combined administration of low dose atorvastatin and vitamin E on inflammatory markers and endothelial function in patients with heart failure. *Eur. J. Hear. Fail.* **2005**, *7*, 1126–1132. [CrossRef] [PubMed]
143. Emami, M.R.; Safabakhsh, M.; Alizadeh, S.; Asbaghi, O.; Khosroshahi, M.Z. Effect of vitamin E supplementation on blood pressure: A systematic review and meta-analysis. *J. Hum. Hypertens.* **2019**, *33*, 499–507. [CrossRef] [PubMed]
144. Gates, P.E.; Boucher, M.L.; Silver, A.E.; Monahan, K.D.; Seals, D.R. Impaired flow-mediated dilation with age is not explained by L-arginine bioavailability or endothelial asymmetric dimethylarginine protein expression. *J. Appl. Physiol.* **2007**, *102*, 63–71. [CrossRef]
145. Shiraseb, F.; Asbaghi, O.; Bagheri, R.; Wong, A.; Figueroa, A.; Mirzaei, K. The effect of L-arginine supplementation on blood pressure in adults: A systematic review and dose-response meta-analysis of randomized clinical trials. *Adv. Nutr. Int. Rev. J.* **2021**. [CrossRef] [PubMed]
146. Whyte, J. Rehabilitation effectiveness: The state of the science and a hope for the future. *Am. J. Phys. Med. Rehabil.* **2007**, *86*, 835–837. [CrossRef]
147. Kachur, S.; Lavie, C.J.; Morera, R.; Ozemek, C.; Milani, R.V. Exercise training and cardiac rehabilitation in cardiovascular disease. *Expert Rev. Cardiovasc. Ther.* **2019**, *17*, 585–596. [CrossRef]
148. Stucki, G.; Kroeling, P. Physical therapy and rehabilitation in the management of rheumatic disorders. *Best Pr. Res. Clin. Rheumatol.* **2000**, *14*, 751–771. [CrossRef]
149. Sahin, H.; Varol, Y.; Naz, I.; Aksel, N.; Tuksavul, F.; Ozsoz, A. The effect of pulmonary rehabilitation on COPD exacerbation frequency per year. *Clin. Respir. J.* **2018**, *12*, 165–174. [CrossRef]
150. McCarthy, B.; Casey, D.; Devane, D.; Murphy, K.; Murphy, E.; Lacasse, Y. Pulmonary rehabilitation for chronic obstructive pulmonary disease. *Cochrane Database Syst. Rev.* **2015**, *2*, CD003793. [CrossRef]
151. Anderson, L.; Thompson, D.R.; Oldridge, N.; Zwisler, A.D.; Rees, K.; Martin, N.; Taylor, R.S. Exercise-based cardiac rehabilitation for coronary heart disease. *Cochrane Database Syst. Rev.* **2016**, *1*, CD001800. [CrossRef]
152. Heran, B.S.; Chen, J.M.; Ebrahim, S.; Moxham, T.; Oldridge, N.; Rees, K.; Thompson, D.R.; Taylor, R.S. Exercise-based cardiac rehabilitation for coronary heart disease. *Cochrane Database Syst. Rev.* **2011**, CD001800. [CrossRef]
153. Smith, E.E.; Markus, H.S. New treatment approaches to modify the course of cerebral small vessel diseases. *Stroke* **2020**, *51*, 38–46. [CrossRef] [PubMed]
154. Soares, R.N.; Murias, J.M.; Saccone, F.; Puga, L.; Moreno, G.; Resnik, M.; De Roia, G.F. Effects of a rehabilitation program on microvascular function of CHD patients assessed by near-infrared spectroscopy. *Physiol. Rep.* **2019**, *7*, e14145. [CrossRef] [PubMed]
155. Ishikawa, K.; Ohta, T.; Zhang, J.; Hashimoto, S.; Tanaka, H. Influence of age and gender on exercise training-induced blood pressure reduction in systemic hypertension. *Am. J. Cardiol.* **1999**, *84*, 192–196. [CrossRef]
156. Sinoway, L.I.; Musch, T.I.; Minotti, J.R.; Zelis, R. Enhanced maximal metabolic vasodilatation in the dominant forearms of tennis players. *J. Appl. Physiol.* **1986**, *61*, 673–678. [CrossRef] [PubMed]
157. Mehra, V.M.; Gaalema, D.E.; Pakosh, M.; Grace, S.L. Systematic review of cardiac rehabilitation guidelines: Quality and scope. *Eur. J. Prev. Cardiol.* **2020**, *27*, 912–928. [CrossRef]
158. Tanaka, S.; Sanuki, Y.; Ozumi, K.; Harada, T.; Tasaki, H. Heart failure with preserved vs reduced ejection fraction following cardiac rehabilitation: Impact of endothelial function. *Hear. Vessel.* **2018**, *33*, 886–892. [CrossRef]
159. Legallois, D.; Belin, A.; Nesterov, S.V.; Milliez, P.; Parienti, J.J.; Knuuti, J.; Abbas, A.; Tirel, O.; Agostini, D.; Manrique, A. Cardiac rehabilitation improves coronary endothelial function in patients with heart failure due to dilated cardiomyopathy: A positron emission tomography study. *Eur. J. Prev. Cardiol.* **2016**, *23*, 129–136. [CrossRef]
160. Cesari, F.; Marcucci, R.; Gori, A.M.; Burgisser, C.; Francini, S.; Sofi, F.; Gensini, G.F.; Abbate, R.; Fattirolli, F. Impact of a cardiac rehabilitation program and inflammatory state on endothelial progenitor cells in acute coronary syndrome patients. *Int. J. Cardiol.* **2013**, *167*, 1854–1859. [CrossRef]

161. Guo, Y.; Ledesma, R.A.; Peng, R.; Liu, Q.; Xu, D. The beneficial effects of cardiac rehabilitation on the function and levels of endothelial progenitor cells. *Hear. Lung Circ.* **2017**, *26*, 10–17. [CrossRef] [PubMed]
162. Merlo, C.; Bernardi, E.; Bellotti, F.; Pomidori, L.; Cogo, A. Supervised exercise training improves endothelial function in COPD patients: A method to reduce cardiovascular risk? *ERJ Open Res.* **2020**, *6*. [CrossRef] [PubMed]
163. Ross, M.D.; Malone, E.; Florida-James, G. Vascular ageing and exercise: Focus on cellular reparative processes. *Oxidative Med. Cell. Longev.* **2016**, *2016*, 3583956. [CrossRef] [PubMed]
164. Finks, S.W.; Rumbak, M.J.; Self, T.H. Treating hypertension in chronic obstructive pulmonary disease. *N. Engl. J. Med.* **2020**, *382*, 353–363. [CrossRef] [PubMed]
165. Slivnick, J.; Lampert, B.C. Hypertension and Heart Failure. *Hear. Fail. Clin.* **2019**, *15*, 531–541. [CrossRef] [PubMed]
166. Ambrosino, P.; Molino, A.; Calcaterra, I.; Formisano, R.; Stufano, S.; Spedicato, G.A.; Motta, A.; Papa, A.; Di Minno, M.N.D.; Maniscalco, M. Clinical assessment of endothelial function in convalescent COVID-19 patients undergoing multidisciplinary pulmonary rehabilitation. *Biomedicines* **2021**, *9*, 614. [CrossRef]

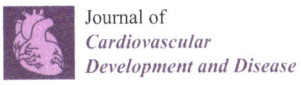

Article

Effectiveness of High-Intensity Interval Training and Continuous Moderate-Intensity Training on Blood Pressure in Physically Inactive Pre-Hypertensive Young Adults

Anil T John [1,2,†], Moniruddin Chowdhury [3,4,†], Md. Rabiul Islam [5], Imtiyaz Ali Mir [1,6,*], Md Zobaer Hasan [7,8], Chao Yi Chong [9], Syeda Humayra [10] and Yukihito Higashi [11,12]

1. Faculty of Health Sciences, Lincoln University College, Petaling Jaya 47301, Selangor, Malaysia; anil1452@gmail.com
2. College of Physiotherapy, Dayananda Sagar University, Bengaluru 560111, India
3. Faculty of Medicine, AIMST University, Bedong 08100, Kedah, Malaysia; moniruc@yahoo.com
4. Department of Public Health, Daffodil International University, Dhaka 1341, Bangladesh
5. Department of Public Health, Independent University Bangladesh, Dhaka 1229, Bangladesh; rabiulislamjuphi@gmail.com
6. Department of Physiotherapy, Faculty of Medicine & Health Sciences, Universiti Tunku Abdul Rahman, Kajang 43000, Selangor, Malaysia
7. School of Science, Monash University Malaysia, Bandar Sunway 47500, Selangor, Malaysia; mdzobaer.hasan@monash.edu
8. General Educational Development, Daffodil International University, Dhaka 1341, Bangladesh
9. Faculty of Medicine & Health Sciences, Universiti Tunku Abdul Rahman, Kajang 43000, Selangor, Malaysia; chaoyichong41@gmail.com
10. Department of Public Health, Faculty of Allied Health Sciences, Daffodil International University, Dhaka 1341, Bangladesh; syedahumayra@gmail.com
11. Department of Regeneration & Medicine, Research Center for Radiation Genome Medicine, Research Institute for Radiation Biology & Medicine, Hiroshima University, Hiroshima 739-8511, Japan; yhigashi@hiroshima-u.ac.jp
12. Division of Regeneration & Medicine, Hiroshima University Hospital, Hiroshima 739-8511, Japan
* Correspondence: imtiyaz2204@gmail.com
† These authors contributed equally to this work.

Abstract: The likelihood of pre-hypertensive young adults developing hypertension has been steadily increasing in recent years. Despite the fact that aerobic exercise training (AET) has demonstrated positive results in lowering high blood pressure, the efficacy of different types of AET among pre-hypertensive young adults has not been well-established. The objective of this study was to evaluate the effectiveness of high-intensity interval training (HIIT) and continuous moderate-intensity training (CMT) on the blood pressure (BP) of physically inactive pre-hypertensive young adults. In total, 32 adults (age 20.0 ± 1.1 years and BMI 21.5 ± 1.8) were randomly assigned to three groups: HIIT, CMT and control (CON). The HIIT and CMT groups participated in 5 weeks of AET, while the CON group followed a DASH diet plan only. The HIIT protocol consisted of a 1:4 min work to rest ratio of participants, at an 80–85% heart rate reserve (HR-reserve) and a 40–60% HR-reserve, respectively, for 20 min; the CMT group exercised at 40–60% of their HR-reserve continuously for 20 min. In both the HIIT and CMT groups, systolic blood pressure (SBP) (3.8 ± 2.8 mmHg, $p = 0.002$ vs. 1.6 ± 1.5 mmHg, $p = 0.011$) was significantly reduced, while significant reductions in the diastolic blood pressure (DBP) (2.9 ± 2.2 mmHg, $p = 0.002$) and mean arterial pressure (MAP) (3.1 ± 1.6 mmHg, $p < 0.0005$) were noted only in the HIIT group. No significant differences in SBP (−0.4 ± 3.7 mmHg, $p = 0.718$), DBP (0.4 ± 3.4 mmHg, $p = 0.714$), or MAP (0.1 ± 2.5 mmHg, $p = 0.892$) were observed in the CON group. Both HIIT and CMT decreased BP in physically inactive pre-hypertensive young adults; however, HIIT yielded more beneficial results in terms of reducing the SPB, DBP and MAP.

Keywords: high-intensity interval training; continuous aerobic training; systolic blood pressure; diastolic blood pressure; pre-hypertension

---

Citation: John, A.T.; Chowdhury, M.; Islam, M.R.; Mir, I.A.; Hasan, M.Z.; Chong, C.Y.; Humayra, S.; Higashi, Y. Effectiveness of High-Intensity Interval Training and Continuous Moderate-Intensity Training on Blood Pressure in Physically Inactive Pre-Hypertensive Young Adults. *J. Cardiovasc. Dev. Dis.* **2022**, *9*, 246. https://doi.org/10.3390/jcdd9080246

Academic Editor: Fabio Angeli

Received: 31 May 2022
Accepted: 25 July 2022
Published: 3 August 2022

Publisher's Note: MDPI stays neutral with regard to jurisdictional claims in published maps and institutional affiliations.

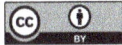

Copyright: © 2022 by the authors. Licensee MDPI, Basel, Switzerland. This article is an open access article distributed under the terms and conditions of the Creative Commons Attribution (CC BY) license (https://creativecommons.org/licenses/by/4.0/).

1. Introduction

Hypertension is considered to be one of the main precursors of cardiovascular diseases (CVDs) and has been linked to 7.7 million deaths globally [1,2]. The Seventh report of the Joint National Committee on Prevention, Detection, Evaluation, and Treatment of High Blood Pressure (JNC7) defined pre-hypertension as a systolic blood pressure (SBP) of 120 mmHg to 139 mmHg and a diastolic blood pressure (DBP) of 80 mmHg to 89 mmHg [3]. Pre-hypertensive people are at an increased risk of acquiring hypertension, and it has been estimated that those with blood pressure (BP) readings between 130 and 139/80 and 89 mmHg are twice as likely to develop hypertension than those with lower readings [4]. Modifiable risk factors of high BP can be controlled by active engagement in physical exercises [3,5]. To prevent the progressive rise in BP and cardiovascular diseases, the control of pre-hypertension and lifestyle modifications require special attention [6].

Studies have suggested that physical exercise is associated with substantial improvements in insulin sensitivity, augmented autonomic nervous system function and decreased vasoconstriction, which may prevent a pathological rise in BP [7,8]. Physical activity (PA) improves the release of growth factors from skeletal muscles into the bloodstream, stimulates angiogenesis, facilitates neurogenesis and induces endothelial cell proliferation with endothelial cell membrane permeability, thus leading to a substantial reduction in BP and the attenuation of hypertension symptoms [9–11].

Worldwide, 9% of premature mortality contributing to approximately 5.3 million deaths in 2008 occurred due to physical inactivity [12]. Regular PA is a well-established intervention for the prevention and treatment of several chronic diseases [13], and it has shown a significant effect on BP reduction [14]. Physical exercise has also been shown to improve various factors involved in the pathophysiology of hypertension [15–18], which can extenuate BP in both hypertensive and non-hypertensive adults [15,19]. Continuous moderate-intensity training (CMT) for at least 30 min or more is traditionally recommended for the prevention and treatment of high BP [13,20].

High-intensity interval training (HIIT) has been documented as a safe and effective training method for cardiac rehabilitation [21]. HIIT can be defined as a short burst of maximal effort interspersed by a few minutes of rest or active recovery, and it has been reported to be more effective than CMT for improving cardiorespiratory fitness in different populations [16–18,22–24]. HIIT, which consists of several bouts of high-intensity exercise (85–95% of HRmax) lasting 1 to 4 min interspersed with intervals of rest or active recovery [15,17,18], has been found to improve endothelial function and its markers [16,18], insulin sensitivity [18], markers of sympathetic activity [16,17], arterial stiffness [15,16], blood glucose and lipoproteins [18]. Despite these favorable outcomes, the efficacy of HIIT in reducing BP among pre-hypertensive young adults is not well established [25]. In addition, there is a scarcity of current literature comparing HIIT and CMT on BP in this particular population. Therefore, the primary purpose of this study was to determine the effects of HIIT and CMT on the BP of physically inactive pre-hypertensive young adults, and then to explore which type of exercise training is more efficient in lowering the BP of this population. To the best of the authors' knowledge, this is the very first study to target pre-hypertensive young adults in Malaysia.

2. Materials and Methods

2.1. Study Setting and Subjects

This 5-week randomized–controlled trial was conducted in the Physiotherapy Centre at the Faculty of Medicine and Health Sciences in University Tunku Abdul Rahman, Sungai Long Kajang, Malaysia. G*power (F test) was used to calculate the sample size, based on the power analysis; a total of 42 participants were required for this study. The study subjects were reached through university portal, emails and posters for voluntary participation. Participants were recruited by convenience sampling as the study population required young adults with pre-hypertension. A total of 87 subjects were initially screened, out of which only 32 adults fit the eligibility criteria after they were administered the International Physical Activity Questionnaires (IPAQ), Physical Activity Readiness Questionnaire (PAR-Q+) and measurement of body mass index (BMI). Using the computer-generated numbers, study participants (22 males and 10 females) were randomly allocated to 3 groups: the HIIT group, CMT group and the control (CON) group.

Inclusion criteria comprised both genders (unmarried), aged between 18 and 25 years old, who were physically inactive with an SBP between 120 and 139 mmHg and/or DBP between 80 and 89 mmHg. Participants with a known history of respiratory illnesses, cardiovascular diseases, diabetes mellitus, overweight/obesity, psychological disorders, or musculoskeletal problems; those taking anti-hypertensive medications; and active smokers were excluded from this study.

The protocol was based on the Helsinki Declaration Accord (World Medical Association for Human Subjects). Moreover, prior ethical clearance was obtained from the Universiti Tunku Abdul Rahman's Scientific and Ethical Review Committee (U/SERC/77/20). Written informed consent was obtained from each participant after debriefing them about the benefits of the study, potential risks of muscle soreness, strict maintenance of data confidentiality and right to withdraw at any point from the study.

2.2. Body Mass Index and Blood Pressure Measurement

In addition to assessing BMI during the screening process, it was also measured at baseline to ensure no abrupt changes in body weight before study initiation and that participants were within the normal BMI range (18.5–24.9). BMI was recorded by measuring the participants' body weight in kilograms and dividing it by their height squared (kg/m^2). The procedure was carried out early in the morning (8:30 am–9:00 am) using a calibrated seca 284 EMR (Hamburg, Germany) wireless measuring station for weight and height. Before measuring the BMI, participants were instructed to remove any excess clothing, and to stand upright and barefooted on the measuring machine. An average of 3 measurements for both weight and height were calculated to assess the BMI score.

Following the standard procedure, participants' BP from the right brachial artery was measured using an automated digital BP monitor (OMRON SEM-1, Kyoto, Kansai Japan) in the morning between 9:15 am and 10:15 am after 5 min of rest in a chair [26,27]. Each participant's right arm was supported on the table at heart level, and both SPB and DBP were measured 3 times with a 5 min interval between each measurement in order to obtain the most accurate result. If the differences between any of the 3 SBP and/or DBP readings were higher than 5 mmHg, the measurement was taken again after a 5 min interval, and the average reading with the least differences was taken into consideration. BP was measured at baseline before beginning the intervention and at the end of the 5-week intervention. The post-test measurement of BP was carried out in a similar way as recorded at baseline. In addition, the mean arterial pressure (MAP) was also estimated at baseline and at the end of intervention with the following formula:

$$MAP = DBP + 1/3(SBP - DBP)$$

2.3. Exercise Intervention Protocol

Before the first exercise session, the subjects' heart rate (HR) was measured using a calibrated pulse oximeter (GIMA: Oxy-5-Plus Oximeter, Italy). The exercise HR (HRmax) of the participants in the HIIT and CMT groups was calculated using the newest age-based formula, [$HRmax = 211 - (0.64 * age)$]. The exercise HR was then calculated using the Karvonen formula [Exercise HR = % of target intensity (HRreserve) + HRrest]. To prevent delayed-onset muscle soreness (DOMS) and to acclimatize all the physically inactive participants in both exercise groups to the exercise regimen, a 1-week familiarization period was provided with a total of 3 exercise sessions on alternate days. Participants in both the experimental groups performed a 5 min warm-up session followed by 20 min of continuous running on a treadmill (BH LK-G6700 Pro Action, St. Charles, MI, USA) without inclination at 40–60% of their HR-reserve. Before ending the exercise session, a 5 min cool-down was performed by all participants by walking on the same treadmill at their own comfortable pace. A pulse oximeter (GIMA: Oxy-5-Plus Oximeter, Gessate, Milan, Italy) was placed on the participants' index finger during the PA to monitor their exercise HR, in addition to using the treadmill's inbuilt heart rate monitor. Differences in the exercise HR in both the monitoring methods were negligible throughout the training protocol. After the familiarization period of 1 week, the HIIT group underwent 4 weeks of HIIT (3 times per week on alternate days excluding the weekends) consisting of 20 min of treadmill (BH LK-G6700 Pro Action, St. Charles, MI, USA) running with a 1:4 min work to rest ratio, an upper HR target at 80–85% of HR-reserve, and a lower HR target at 40–60% of HR-reserve. The CMT group continued with 4 weeks of the same exercise protocol on the treadmill, which was carried out in the familiarization period at an intensity of 40–60% of their HR-reserve. Exercise HR during these 4 weeks of aerobic exercise training (AET) for both groups were monitored in the same way as stated above in the familiarization program. The indication for the termination of the exercise sessions was in accordance with ACSM's guidelines. It was not feasible to blind the participants or therapists, as they both knew the type of intervention being received and delivered, respectively, but outcome assessors were blinded to control the detection bias.

The CON group did not participate in any exercise program; they were instructed to follow a Dietary Approaches to Stop Hypertension (DASH) diet and restrict their sodium intake (<100 mmol/day) according to the JNV VIII guidelines. In addition to the distribution of the guidelines given, participants in the CON group were reminded via telephone calls once weekly about the DASH diet and sodium restrictions to ensure that they were strictly following the guidelines.

All the participants in the 3 groups were instructed not to engage in any other form of PA during these 5 weeks to prevent any extraneous effect on the outcomes. In addition, to avoid the acute post-exercise effects on BP, participants were also instructed not to perform any exercise 24 h prior to the post-test BP measurement. In accordance with the CONSORT statement, a detailed description of this clinical trial is shown in Figure 1 below.

2.4. Statistical Analysis

The data were processed using the Statistical Package for Social Science (SPSS) version 26.0. The Shapiro–Wilk test was first performed to check the normality assumption of data as it is required to fulfil the conditions of a paired sample t-test. The Shapiro–Wilk test (Table 1) demonstrated that data were normally distributed ($p > 0.05$) in all 3 groups with respect to the SBP, DBP and MAP at baseline; therefore, these outcome measures were compared using the paired sample t-test to determine within-group differences. To evaluate between-group differences, a one-way ANOVA test was carried out. The conditions to conduct the one-way ANOVA test were fulfilled, in which each group represented the qualitative variables, and the dependent variables, SBP, DBP and MAP, were quantitative variables. A post hoc test was further employed to assess which group differed significantly from the other two groups after performing the one-way ANOVA test. Results are presented as the mean ± SD for all the outcome measures. All reported probability values were 2-sided, and a p-value of <0.05 was considered statistically significant.

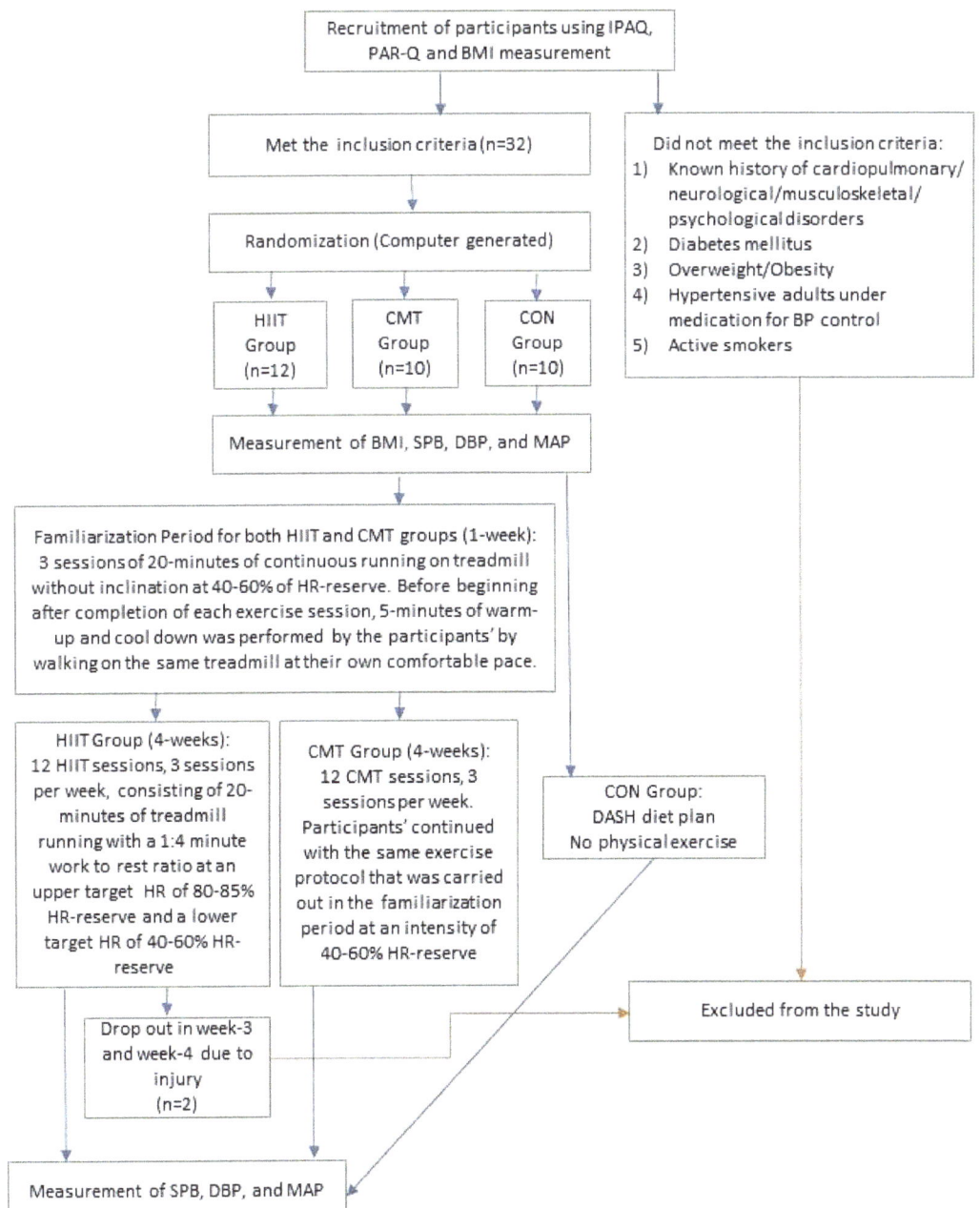

Figure 1. Flowchart of Trial: IPAQ = International Physical Activity Questionnaire; PAR-Q = Physical Activity Readiness Questionnaire; BMI = Body Mass Index; SBP = Systolic Blood Pressure; DBP = Diastolic Blood Pressure; MAP = Mean Arterial Pressure; HIIT = High Intensity Interval Training; CMT = Continuous Moderate-intensity Training; CON = Control; HR-reserve = Heart Rate Reserve.

Table 1. Test of normality at baseline for SBP, DBP and MAP among 3 groups.

	Group	Statistic	p-Value
Pre-SBP mean	HIIT Group	0.960	0.780
	CMT Group	0.981	0.972
	CON Group	0.853	0.063
Pre-DBP mean	HIIT Group	0.970	0.890
	CMT Group	0.912	0.294
	CON Group	0.874	0.112
Pre-MAP mean	HIIT Group	0.989	0.995
	CMT Group	0.921	0.365
	CON Group	0.923	0.387

Shapiro–Wilk Test; Level of Significance: $p < 0.05$.

3. Results

3.1. Descriptive Statistics

At the beginning of this study, 32 participants were randomly assigned to the HIIT (6 males and 6 females), CMT (6 males and 4 females) and CON groups (10 males). Two participants dropped out of the HIIT group (both males) during the third and fourth weeks of training due to musculoskeletal injury. The mean ages of the participants in the HIIT, CMT and CON groups were 21 ± 0.8, 19 ± 1.3 and 21 ± 1.0, respectively. Similarly, the mean BMIs measured at baseline were 20.8 ± 1.9, 21.7 ± 1.6 and 22.0 ± 1.9 for the HIIT, CMT and CON groups, respectively. The BMI of the CON group was slightly higher than that of the other two groups, which was most probably due to the fact that all the participants in the CON group were males.

3.2. Comparison within the Groups

Table 2 depicts that the CON group had the highest baseline and post-intervention SBP mean values of 127.93 ± 5.09 mmHg and 128.37 ± 5.32 mmHg, respectively. The HIIT group had the highest baseline DBP (78.57 ± 5.36 mmHg), and CMT group had greater post-test DBP (75.73 ± 4.26). At baseline, the MAP was highest in the CMT group (93.20 ± 2.89) and greater in the CON group (91.86 ± 4.18) post-test.

Table 2. All groups' SBP, DBP and MAP mean (X) with standard deviation (SD).

	HIIT Group X ± SD		CMT Group X ± SD		CON Group X ± SD	
	Pre-Test	Post-Test	Pre-Test	Post-Test	Pre-Test	Post-Test
SBP (mmHg)	122.76 ± 2.65	119 ± 3.91	125.23 ± 3.76	123.67 ± 3.98	127.93 ± 5.09	128.37 ± 5.32
DBP (mmHg)	78.57 ± 5.36	75.63 ± 4.86	77.23 ± 4.54	75.73 ± 4.26	74.00 ± 6.23	73.60 ± 5.78
MAP (mmHg)	93.14 ± 3.46	90.09 ± 2.57	93.20 ± 2.89	91.71 ± 3.08	91.98 ± 4.62	91.86 ± 4.18

Table 3 illustrates the results of the paired sample t-test. In the CON group, a mean difference of -0.43 (p-value = $0.718 > 0.05$) for the SPB was observed, indicating a non-significant difference between the pre-SBP and post-SBP. For the DBP, a mean difference of 0.40 (p-value = $0.714 > 0.05$) was found, showing no significant difference between the pre-DBP and post-DBP for CON group. Similarly, the MAP did not exhibit any significant difference (mean = 0.11, p-value = 0.892). For the CMT group, a mean difference of 1.57 (p-value = $0.011 < 0.05$) was observed in terms of SBP, which was statistically significant. However, for the DBP, the mean difference between the pre- and post-tests was 1.50 (p-value = $0.161 > 0.05$), depicting a non-significant difference between the pre-DBP and post-DBP in the CMT group. The MAP in the CMT group showed an insignificant reduction in the mean (1.49, p-value = 0.054). A mean difference of 3.76 (p-value = $0.002 < 0.05$) was found in the HIIT group for the SBP and 2.93 (*p*-value = 0.002 < 0.05) for the DBP, indicating a statistically significant difference between the pre- and post-tests of both the SPB and DPB, respectively, in the HIIT group. A similar result was noticed found in MAP, with a significant mean difference of 3.05 (*p*-value < 0.0005).

Table 3. Paired sample t-tests for SBP, DBP and MAP among the 3 groups.

	Groups	Paired Differences				
		Mean	Std. Deviation	t	df	*p*-Value
	CON Group					
Pair 1	Pre-SBP mean–post-SBP mean	−0.43	3.68	−0.37	9	0.718
Pair 2	Pre-DBP mean–post-DBP mean	0.40	3.35	0.38	9	0.714
Pair 3	Pre-MAP mean–post-MAP mean	0.11	2.50	0.14	9	0.892
	CMT Group					
Pair 1	Pre-SBP mean–post-SBP mean	1.57	1.54	3.22	9	0.011
Pair 2	Pre-DBP mean–post-DBP mean	1.50	3.10	1.53	9	0.161
Pair 3	Pre-MAP mean–post-MAP mean	1.49	2.12	2.22	9	0.054
	HIIT Group					
Pair 1	Pre-SBP mean–post-SBP mean	3.76	2.83	4.20	9	0.002
Pair 2	Pre-DBP mean–post-DBP mean	2.93	2.23	4.16	9	0.002
Pair 3	Pre-MAP mean–post-MAP mean	3.05	1.64	5.90 *	9	<0.0005

Paired sample *t*-test was performed; * Indicates statistically significant at 5% level of significance.

3.3. Comparison between the Groups

For the SBP, the F-test (one-way ANOVA) result was 5.02 (*p*-value = 0.014 < 0.05) (Table 4). Therefore, it can be concluded that there were significant differences in the mean SBP across the three groups. However, for the DBP, the F-test statistic was 1.87 (*p*-value = 0.173 > 0.05), indicating a non-significant difference among the three groups. The MAP F-test was 4.76 (*p*-value = 0.017 < 0.05), showing a significant difference between the 3 groups.

Table 4. Comparison of SBP, DBP and MAP mean difference across the 3 groups.

		ANOVA				
		Sum of Squares	df	Mean Square	F	*p*-Value
SBP	Between Groups	69.72	2	34.86	5.02 *	0.014
	Within Groups	187.53	27	6.95		
	Total	257.25	29			
DBP	Between Groups	32.25	2	16.12	1.87	0.173
	Within Groups	232.47	27	8.61		
	Total	264.71	29			
MAP	Between Groups	43.08	2	21.54	4.76 *	0.017
	Within Groups	122.13	27	4.52		
	Total	165.21	29			

One-way ANOVA test was performed; * Indicates statistically significant at 5% level of significance.

Since the one-way ANOVA test showed significant differences in SBP and MAP across the three groups, a post hoc test (Tukey test) was performed to investigate which pairs of the groups were different in terms of the mean SBP and mean MAP. We found that the SBP mean difference in the HIIT and CMT groups was statistically insignificant (p-value = 0.282 > 0.05) (Table 5). However, we noticed a significant SBP mean difference between the HIIT group and the CON group (p-value = 0.010 < 0.05), but the SBP mean difference between the CMT and CON groups was statistically insignificant (p-value = 0.258 > 0.05). The MAP did not show any significant mean difference between the HIIT and CMT groups (p-value = 0.244 > 0.05) and between the CMT and CON groups (p-value = 0.337 > 0.05). However, a significant mean difference in MAP was seen between the HIIT and CON groups (p-value = 0.013 < 0.05). Hence, it can be deduced that HIIT is more effective in reducing the SBP, DBP and MAP compared to the CMT.

Table 5. Post hoc test (Tukey test).

Dependent Variable	(I) Group	(J) Group	Mean Difference (I-J)	p-Value
SBP	HIIT	CMT	−1.83	0.282
		CON	−3.73 *	0.010
	CMT	HIIT	1.83	0.282
		CON	−1.90	0.258
	CON	HIIT	3.73 *	0.010
		CMT	1.90	0.258
MAP	HIIT	CT	−1.57	0.244
		CON	−2.93 *	0.013
	CMT	HIIT	1.56	0.244
		CON	−1.37	0.337
	CON	HIIT	2.93 *	0.013
		CMT	1.37	0.337

Post hoc (Tukey) test was performed; * Indicates statistically significant at 5% level of significance.

4. Discussion

Earlier studies [28,29] broadly supported the improved cardiopulmonary benefits of HIIT over CMT. Nevertheless, no previous study has conspicuously explored HIIT and CMT outcomes in the pre-hypertensive young population by incorporating a comparator CON group with the DASH protocol. Thus, the research provided valuable insights into the field of physical therapy and significantly contributed to the current body of scientific literature. This study showed the beneficial effects of HIIT and CMT on the resting BP of physically inactive young adults with pre-hypertension. It is evident from the findings of the current study that both HIIT and CMT can reduce SBP significantly among pre-hypertensive young adults. The positive role of exercise training on BP can be perceived through its action on sympathetic activity, enhanced endothelial function and decreased oxidative stress, which cumulatively contributes to the prevention and treatment of hypertension [30]. In addition, PA may be accountable for reducing exercise-induced oxidative stress by producing an increased level of antioxidants, attenuating vascular and cardiac sympathetic activity, reducing serum vasoconstrictor factor levels and increasing endothelial dilating factors, which that consequently helps in lowering the peripheral vascular resistance and subsequently leads to improved BP [16,31]. A previous meta-analysis revealed that the two most prominent intervention protocols HIIT and CMT were effective in reducing SBP in adults with pre- to established hypertension [25]. Our findings correlate with a study that compared the effects of continuous and interval training in the management of hypertension, wherein researchers found a SBP reduction in both experimental groups (−16.4 ± 13.2 mmHg and −13.9 ± 12.6 mmHg, respectively) [32]. Similar results were also derived from the systematic review by Punia S et al. [33]. Our study revealed significant reductions in SBP after conducting 5 weeks of an AET (HIIT and CMT) program. Therefore, in addition to lowering SBP among the hypertensive population, HIIT and CMT can be useful tools in reducing the SBP among pre-hypertensive young adults.

The current study demonstrated a significant reduction in DBP among the participants undergoing the HIIT exercise protocol, whereas a non-significant reduction in DBP was observed among the CMT and control groups. In [34], it is suggested that HIIT demonstrated greater improvements in the endothelial function and arterial stiffness compared to CMT. This explains the increased BP reduction in the HIIT group as endothelium plays a pivotal role in the homeostasis and maintenance of vascular tonus, which may be a contributing factor in BP reduction. A recent randomized clinical trial also revealed similar results, where the authors found a significant reduction in SBP but a non-significant reduction in DBP [35]. Although the decrease in the DBP of the CMT group was statistically non-significant in this study, if given a longer intervention period, there would be a more obvious result, as most studies have confirmed a significant reduction in DBP following 8 or more weeks of continuous exercise in hypertensive and normotensive adults [32,36]. Interestingly, in the current study, within a time frame of 5 weeks, HIIT was shown to be effective in reducing DBP significantly. Therefore, HIIT could be a better option in controlling the DBP of pre-hypertensive young adults.

MAP measures the pressure necessary for the adequate perfusion of the organs of the whole body. Therefore, it could be a better indicator of perfusion than SBP. High MAP can be detrimental, leading to morbid conditions such as ventricular hypertrophy, myocardial infarction and stroke. HIIT intervention in this current study also demonstrated significantly greater reductions in the MAP in comparison to CMT (3.05 vs. 1.49). Similar findings were reported in past studies, wherein HIIT led to notable reductions in the MAP among pre-hypertensive subjects [37] and sedentary individuals [38,39]. Overall, the HIIT exercise resulted in a significant BP reduction and a favorable alteration in MAP, thus showing a positive cardiovascular response post-intervention. However, further studies are required to evaluate the potential mechanisms contributing to these physiological responses and changes in the pre-hypertensive population.

HIIT interventions are considered to be more effective and time-efficient interventions for BP and aerobic capacity level improvements as compared to other exercises [40]. Wahl P et al. [41] found that HIIT stimulated a transient increase in the circulating levels of vascular endothelial growth factor and hepatocyte growth factor. Thus, it can be postulated that HIIT intervention reduces BP by actively promoting and stimulating the angiogenic factors. A study comparing HIIT and CMT [16] showed that HIIT is far superior in lowering BP compared to CMT due to three factors: improving cardiorespiratory fitness, hormonal response and nitric oxide response, which is a mediator of vasodilation in blood vessels that plays a major role in BP control. It has been stated that HIIT interventions that last for 4–12 weeks are able to produce a larger decrease in SPB (−3.63 mmHg) than other forms of exercise [40]. Previous studies [16–18] also support the finding that HIIT is superior to CMT in improving cardiorespiratory fitness and reducing BP among normotensive and hypertensive individuals, but its efficacy in reducing BP among the pre-hypertensive population requires further investigation. In the current study, there was a significant difference in the mean SBP across the three groups, HIIT, CMT and CON, as revealed by the ANOVA test. Further analysis via a post hoc test demonstrated a significant mean difference in the SBP between the HIIT group and CON group (p-value = 0.010 < 0.05). However, there was an insignificant mean difference in the SBP between the CMT and CON group participants (p-value = 0.282 > 0.05). Additionally, HIIT was found to be effective in reducing the DBP significantly (p-value = 0.002 < 0.05). Although PA has been associated with reduced BP, there can be some variations due to different training modalities, exercise prescriptions, intensities, frequencies and durations of intervention [34]. Nevertheless, the current study clearly demonstrates that HIIT is superior to CMT in controlling the progression of pre-hypertension towards hypertension in Malaysian young adults.

Studies by Stephen PJ et al. [42] and Paula TP et al. [43] revealed that the DASH diet and sodium restriction have significant effect on the reduction in SBP, DBP and HR among hypertensive patients. A recent meta-analysis also revealed similar observations [44]. Therefore, a possible reason that there was no reduction in SPB or DBP in the CON group could be non-adherence to the diet protocol, even after weekly reminders via phone calls to the participants to ensure that they were strictly adhering to the regimen. Although HIIT and CMT groups were not instructed to follow the DASH diet and sodium restriction as the researchers aimed to determine the effectiveness of HIIT and CMT solely, a significant SBP reduction and a non-significant DBP reduction were observed among the participants of the CMT group, whereas in the HIIT group, both SBP and DBP were significantly reduced after 5 weeks. In conclusion, the study results indicate a higher efficacy of HIIT over CMT even in the absence of the DASH diet to control the resting BP in the pre-hypertensive young adults.

5. Strengths, Limitations and Recommendations

Due to the time constraint and limited resources, the researchers were only able to recruit 32 participants for this research. However, this was a hypothesis-generating study and differed methodologically; therefore, even with the limited sample size, this research provided a deeper insight into the cardioprotective role of exercise training in BP. Second, the HIIT and CMT groups each consisted of only 4 and 6 females in the respective groups, whereas the CON group consisted of all males. This is due to the fact that during the screening process, many female participants were under hypotensive or normotensive categories, and after screening, eligible participants were divided randomly into three groups. The dietary intake of the participants in the CON group may have also played a significant role regarding controlling BP, since it was not possible to directly observe and monitor their adherence to the DASH diet and sodium restriction. Therefore, future studies with a larger sample size, a longer intervention duration, and the stringent control of the DASH diet plan are highly recommended. Furthermore, HIIT with the DASH diet plan could be a better approach towards controlling pre-hypertension in a short period of time.

6. Conclusions

HIIT can effectively reduce both the SBP and DBP of healthy, physically inactive pre-hypertensive young adults, but CMT reduced only the SBP in this study. Therefore, HIIT could be a promising alternative intervention in BP reduction and thus could be functional in preventing the progression of pre-hypertension towards hypertension among physically inactive young adults.

Author Contributions: The conceptualization process involved I.A.M. and A.T.J. Study design was carried out by I.A.M., M.C. and A.T.J. Data collection was performed by C.Y.C. and I.A.M. Data analyses and interpretation were performed by A.T.J., I.A.M., M.C., M.R.I., M.Z.H. and Y.H. Manuscript drafting and critical review were performed by A.T.J., I.A.M., M.C., M.R.I., M.Z.H., S.H. and Y.H. All authors have read and agreed to the published version of the manuscript.

Funding: This research received no external funding.

Institutional Review Board Statement: This study was conducted according to the Helsinki Declaration Accord. In addition, prior ethical clearance was obtained from the Universiti Tunku Abdul Rahman's Scientific and Ethical Review Committee (U/SERC/77/20).

Informed Consent Statement: Written informed consent was obtained from all participants involved in the study.

Data Availability Statement: Not applicable.

Acknowledgments: We express our gratitude to the participants of this research and our nursing staff for helping us with the measurement of outcome variables.

Conflicts of Interest: The authors have no conflict of interest.

References

1. Chow, C.K.; Teo, K.K.; Rangarajan, S.; Islam, S.; Gupta, R.; Avezum, A.; Bahonar, A.; Chifamba, J.; Dagenais, G.; Diaz, R.; et al. Prevalence, awareness, treatment, and control of hypertension in rural and urban communities in high-, middle-, and low-income countries. *JAMA* **2013**, *310*, 959–968. [CrossRef]
2. Mozaffarian, D.; Benjamin, E.J.; Go, A.S.; Arnett, D.K.; Blaha, M.J.; Cushman, M.; Das, S.R.; Ferranti, S.; Després, J.P.; Fullerton, H.J.; et al. Executive summary: Heart disease and stroke statistics-2016 update: A report from the american heart association. *Circulation* **2016**, *133*, 447–454. [CrossRef] [PubMed]
3. Chobanian, A.V.; Bakris, G.L.; Black, H.R.; Cushman, W.C.; Green, L.A.; Izzo, J.L., Jr.; Jones, D.W.; Materson, B.J.; Oparil, S.; Wright, J.T., Jr.; et al. The seventh report of the joint national committee on prevention, detection, evaluation, and treatment of high blood pressure: The jnc 7 report. *JAMA* **2003**, *289*, 2560–2571. [CrossRef] [PubMed]
4. Vasan, R.S.; Larson, M.G.; Leip, E.P.; Evans, J.C.; O'Donnell, C.J.; Kannel, W.B.; Levy, D. Impact of high-normal blood pressure on the risk of cardiovascular disease. *N. Engl. J. Med.* **2001**, *345*, 1291–1297. [CrossRef] [PubMed]
5. He, J.; Whelton, P.K.; Appel, L.J.; Charleston, J.; Klag, M.J. Long-term effects of weight loss and dietary sodium reduction on incidence of hypertension. *Hypertension* **2000**, *35*, 544–549. [CrossRef] [PubMed]
6. Nytrøen, K.I.; Rolid, K.; Andreassen, A.K.; Yardley, M.; Gude, E.; Dahle, D.O.; Bjørkelund, E.; Relbo, A.; Grov, I.; Philip, W.J.; et al. Effect of high-intensity interval training in de novo heart transplant recipients in Scandinavia: One-year follow-up of the HITTS randomized, controlled study. *Circulation* **2019**, *139*, 2198–2211. [CrossRef]
7. Silva, M.I.C.; Mostarda, C.T.; Moreira, E.D.; Silva, K.A.S.; Santos, F.; Angelis, K.; Farah, V.M.A.; Irigoyen, M.C. Preventive role of exercise training in autonomic, hemodynamic and metabolic parameters in rats under high risk of metabolic syndrome development. *J. Appl. Physiol.* **2013**, *114*, 786–791. [CrossRef] [PubMed]
8. Araujo, A.J.S.D.; Santos, A.C.V.D.; Souza, K.D.S.; Aires, M.B.; Filho, V.J.S.; Fioretto, E.T.; Mota, M.M.; Santos, M.R.V. Resistance training controls arterial blood pressure in rats with l-name-induced hypertension. *Arq. Bras. Cardiol.* **2013**, *100*, 339–346. [CrossRef] [PubMed]
9. Bell, T.P.; McIntyre, K.A.; Hadley, R. Effect of long-term physical exercise on blood pressure in african americans. *Int. J. Exerc. Sci.* **2014**, *7*, 3. [CrossRef]
10. Diaz, K.M.; Shimbo, D. Physical Activity and the Prevention of Hypertension. *Curr. Hypertens. Rep.* **2013**, *15*, 659–668. [CrossRef]
11. Cornelissen, V.A.; Smart, N.A. Exercise Training for Blood Pressure: A Systematic Review and Meta-analysis. *J. Am. Heart Assoc.* **2013**, *2*, e004473. [CrossRef]
12. Lee, I.M.; Shiroma, E.J.; Lobelo, F.; Puska, P.; Blair, S.N.; Katzmarzyk, P.T.; Lancet Physical Activity Series Working Group. Effect of physical inactivity on major non-communicable diseases worldwide: An analysis of burden of disease and life expectancy. *Lancet* **2012**, *380*, 219–229. [CrossRef]
13. Haskell, W.L.; Lee, I.M.; Pate, R.R.; Powell, K.E.; Blair, S.N.; Franklin, B.A.; Macera, C.A.; Heath, G.W.; Thompson, P.D.; Bauman, A. Physical activity and public health: Updated recommendation for adults from the american college of sports medicine and the american heart association. *Circulation* **2007**, *116*, 1081. [CrossRef] [PubMed]
14. Hambrecht, R.; Fiehn, E.; Weigl, C.; Gielen, S.; Hamann, C.; Kaiser, R.; Yu, J.; Adams, V.; Niebauer, J.; Schuler, G. Regular physical exercise corrects endothelial dysfunction and improves exercise capacity in patients with chronic heart failure. *Circulation* **1998**, *24*, 2709–2715. [CrossRef] [PubMed]
15. Guimarães, G.V.; Ciolac, E.G.; Carvalho, V.O.; D'Avila, V.M.; Bortolotto, L.A.; Bocchi, E.A. Effects of continuous vs. Interval exercise training on blood pressure and arterial stiffness in treated hypertension. *Hypertens. Res.* **2010**, *33*, 627. [CrossRef]
16. Ciolac, E.G.; Bocchi, E.A.; Bortolotto, L.A.; Carvalho, V.O.; Greve, J.; Guimaraes, G.V. Effects of high-intensity aerobic interval training vs. Moderate exercise on hemodynamic, metabolic and neuro-humoral abnormalities of young normotensive women at high familial risk for hypertension. *Hypertens. Res.* **2010**, *33*, 836. [CrossRef]
17. Ciolac, E.G.; Bocchi, E.A.; Greve, J.M.; Guimarães, G.V. Heart rate response to exercise and cardiorespiratory fitness of young women at high familial risk for hypertension: Effects of interval vs continuous training. *Eur. J. Cardiovasc. Prev. Rehabil.* **2011**, *18*, 824–830. [CrossRef]
18. Tjønna, A.E.; Lee, S.J.; Rognmo, Ø.; Stølen, T.O.; Bye, A.; Haram, P.M.; Loennechen, J.P.; Al-Share, Q.Y.; Skogvoll, E.; Slørdahl, S.A.; et al. Aerobic interval training versus continuous moderate exercise as a treatment for the metabolic syndrome: A pilot study. *Circulation* **2008**, *118*, 346–354. [CrossRef]
19. Ciolac, E.G.; Guimarães, G.V.; Bortolotto, L.A.; Doria, E.L.; Bocchi, E.A. Acute effects of continuous and interval aerobic exercise on 24-h ambulatory blood pressure in long-term treated hypertensive patients. *Int. J. Cardiol.* **2009**, *133*, 381–387. [CrossRef]
20. Pescatello, L.M.; Franclin, B.A.; Fagard, R.; Faqquhar, W.B. Exercise and hypertension. *Med. Sci. Sports Exerc.* **2004**, *36*, 533–553. [CrossRef] [PubMed]
21. Guiraud, T.; Nigam, A.; Gremeaux, V.; Meyer, P.; Juneau, M.; Bosquet, L. High-intensity interval training in cardiac rehabilitation. *Sports Med.* **2012**, *42*, 587–605. [CrossRef] [PubMed]
22. Gillen, J.B.; Gibala, M.J. Is high-intensity interval training a time-efficient exercise strategy to improve health and fitness? *Appl. Physiol. Nutr. Metab.* **2013**, *39*, 409–412. [CrossRef] [PubMed]
23. Helgerud, J.; Hoydal, K.; Wang, E.; Karlsen, T.; Berg, P.; Bjerkaas, M.; Simonsen, T.; Helgesen, C.; Hjorth, N.; Bach, R.; et al. Aerobic high-intensity intervals improve v o2max more than moderate training. *Med. Sci. Sports Exerc.* **2007**, *39*, 665–671. [CrossRef] [PubMed]

24. Wisløff, U.; Støylen, A.; Loennechen, J.P.; Bruvold, M.; Rognmo, Ø.; Haram, P.M.; Tjønna, A.E.; Helgerud, J.; Slørdahl, S.A.; Lee, S.J.; et al. Superior cardiovascular effect of aerobic interval training versus moderate continuous training in heart failure patients: A randomized study. *Circulation* **2007**, *115*, 3086–3094. [CrossRef] [PubMed]
25. Costa, E.C.; Hay, J.L.; Kehler, D.S.; Boreskie, K.F.; Arora, R.C.; Umpierre, D.; Szwajcer, A.; Duhamel, T.A. Effects of high-intensity interval training versus moderate-intensity continuous training on blood pressure in adults with pre-to established hypertension: A systematic review and meta-analysis of randomized trials. *Sports Med.* **2018**, *48*, 2127–2142. [CrossRef] [PubMed]
26. Cicolini, G.; Pizzi, C.; Palma, E.; Bucci, M.; Schioppa, F.; Mezzetti, A.; Manzoli, L. Differences in blood pressure by body position (supine, Fowler's, and sitting) in hypertensive subjects. *Am. J. Hypertens.* **2011**, *24*, 1073–1079. [CrossRef] [PubMed]
27. Manzoli, L.; Simonetti, V.; D'Errico, M.M.; De Vito, C.; Flacco, M.E.; Forni, C.; La Torre, G.; Liguori, G.; Messina, G.; Mezzetti, A.; et al. (In) accuracy of blood pressure measurement in 14 Italian hospitals. *J. Hypertens.* **2012**, *30*, 1955–1960. [CrossRef]
28. Silva, B.N.C.; Petrella, A.F.; Christopher, N.; Marriott, C.F.; Gill, D.P.; Owen, A.M.; Petrella, R.J. The benefits of high-intensity interval training on cognition and blood pressure in older adults with hypertension and subjective cognitive decline: Results from the heart & mind study. *Front. Aging. Neurosci.* **2021**, *13*, 643809.
29. Keteyian, S.J.; Hibner, B.A.; Bronsteen, K.; Kerrigan, D.; Aldred, H.A.; Reasons, L.M.; Saval, M.A.; Brawner, C.A.; Schairer, J.R.; Thompson, T.M. Greater improvement in cardiorespiratory fitness using higher-intensity interval training in the standard cardiac rehabilitation setting. *J. Cardiopulm. Rehabil. Prev.* **2014**, *34*, 98–105. [CrossRef]
30. Nasi, M.; Patrizi, G.; Pizzi, C.; Landolfo, M.; Boriani, G.; Dei Cas, A.; Cicero, A.F.; Fogacci, F.; Rapezzi, C.; Sisca, G. The role of physical activity in individuals with cardiovascular risk factors: An opinion paper from Italian Society of Cardiology-Emilia Romagna-Marche and SIC-Sport. *J. Cardiovasc. Med.* **2019**, *20*, 631–639. [CrossRef]
31. Facioli, T.D.P.; Buranello, M.C.; Regueiro, E.M.G.; Basso-Vanelli, R.P.; Durand, M.D.T. Effect of physical training on nitric oxide levels in patients with arterial hypertension: An integrative review. *Int. J. Cardiovasc. Sci.* **2021**, *35*, 253–264. [CrossRef]
32. Lamina, S. Effects of continuous and interval training programs in the management of hypertension: A randomized controlled trial. *J. Clin. Hypertens.* **2010**, *12*, 841–849. [CrossRef] [PubMed]
33. Punia, S.; Kulandaivelan, S.; Singh, V.; Punia, V. Effect of aerobic exercise training on blood pressure in indians: Systematic review. *Int. J. Chronic Dis.* **2016**. [CrossRef]
34. Leal, J.M.; Galliano, L.M.; Del Vecchio, F.B. Effectiveness of high-intensity interval training versus moderate-intensity continuous training in hypertensive patients: A systematic review and meta-analysis. *Curr. Hypertens. Rep.* **2020**, *22*, 1–3. [CrossRef] [PubMed]
35. Olea, M.A.; Mancilla, R.; Martínez, S.; Díaz, E. Effects of high intensity interval training on blood pressure in hypertensive subjects. *Rev. Med. Chil.* **2017**, *145*, 1154–1159. [CrossRef] [PubMed]
36. Skutnik, B.C.; Smith, J.R.; Johnson, A.M.; Kurti, S.P.; Harms, C.A. The effect of low volume interval training on resting blood pressure in pre-hypertensive subjects: A preliminary study. *Phys. Sportsmed.* **2016**, *44*, 177–183. [CrossRef] [PubMed]
37. Skutnik, B.C. The Effects of High Intensity Interval Training on Resting Mean Arterial Pressure and C-Reactive Protein Content in Prehypertensive Subjects. Ph.D. Thesis, Kansas State University, Manhattan, KS, USA, 2013.
38. Grace, F.; Herbert, P.; Elliott, A.D.; Richards, J.; Beaumont, A.; Sculthorpe, N.F. High intensity interval training (HIIT) improves resting blood pressure, metabolic (MET) capacity and heart rate reserve without compromising cardiac function in sedentary aging men. *Exp. Gerontol.* **2018**, *109*, 75–81. [CrossRef]
39. Muth, B.J. Cardiovascular Effects of High-Intensity Interval Training and Moderate-Intensity Continuous Training in Sedentary Individuals. Ph.D. Thesis, University of Delaware, Newark, DE, USA, 2018.
40. García-Hermoso, A.; Cerrillo-Urbina, A.J.; Herrera-Valenzuela, T.; Cristi-Montero, C.; Saavedra, J.M.; Martínez-Vizcaíno, V. Is high-intensity interval training more effective on improving cardiometabolic risk and aerobic capacity than other forms of exercise in overweight and obese youth? A meta-analysis. *Obes. Rev.* **2016**, *17*, 531–540. [CrossRef]
41. Wahl, P.; Jansen, F.; Achtzehn, S.; Schmitz, T.; Bloch, W.; Mester, J.; Werner, N. Effects of high intensity training and high volume training on endothelial microparticles and angiogenic growth factors. *PLoS ONE* **2014**, *9*, e96024. [CrossRef]
42. Juraschek, S.P.; Miller, E.R.; Weaver, C.M.; Appel, L.J. Effects of Sodium Reduction and the DASH Diet in Relation to Baseline Blood Pressure. Randomized Controlled Trial. *J. Am. Coll. Cardiol.* **2017**, *70*, 2841–2848. [CrossRef]
43. Paula, T.P.; Viana, L.V.; Neto, A.T.; Leitao, C.B.; Gross, J.L.; Azevedo, M.J. Effects of the DASH Diet and Walking on Blood Pressure in Patients with Type 2 Diabetes and Uncontrolled Hypertension: A Randomized Controlled Trial. *J. Clin. Hypertens.* **2015**, *17*, 895–901. [CrossRef] [PubMed]
44. Filippou, C.D.; Tsioufis, C.P.; Thomopoulos, C.G.; Mihas, C.C.; Dimitriadis, K.S.; Sotiropoulou, L.I.; Chrysochoou, C.A.; Nihoyannopoulos, P.I.; Tousoulis, D.M. Dietary Approaches to Stop Hypertension (DASH) Diet and Blood Pressure Reduction in Adults with and without Hypertension: A Systematic Review and Meta-Analysis of Randomized Controlled Trials. *Adv. Nutr.* **2020**, *11*, 1150–1160. [CrossRef] [PubMed]

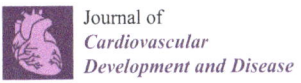

Journal of
Cardiovascular
Development and Disease

Review

Artificial Intelligence in Hypertension Management: An Ace up Your Sleeve

Valeria Visco [1], Carmine Izzo [1], Costantino Mancusi [2], Antonella Rispoli [1], Michele Tedeschi [1], Nicola Virtuoso [3], Angelo Giano [1], Renato Gioia [1], Americo Melfi [3], Bianca Serio [4], Maria Rosaria Rusciano [1], Paola Di Pietro [1], Alessia Bramanti [1], Gennaro Galasso [1], Gianni D'Angelo [5], Albino Carrizzo [1,6], Carmine Vecchione [1,6] and Michele Ciccarelli [1,*]

1. Department of Medicine, Surgery and Dentistry, University of Salerno, 84081 Baronissi, Italy
2. Department of Advanced Biomedical Sciences, Federico II University of Naples, 80138 Naples, Italy
3. Cardiology Unit, University Hospital "San Giovanni di Dio e Ruggi d'Aragona", 84131 Salerno, Italy
4. Hematology and Transplant Center, University Hospital "San Giovanni di Dio e Ruggi d'Aragona", 84131 Salerno, Italy
5. Department of Computer Science, University of Salerno, 84084 Fisciano, Italy
6. Vascular Physiopathology Unit, IRCCS Neuromed, 86077 Pozzilli, Italy
* Correspondence: mciccarelli@unisa.it

Abstract: Arterial hypertension (AH) is a progressive issue that grows in importance with the increased average age of the world population. The potential role of artificial intelligence (AI) in its prevention and treatment is firmly recognized. Indeed, AI application allows personalized medicine and tailored treatment for each patient. Specifically, this article reviews the benefits of AI in AH management, pointing out diagnostic and therapeutic improvements without ignoring the limitations of this innovative scientific approach. Consequently, we conducted a detailed search on AI applications in AH: the articles (quantitative and qualitative) reviewed in this paper were obtained by searching journal databases such as PubMed and subject-specific professional websites, including Google Scholar. The search terms included artificial intelligence, artificial neural network, deep learning, machine learning, big data, arterial hypertension, blood pressure, blood pressure measurement, cardiovascular disease, and personalized medicine. Specifically, AI-based systems could help continuously monitor BP using wearable technologies; in particular, BP can be estimated from a photoplethysmograph (PPG) signal obtained from a smartphone or a smartwatch using DL. Furthermore, thanks to ML algorithms, it is possible to identify new hypertension genes for the early diagnosis of AH and the prevention of complications. Moreover, integrating AI with omics-based technologies will lead to the definition of the trajectory of the hypertensive patient and the use of the most appropriate drug. However, AI is not free from technical issues and biases, such as over/underfitting, the "black-box" nature of many ML algorithms, and patient data privacy. In conclusion, AI-based systems will change clinical practice for AH by identifying patient trajectories for new, personalized care plans and predicting patients' risks and necessary therapy adjustments due to changes in disease progression and/or therapy response.

Keywords: hypertension; artificial intelligence; machine learning; blood pressure; deep learning; deep neural networks; big data; wearable technology; digital health; photoplethysmograph

Citation: Visco, V.; Izzo, C.; Mancusi, C.; Rispoli, A.; Tedeschi, M.; Virtuoso, N.; Giano, A.; Gioia, R.; Melfi, A.; Serio, B.; et al. Artificial Intelligence in Hypertension Management: An Ace up Your Sleeve. *J. Cardiovasc. Dev. Dis.* **2023**, *10*, 74. https://doi.org/10.3390/jcdd10020074

Academic Editor: John Lynn Jefferies

Received: 27 December 2022
Revised: 5 February 2023
Accepted: 7 February 2023
Published: 9 February 2023

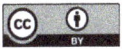

Copyright: © 2023 by the authors. Licensee MDPI, Basel, Switzerland. This article is an open access article distributed under the terms and conditions of the Creative Commons Attribution (CC BY) license (https://creativecommons.org/licenses/by/4.0/).

1. Introduction

Arterial hypertension (AH) is a global public health problem, and its treatment is primarily aimed at reducing associated cardiovascular (CV) morbidity and mortality [1,2]. AH affected more than 1.13 billion individuals in 2015, and the prevalence appears to affect approximately 35–45% of Campo's overall population [3]. Moreover, AH is the most significant contributor to the global burden of CV diseases and represents a heavy socio-economic burden for many countries [4,5]; indeed, even moderate elevations in arterial blood pressure (BP) are associated with a significant reduction in life expectancy [6]. Furthermore, current data suggest that over 14 million people are unaware of their abnormal BP level; consequently, they are not receiving appropriate medication for it, nor do they engage in other interventions to maintain BP in the normal range [7]. Regardless of guidelines, BP control in hypertensive patients in treatment is insufficient due to many factors, including poor adherence to therapy [8]. Moreover, the definition of "hypertension" recapitulates several different sub-phenotypes influenced by multiple variables: gender, BMI, lifestyle conditions, and so on [9]. Furthermore, the pharmacological therapy used to treat essential AH has remained substantially unchanged in the last 20 years and is mainly focused on regulating vascular resistance [1,10]. Therefore, there is an evident gap in the knowledge required to deepen the multifaced aspects of AH and prompt the research and development of novel approaches.

In this scenario, the possibility of collecting, storing, and analyzing multiple pieces of information from a single patient in the form of electronic health records (EHRs) requires revising the conventional healthcare model of AH management using new technologies or monitoring techniques [11,12]. In this context, artificial intelligence (AI) is a technological method that has been in development in recent years [13–15], and, if used appropriately, it could have surprising results in developing predictive models of AH, formulating the diagnosis, stratifying patients, and identifying the most effective therapy (Table 1).

Table 1. AI application in hypertension management.

	Applications	Benefits
Measuring BP	Estimate BP by analyzing PPG signal with ML and DL algorithms.	Self-monitoring BP for hypertension
Predicting AH development	Predict the risk of developing AH by using genetics, medical data, and behavioral, environmental, and socioeconomic factors.	Timely intervention
Diagnosing AH	Accurately diagnosing AH by using CV risk factors, anthropometric data, vital signs, and laboratory data.	Precision diagnosis
Predicting AH treatment success	Identify factors contributing to treatment success.	Personalized treatment plan
Predicting AH prognosis	Stratify patients and predict CV outcomes.	Treatment plan adjustment

AI: artificial intelligence; BP: blood pressure; PPG: photoplethysmograph; ML: machine learning; DL: deep learning; AH: arterial hypertension; CV: cardiovascular.

Specifically, accurate BP estimation is essential because BP is a risk factor for many clinical CV events, including stroke and dementia, and therefore can be integrated into several models for risk stratification [16,17]; moreover, in the computational simulation of CV disease, BP can influence the value of focal hemodynamic metrics, e.g., fractional flow [18]; consequently, patient-specific BP values can improve the accuracy of simulation results and have been applied in some recent models [19,20].

Therefore, AI-based systems might change clinical practice for AH by identifying patient trajectories for new, personalized care plans and predicting patients' risks and necessary therapy adjustments due to changes in disease progression and/or therapy response. Accordingly, a basic knowledge of this science is essential because AI might change medical practice jobs: tiring and routine tasks could be completed by computers to free up time and allow cardiologists to carry out more difficult and sensitive tasks. Therefore, in this review, we describe multiple applications of AI, encompassing diagnostic, prognostic, and therapeutic issues currently unsolved in managing AH (Tables S1–S4).

Overall, this manuscript aims to provide a complete picture of the state of the art of AI in AH (primary and secondary) management, analyzing every aspect of the diagnosis, treatment, and patient follow-up, without neglecting the limitations and all of the possible tools to overcome them.

2. The Principles of AI

AI is a wide-ranging branch of computer science concerned with building smart machines capable of increasing their knowledge through an automatic learning process that typically requires human intelligence [21–23]. Therefore, AI is an interdisciplinary science with multiple approaches that incorporate reasoning (making inferences using data), natural language processing (ability to read and understand human languages), planning (ability to act autonomously and flexibly to create a sequence of actions to achieve a final goal), and machine learning (ML) (algorithms that develop automatically through experience) [21]. Specifically, AI based on ML techniques [15] is used to perform predictive analyses by examining mechanisms and associations among given variables from training datasets, which may consist of a variety of data inputs, including wearable devices, multi-omics, and standardized EHRs [10,24]. Essentially, in ML, the rules would be learned by algorithms directly from a set of data rather than being encoded by hand [25]; consequently, by using specific algorithms, ML can establish complex relationships among data, rules governing a system, behavioral patterns, and classification schemes [15]. The classic ML process begins with data acquisition, continues with feature extraction, algorithm selection, and model development, and leads to model evaluation and application [26] (Figure 1). Supervised and unsupervised learning are the most popular approaches employed in ML. Supervised learning is used to predict unknown outputs from a known labeled dataset, hypotheses, and appropriate algorithms, such as an artificial neural network (ANN), support vector machine (SVM), and K-nearest neighbor. The choice of the technique depends on the dataset's features, number of variables, learning curve, training, and computation time [27,28]. Specifically, supervised learning provides predictions from big data analytics but requires manually labeled datasets and biases that can arise from the dataset itself or the algorithms [24].

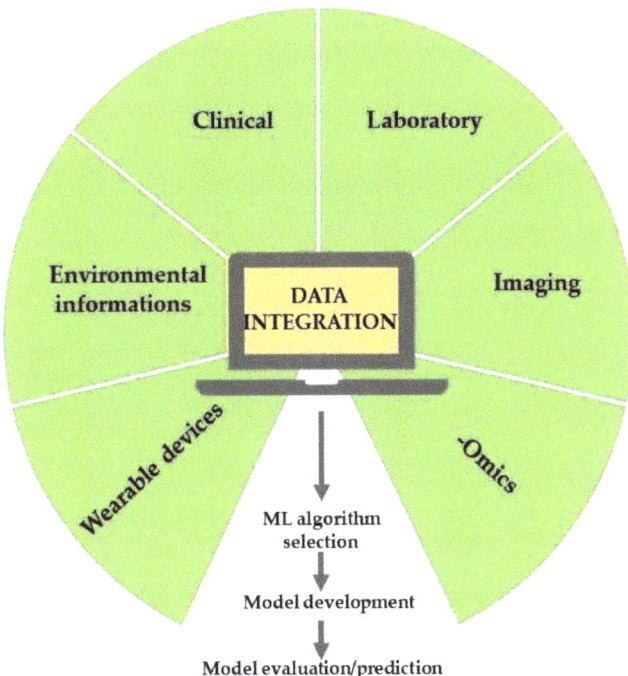

Figure 1. The typical ML workflow in healthcare research.

On the other hand, in unsupervised learning techniques, there is no information on the features to be predicted; consequently, these techniques must learn from the relationships among the elements of a dataset and classify them without basing them on categories or labels [22]. Therefore, they look for structures, patterns, or characteristics in the source data that can be reproduced in new datasets [15]. ML mainly mimics the nervous system's structure by creating ANNs, which are networks of units called artificial neurons structured into layers [29]. The system learns to generate patterns from data entered in the training session [29]. A specific ANN, consisting of more layers that allow for improved predictions from data, is known as a deep neural network (DNN). Its performance could be enhanced as the dimension of the training dataset rises [25]. Still, it largely depends on the distribution gap between training and test datasets: a highly divergent test dataset would test an ML prediction model on a feature space that it was not trained on, resulting in poor testing and results; additionally, a highly overlapping test dataset would not test the model for its generalization ability [30]. Specifically, DL employs algorithms such as DNNs and convolutional neural networks (CNNs) [15]. Nevertheless, regardless of its capability of using unlabeled datasets, unsupervised learning still has some limitations, such as the generalizability of cluster patterns identified from a cohort of patients, which can lead to overfitting to the training dataset, and the need to be validated in different large datasets [24]. In the real world, AI can provide tools to improve and extend the effectiveness of clinical interventions [15]. For example, incorporating AI into hypertension management could improve every stage of patient care, from diagnosis to therapy; consequently, the clinical practice could become more efficient and effective.

3. Methods

We conducted a detailed search on AI applications in AH. The research includes topics ranging from big data to complex technology-based interventions. Specifically, the articles reviewed in this paper were obtained by searching journal databases such as PubMed and subject-specific professional websites, including Google Scholar. The search terms included artificial intelligence, artificial neural network, deep learning, machine learning, big data, arterial hypertension, blood pressure, blood pressure measurement, CV disease, and personalized medicine. The inclusion criteria focus on articles directly or indirectly related to the topic of AI and AH. Specifically, both quantitative (measurable data) and qualitative (reasons, opinions, and motivations) reports were reviewed.

The authors independently screened titles and abstracts; subsequently, full texts were sourced for relevant articles. The reference lists of included trials and meta-analyses were also reviewed for significant articles.

4. AI in the Measurement of Blood Pressure

The commonly used methods for BP monitoring are either non-invasive inflatable cuff-based oscillometric or invasive arterial line manometric measurement. The former takes intermittent measures because a pause of at least 1–2 min between two BP measurements is necessary to avoid errors in the measurement [31,32]; moreover, the inflation of the cuff may disturb the patient, and the consequences of these disturbances are alterations in BP [33]. On the other hand, invasive arterial line manometric measurement has an elevated risk of complications; consequently, these unsolved issues drive the search for new non-invasive BP monitoring techniques.

In this scenario, AI algorithms could help improve precision, accuracy, and reproducibility in diagnosing and managing AH using emerging wearable technologies. Alternatives for monitoring BP are cuff-based devices (such as volume-clamp devices or wrist-worn inflatable cuffs) and cuffless devices that use mechanical and optical sensors to determine features of the blood pulse waveform shape (for example, tonometry [34], photoplethysmography [35], and capacitance [32]). In particular, cuffless blood pressure monitoring has been evaluated using a two-step algorithm with a single-channel photoplethysmograph (PPG). This system achieved an AAMI/ISO standard accuracy in all blood pressure categories except systolic hypotension [36]. Independently of the acquisition method, the received signals are preprocessed and sent for feature extraction and selection. Subsequently, the signals and the gathered data can be used to feed ML to obtain systolic BP (SBP) and diastolic BP (DBP) estimations from the raw signals [35] (Figure 2).

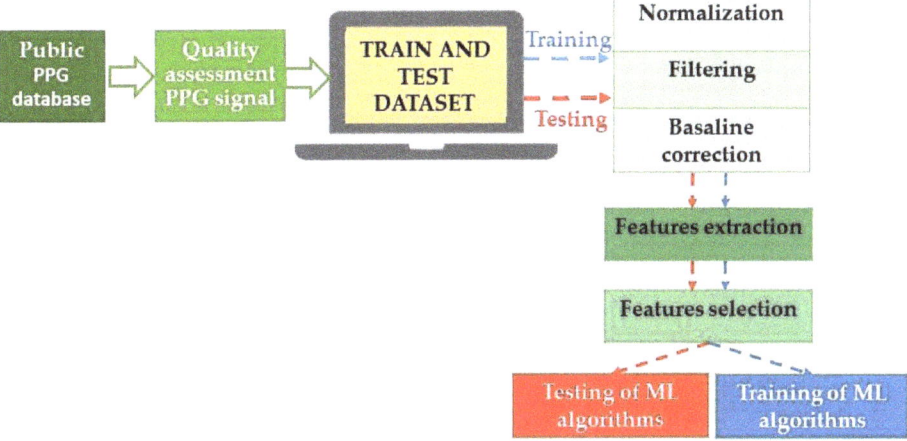

Figure 2. Block diagram of the blood pressure estimation process using ML techniques. In detail, the raw signals are prepared through normalization, the correction of baseline wandering due to respiration, and finally, signal filtration. Specifically, to construct a dataset for BP estimation models, it is necessary to accurately extract the features of the original waveform (and underlying demographic and statistical data) and select effective features, improving the generalization and reducing the risk of overfitting the algorithms. PPG: photoplethysmograph; ML: machine learning.

Since the volume and distension of arteries can be related to the pressure in the arteries, the PPG signal produces pulse waveforms that are similar to pressure waveforms created by tonometry. PPG offers the added advantage that it can be measured continuously using miniature, inexpensive, and wearable optical electronics [37]. However, PPG signal measurements are not without technical challenges; indeed, they require noise elimination, multisite measurement, multiphotodector development, event detection, event visualization, different models, the accurate positioning of sensors, and the calculation of propagation distances, without neglecting the impact of the variable PEP time on the pulse wave velocity timing [37]. Moreover, there are several PPG-based methods for estimating BP: the PPG signal alone and its derivate, ECG and PPG signals, BCG and PPG signals, and PCG and PPG signals; each has advantages and limitations [38–42], which, however, are beyond this discussion.

ML Algorithms in BP Estimation

To adapt to the nonlinearity of the dataset and to create a relationship between features and estimated BP, there are different ML approaches [43]:

1. Gaussian Process Regression: A Bayesian regression approach gives a probability distribution over all possible values [35,44].
2. Ensemble trees: The idea is to pull together a set of weak learners to create a strong learner [45].
3. Multivariate Linear Regression: It is a method to analyze the correlation, correlation direction, and strength between multiple independent variables and the dependent variable [33,46,47].

4. Support vector regression: It is a non-parametric algorithm that uses a kernel function (a class of algorithms for pattern analysis, whose general task is to find and study relations in datasets) [48–51].
5. Random forest, gradient boosting, and adaptive boosting regression [48,49].
6. CNN [52,53].

After hyper-parameter optimization, it is necessary to evaluate the performance of ML algorithms through the correlation between the acquired predicted data and the ground-truth data. The difference between reference and estimated BP could be considered using the following criteria: the mean absolute error, mean squared error, and correlation coefficient [35]. The role of parameter optimization is to lower the value of the predicted error. The mean absolute and standard deviations are the model's predictive performance indicators.

Specifically, these AI-based systems could help continuously monitor BP using wearable technologies and improve AH management and outcomes [33,50]. Starting from the input (raw signals), we can reach the output (estimated SBP and DBP) through the algorithms of ML [24]. In particular, BP can be estimated from a PPG signal obtained from a smartphone or a smartwatch by using DL [54,55].

Moreover, future studies on AI and wearable devices need to confirm the above results and provide conclusive clinical data to support using a combination of AI and wearable-device-obtained data to correctly perform BP measurements, which may offer an alternative to current oscillometric methods [24].

5. Use of AI for the Prediction of Undiagnosed Hypertension

AH is generally asymptomatic or variably occurs with symptoms such as headache, dizziness, tinnitus, and nosebleeds in a minority of patients. For this reason, it is not always possible to readily identify and predict this disease.

The goal should be to implement primary and secondary prevention methods. This task could greatly benefit AI implementation, featuring the individual identification of each patient's previous and new CV risk factors and treating modifiable risk factors. AI can predict the patient's risk of AH development thanks to different algorithm settings with big sets of data. Predicting AH onset has been attempted in the last decade with progressively greater precision thanks to technological advancements.

Accordingly, risk factors for AH, such as low levels of education, a sedentary job, a family history of AH, demographic data, routine blood tests, BMI, waist and hip circumference and ratio, diet, physical exercise, and salt and alcohol intake, showed effectiveness in predicting elevated SBP using ML techniques [56–58], for instance, an ANN [59]. On the other hand, AI techniques are also emerging in gene expression analysis; specifically, it is possible to improve AH predictive models by integrating data from a combination of gene expression and next-generation sequencing in ML analysis [60]. Furthermore, thanks to ML algorithms, it is possible to identify new hypertension genes; accordingly, Li et al. [61] analyzed gene expression in hypertensive patients, thus identifying 177 new hypertension genes thanks to ML algorithm development: this was then integrated with environmental factors in evaluating the risk of AH [53,62].

Furthermore, health risk prediction using a DL architecture appears suitable for extensive complex datasets, as shown by Maxwell et al. [63]. Using physical examination records of 110,300 patients, it was possible to examine, classify, and learn each risk factor contributing to chronic diseases such as AH, diabetes, and liver steatosis [63].

With the same principle, Ye et al. [56] validated an accurate 1-year risk prediction model for the incidence of essential AH. In this retrospective and prospective study, risk factors (type 2 diabetes, dyslipidemias, CV diseases, etc.) were calculated, evaluated, and stratified, yielding an accuracy of 91.7% for the prediction of the AH incidence at 1 year, with 87% in the prospective cohort (validation) [56].

Furthermore, the AI risk assessment of AH development can also benefit from cardiorespiratory fitness data obtained from treadmill exercise stress testing [64]. Overall, AI has the potential to increase efficacy by aggregating immense volumes of information, virtually predicting the risk of AH and consequently preventing or delaying the development of this disease by directing early interventions [24].

Making the AH diagnosis using validated guidelines [65,66] is an easy task for AI. Using inputs such as BP, comorbidities, demographic data, and routine blood tests, the accuracy can reach 92.85% with an ANN [67]. With a similar dataset (age, BP, BMI, serum lipoproteins profile, smoking habit, and exercise), using ML, the accuracy is estimated at 82% [68].

The most common example of AI for AH diagnosis, and probably still the most accurate, is twenty-four-hour ambulatory BP monitoring (ABPM) [69]. Thanks to direct and regular interval BP measurements and a relatively easy algorithm, ABPM software can identify and classify AH. ABPM is particularly useful in correctly evaluating white coats and masked AH [70,71].

New approaches based on ANNs try to estimate BP for AH diagnosis in healthy individuals using factors such as BMI, age, exercise, smoking, and alcohol consumption, although with limited accuracy and efficacy [68]. An interesting method for SBP prediction is the use of retinal fundus images. This factor was used by Poplin et al. [72], who showed that DL could be used in this case, even if the BP error was 11.23 mmHg, clearly not accurate enough to be of diagnostic use.

The ability of AI to diagnose AH is dependent on its accuracy. Further studies will identify more methods of BP prediction for the early diagnosis of AH and complication prevention. Looking at the world around us, AI's future in AH diagnosis and management probably lies in systems that can constantly retrieve vital signs, such as smartphones, smartwatches, and all of the relative accessories [73].

6. Targeting AH by AI

Optimizing pharmacological therapy to achieve the optimal control of BP levels represents a tough challenge for physicians. The management of AH is based on evidence-based medicine and expert opinions; BP control rates remain poor worldwide and are far from satisfactory across Europe [74].

Specifically, the importance of AI in this field is in the robust identification of modifiable factors that impact the evolution of AH; moreover, this new instrument could support the choice of the most appropriate management of AH. Indeed, most hypertensive patients need medication and lifestyle changes to achieve optimal BP control, and AI is helpful due to its better capability of identifying the best combination therapy compared to standard analysis [74].

Several works discussed and analyzed the opportunity of using AI to evaluate the impacts of different factors on BP values. Koren et al. applied ANN and decision trees to identify parameters contributing to Campo's success in his AH drug treatment [75]. Indeed, ML algorithms allow better real-world data analysis, identifying patterns and trends not easily recognized with classical experimental or observational approaches. Randomized trials usually compare the effectiveness of a drug to a placebo or, at best, to an already-approved compound. However, evaluating the differences between and advantages of drug combinations, frequently necessary for AH treatment, is a more complex task [75] that AI could fulfill. Here, we provide some previous experience and approaches; for example, the computer was presented with a training dataset in the first training phase, and for each instance, it was given the correct classification. Specifically, the appropriate classification of the algorithm was divided into two reference categories: "treatment success", defined as BP lower than 140/90 mmHg within 90 days after starting therapy, and "treatment failure" in any other case. Finally, AI decision trees and ANN compared various classes of antihypertensives in patients: beta-blockers alone or in combination were the most effective [75]. In another study, ML methods predicted individual treatment effects of intensive BP therapy [76]; notably, the results revealed an improvement in the discrimination and calibration of individualized medications from clinical trial data. Moreover, Ye X. et al. [77] demonstrated the potential of using predictive models to select optimal AH treatment pathways; specifically, along with clinical guidelines and guideline-based CDS systems, the LSTM models show the best prediction for achieving the optimal control of BP with different combinations of treatments. ML can also detect adherence to antihypertensive therapy by analyzing data recorded from a smartphone application to promote patients' awareness, self-monitoring, and treatment compliance [78].

Nonetheless, the exploitation of AI in the healthcare field is still in its early phases, and its potential is not entirely explored. Indeed, AI represents the opportunity for a global evaluation of the patient in his or her complexity because it allows the integration of clinical, demographic, biochemical, and instrumental data to develop models that physicians and healthcare providers could use to improve AH management and test new drug therapies using the multi-omics method [79,80].

We are now entering an era in which omics-based technology evolution will start to deliver long-promised elements that may improve the understanding of the complex mechanistic basis of this disease [79]. Accordingly, the key to better disease management will pass through personalized medicine. The key to this is future drug discovery that will be possible thanks to enhanced AI technologies exploiting information integration. Data from sequenced genomes, functional genomics, protein profiling, metabolomics, and bioinformatics may ensure a better comprehensive systems-based analysis for further understanding AH disease's complexities. Integrating AI with omics-based technologies will lead to the definition of the trajectory of the hypertensive patient and the use of the most appropriate drug.

In conclusion, AI can improve intelligent healthcare systems that provide personalized recommendations and treatment approaches [24].

7. Definition of the Hypertensive Patient's Trajectory: Role of AI in AH Prognosis

According to the recent AHA and ESC guidelines [74,81], the evaluation of the prognosis of AH is related to the demographic characteristics, the progression of organ injury, and comorbidities of the patients. Predicting the outcomes of hypertensive patients is significant research work [82].

There are currently several clinical risk scores intended for specific populations and risk groups [83–85]. Nevertheless, most of these scores are based on linear models and might therefore lack specificity and sensitivity in certain subgroups [86]. Moreover, the wide variety of scores may also cause slow adoption in real-world clinical practice [86].

The role of AI concerning the prognostic establishment of AH is due to the utility of ML algorithms trained on large datasets to estimate prognoses and potentially guide medical treatments [87].

The recent focus on AI and ML methods for AH prognosis is related to the critical repercussions of elevated BP for the risk of developing organ damage. Despite commonly used statistical methods, AI systems can process large amounts of complex data. Therefore, AI and ML aim to process a prognostic model that has clinical relevance in managing patients in the real world [88]. The prognostic impact of AH needs the stratification of patients based on their global evaluation with the integration of different parameters, such as the grade and stage of AH, BP control, and concomitant comorbidities. Indeed, AI can stratify patients correctly through the use of classification algorithms (SVM, C4.5 decision tree, random forest (RF), and extreme gradient boosting (XGBoost)); specifically, XGBoost has the best prediction performance [82].

However, the accuracy of the definition of the individual trajectory can be enhanced by a prolonged follow-up [89] and an increase in the number of relevant features, such as genomic variants associated with specific hypertensive phenotypes and different outcomes [61,90].

Moreover, the prognosis determines the frequency and the type of clinical monitoring. Specifically, AI allows the elaboration of new risk stratification to develop novel prognostic layers in favor of personalized medicine with the prospect of efficiently measuring the grade classification of AH [91] and identifying different outcomes' profiles [89]. In conclusion, the clinical advantages of implementing AI systems and their integration into current prognostic stratification might grant the correct identification of classes of outcomes of patients, improving their clinical management.

8. AI in Secondary Arterial Hypertension

The causes of hypertension are multiple, and we must not overlook secondary arterial hypertension; indeed, in 10–15% of cases, the specific cause underlying hypertension can be identified [92]. Specifically, to arrive at the diagnosis of essential hypertension, all causes of secondary hypertension must be ruled out, and the accurate history, thorough examination, and performance of all necessary tests based on the data collected always place the physician and his or her knowledge of internal medicine at the basis of the evaluation of each hypertensive patient. Consequently, diagnosis and patient management must be connected to the clinician, who can use AI to speed up and facilitate his or her task. In any case, AI and ML cannot wholly replace the doctor's role, but they represent a useful tool in his hands. Identifying secondary hypertension in its various subtypes is essential to preventing and targeting the treatment of CV complications. However, screening for secondary hypertension can be time-consuming, expensive, and difficult; consequently, simplified diagnostic tests are urgently required to distinguish between primary and secondary hypertension to address the current underdiagnosis of the latter. In children and adolescents, the most common causes of hypertension are renal parenchymal or vascular disease and aortic coarctation [93]; in adults, earlier studies identified renal parenchymal and vascular diseases as the most common causes of secondary hypertension. Obstructive sleep apnea (OSA) was recognized as an exceedingly common cause of secondary hypertension [94]. Among endocrine causes, we include primary aldosteronism (the most common), thyroid disease (hypo- or hyperthyroidism), hypercortisolism (Cushing's), and finally, phaeochromocytoma [92]. The application of ML methods to the etiological diagnosis of secondary hypertension can be helpful in clinical practice. Accordingly, AI technology should be implemented cautiously; to be a partner of clinicians, there is still a long way to go, but it can serve as a virtual assistant and enable clinicians to promote quality and increase efficiency. Based on EMRs from Fuwai Hospital, five ML prediction models with good performance and applicability to the etiology detection of secondary hypertension were developed by Campo [95], which demonstrated that ML approaches were feasible and effective in diagnosing secondary hypertension. Reel and colleagues [95] showed that the MOmics approach provided better discriminatory power compared to single-omics (monoomics) data analysis and appropriately classified different forms of endocrine hypertension with high sensitivity and specificity, providing potential diagnostic biomarker combinations for diagnosing secondary hypertension subtypes. However, there still needs to be more data in the literature on the application of AI in the field of secondary hypertension; consequently, these innovative and clinically relevant prediction models still require further validation and more clinical tests before being implemented into clinical practice.

9. Limitations of Applying ML in CV Research

Despite the great importance that AI has taken on in the last few years, it is necessary to underline that this system is not free from technical issues and biases (Table S5). The quality of the algorithms underlying AI technology can be affected by some limitations, such as the inconsistent quality of the studies that form the databases at the heart of AI [96].

Specifically, overfitting is a significant issue common to all ML models: this happens when a model has become overly attuned to the training data, such that it does not generalize to new datasets; this is the opposite of underfitting, where the algorithm cannot wholly capture the predictive power of the data. These two issues (over- and underfitting) could be solved by improving the parameters of the model or making modifications to the training set [21].

Moreover, it is also essential to consider the adversarial robustness of a model (ability to resist being fooled), which could be improved by enlarging the training set [97].

Furthermore, many clinicians remain wary of ML because of concerns about the "black-box" nature of many ML algorithms. These models are sufficiently complex that they are not directly interpretable to humans. Subsequently, the lack of interpretability of predictive models can undermine trust in those models, especially in the medical field, in which so many decisions are life-and-death issues [98]. To be trusted, users must comprehend the model outputs [98]. Consequently, the "explainability" technique in ML seeks to imbue humans with a high level of understanding of how an algorithm works and makes decisions without carefully considering each step [99]; however, the nature of explanations as approximations may omit important information about how black-box models work and why they make specific predictions [100].

Another flaw is the lack of discernment of predisposing factors for specific CV diseases from confounding factors. Moreover, it is also possible that, during data analysis processes by specialized clinicians, some may contribute to lowering the accuracy of the databases owing to their biases, thus making their validation even more time-consuming [28].

It would also be necessary for some AI-automated diagnostic CV algorithms to identify CV risk factors that are essential but still not unanimously recognized since, sometimes, there is no consensus among cardiologists. Therefore, it would be desirable to validate data through a clinical consensus before merging them into the AI, though expensive and time-consuming. Another important aspect is the disparity between various racial groups, ethnic minorities, and social classes. Some CV diseases are more represented in some races and/or ethnic minorities and can express themselves with different phenotypes [101].

Prospectively, it will be necessary to render AI accessible to patients and promote awareness, self-monitoring, healthy behaviors, and therapeutic adherence by integrating new technologies, such as wearable devices that can automatically analyze activity levels and give feedback, such as lifestyle and drug dose changes [24].

10. Conclusions

The study of AH needs a revolution, and its future may lie in the favorable convergence of digital data and biotechnological and biomedical sciences and their implementation in healthcare delivery with new delivery models and effective strategies for population health. With AI, we could better understand epigenetic changes relevant to AH onset and progression, potentially classify the risk of AH in individuals, identify the mechanism of poorly controlled AH, and evaluate treatment responses in clinical trials using a multi-omics approach [102]. Furthermore, AI could target healthy individuals who are at higher risk of developing AH and may benefit from lifestyle modifications for the primary prevention of CV disease [24].

In conclusion, AH prediction and management using a combination of AI and wearable technology could potentially be the first real chance for precision CV medicine [102]. Moreover, future AI-enhanced AH care will encourage patient awareness, self-monitoring, healthy behaviors, and treatment adherence, along with developing digital technologies [24]. Therefore, future research needs to focus on precision AH medicine utilizing AI-based technologies to reduce the global burden of AH without neglecting the significant limitations that this approach still has.

Supplementary Materials: The following supporting information can be downloaded at https://www.mdpi.com/article/10.3390/jcdd10020074/s1. Table S1: Major contributions of AI in AH measurement. Table S2: Major contributions of AI in AH prediction and diagnosis. Table S3: Major contributions of AI in AH treatment. Table S4: Major contributions of AI in AH outcome. Table S5: Limitations of applying ML in cardiovascular research Supplementary References [34,35,51,56–61,63,64,68,75–77,82,89,90,103].

Author Contributions: Conceptualization, V.V. and M.C.; data curation, V.V., M.C., C.I., A.R., M.T., A.G., B.S., A.M., M.R.R. and P.D.P.; writing—original draft preparation, V.V., M.C., C.I., A.R., M.T., N.V., R.G., A.G., A.C. and C.V.; writing—review and editing, V.V., M.C., C.I., C.M., G.D., A.B., G.G. and C.V.; supervision, V.V. and M.C. All authors have read and agreed to the published version of the manuscript.

Funding: This work was funded by the project "SOLOMAX—SOciaLNetwOrk of MedicAlEXperiences" (to MC) from the Italian Ministry of Economic Development (MISE).

Institutional Review Board Statement: Not applicable.

Informed Consent Statement: Not applicable.

Data Availability Statement: Not applicable.

Conflicts of Interest: The authors declare no conflict of interest.

References

1. Sorriento, D.; Rusciano, M.R.; Visco, V.; Fiordelisi, A.; Cerasuolo, F.A.; Poggio, P.; Ciccarelli, M.; Iaccarino, G. The Metabolic Role of GRK2 in Insulin Resistance and Associated Conditions. *Cells* **2021**, *10*, 167. [CrossRef]
2. Visco, V.; Finelli, R.; Pascale, A.V.; Giannotti, R.; Fabbricatore, D.; Ragosa, N.; Ciccarelli, M.; Iaccarino, G. Larger Blood Pressure Reduction by Fixed-Dose Compared to Free Dose Combination Therapy of ACE Inhibitor and Calcium Antagonist in Hypertensive Patients. *Transl. Med. UniSa* **2017**, *16*, 17–23.
3. NCD Risk Factor Collaboration. Worldwide trends in blood pressure from 1975 to 2015: A pooled analysis of 1479 population-based measurement studies with 19.1 million participants. *Lancet* **2017**, *389*, 37–55. [CrossRef]
4. Izzo, C.; Vitillo, P.; Di Pietro, P.; Visco, V.; Strianese, A.; Virtuoso, N.; Ciccarelli, M.; Galasso, G.; Carrizzo, A.; Vecchione, C. The Role of Oxidative Stress in Cardiovascular Aging and Cardiovascular Diseases. *Life* **2021**, *11*, 60. [CrossRef]
5. Whitworth, J.A.; World Health Organization; International Society of Hypertension Writing Group. 2003 World Health Organization (WHO)/International Society of Hypertension (ISH) statement on management of hypertension. *J. Hypertens.* **2003**, *21*, 1983–1992. [CrossRef]
6. Pereira da Silva, A.; Matos, A.; Aguiar, L.; Ramos-Marques, N.; Ribeiro, R.; Gil, A.; Gorjao-Clara, J.; Bicho, M. Hypertension and longevity: Role of genetic polymorphisms in renin-angiotensin-aldosterone system and endothelial nitric oxide synthase. *Mol. Cell Biochem.* **2019**, *455*, 61–71. [CrossRef]
7. Wall, H.K.; Ritchey, M.D.; Gillespie, C.; Omura, J.D.; Jamal, A.; George, M.G. Vital Signs: Prevalence of Key Cardiovascular Disease Risk Factors for Million Hearts 2022—United States, 2011–2016. *MMWR Morb. Mortal Wkly. Rep.* **2018**, *67*, 983–991. [CrossRef]
8. O'Brien, E.; Asmar, R.; Beilin, L.; Imai, Y.; Mancia, G.; Mengden, T.; Myers, M.; Padfield, P.; Palatini, P.; Parati, G.; et al. Practice guidelines of the European Society of Hypertension for clinic, ambulatory and self blood pressure measurement. *J. Hypertens.* **2005**, *23*, 697–701. [CrossRef]
9. Visco, V.; Pascale, A.V.; Virtuoso, N.; Mongiello, F.; Cinque, F.; Gioia, R.; Finelli, R.; Mazzeo, P.; Manzi, M.V.; Morisco, C.; et al. Serum Uric Acid and Left Ventricular Mass in Essential Hypertension. *Front. Cardiovasc. Med.* **2020**, *7*, 570000. [CrossRef]
10. Dzau, V.J.; Balatbat, C.A. Future of Hypertension. *Hypertension* **2019**, *74*, 450–457. [CrossRef]
11. De Luca, V.; Tramontano, G.; Riccio, L.; Trama, U.; Buono, P.; Losasso, M.; Bracale, U.M.; Annuzzi, G.; Zampetti, R.; Cacciatore, F.; et al. "One Health" Approach for Health Innovation and Active Aging in Campania (Italy). *Front. Public Health* **2021**, *9*, 658959. [CrossRef]
12. Visco, V.; Finelli, R.; Pascale, A.V.; Mazzeo, P.; Ragosa, N.; Trimarco, V.; Illario, M.; Ciccarelli, M.; Iaccarino, G. Difficult-to-control hypertension: Identification of clinical predictors and use of ICT-based integrated care to facilitate blood pressure control. *J. Hum. Hypertens.* **2018**, *32*, 467–476. [CrossRef]
13. Visco, V.; Esposito, C.; Manzo, M.; Fiorentino, A.; Galasso, G.; Vecchione, C.; Ciccarelli, M. A Multistep Approach to Deal With Advanced Heart Failure: A Case Report on the Positive Effect of Cardiac Contractility Modulation Therapy on Pulmonary Pressure Measured by CardioMEMS. *Front. Cardiovasc. Med.* **2022**, *9*, 874433. [CrossRef]
14. Visco, V.; Esposito, C.; Vitillo, P.; Vecchione, C.; Ciccarelli, M. It is easy to see, but it is better to foresee: A case report on the favourable alliance between CardioMEMS and levosimendan. *Eur. Heart J. Case Rep.* **2020**, *4*, 1–5. [CrossRef]
15. Visco, V.; Ferruzzi, G.J.; Nicastro, F.; Virtuoso, N.; Carrizzo, A.; Galasso, G.; Vecchione, C.; Ciccarelli, M. Artificial Intelligence as a Business Partner in Cardiovascular Precision Medicine: An Emerging Approach for Disease Detection and Treatment Optimization. *Curr. Med. Chem.* **2020**, *28*, 6569–6590. [CrossRef]
16. Zhou, J.; Lee, S.; Wong, W.T.; Waleed, K.B.; Leung, K.S.K.; Lee, T.T.L.; Wai, A.K.C.; Liu, T.; Chang, C.; Cheung, B.M.Y.; et al. Gender-specific clinical risk scores incorporating blood pressure variability for predicting incident dementia. *J. Am. Med. Inform. Assoc.* **2022**, *29*, 335–347. [CrossRef]
17. Tian, X.; Fang, H.; Lan, L.; Ip, H.L.; Abrigo, J.; Liu, H.; Zheng, L.; Fan, F.S.Y.; Ma, S.H.; Ip, B.; et al. Risk stratification in symptomatic intracranial atherosclerotic disease with conventional vascular risk factors and cerebral haemodynamics. *Stroke Vasc. Neurol.* **2022**, svn-2022-001606. [CrossRef]
18. Leng, X.; Lan, L.; Ip, V.H.L.; Liu, H.; Abrigo, J.; Liebeskind, D.S.; Wong, L.K.S.; Leung, T.W. Noninvasive fractional flow in intracranial atherosclerotic stenosis: Reproducibility, limitations, and perspectives. *J. Neurol. Sci.* **2017**, *381*, 150–152. [CrossRef]
19. Zhong, L.; Zhang, J.M.; Su, B.; Tan, R.S.; Allen, J.C.; Kassab, G.S. Application of Patient-Specific Computational Fluid Dynamics in Coronary and Intra-Cardiac Flow Simulations: Challenges and Opportunities. *Front. Physiol.* **2018**, *9*, 742. [CrossRef]

20. Wang, X.; Liu, H.; Xu, M.; Chen, C.; Ma, L.; Dai, F. Efficacy assessment of superficial temporal artery-middle cerebral artery bypass surgery in treating moyamoya disease from a hemodynamic perspective: A pilot study using computational modeling and perfusion imaging. *Acta Neurochir.* 2023. [CrossRef]
21. Padmanabhan, S.; Tran, T.Q.B.; Dominiczak, A.F. Artificial Intelligence in Hypertension: Seeing Through a Glass Darkly. *Circ. Res.* 2021, 128, 1100–1118. [CrossRef]
22. Dorado-Diaz, P.I.; Sampedro-Gomez, J.; Vicente-Palacios, V.; Sanchez, P.L. Applications of Artificial Intelligence in Cardiology. The Future is Already Here. *Rev. Esp. Cardiol. Engl. Ed.* 2019, 72, 1065–1075. [CrossRef]
23. Bonderman, D. Artificial intelligence in cardiology. *Wien. Klin. Wochenschr.* 2017, 129, 866–868. [CrossRef]
24. Chaikijurajai, T.; Laffin, L.J.; Tang, W.H.W. Artificial Intelligence and Hypertension: Recent Advances and Future Outlook. *Am. J. Hypertens.* 2020, 33, 967–974. [CrossRef]
25. Schmidt-Erfurth, U.; Sadeghipour, A.; Gerendas, B.S.; Waldstein, S.M.; Bogunovic, H. Artificial intelligence in retina. *Prog. Retin. Eye Res.* 2018, 67, 1–29. [CrossRef]
26. Johnson, K.W.; Torres Soto, J.; Glicksberg, B.S.; Shameer, K.; Miotto, R.; Ali, M.; Ashley, E.; Dudley, J.T. Artificial Intelligence in Cardiology. *J. Am. Coll. Cardiol.* 2018, 71, 2668–2679. [CrossRef]
27. Bzdok, D.; Krzywinski, M.; Altman, N. Machine learning: Supervised methods. *Nat. Methods* 2018, 15, 5–6. [CrossRef]
28. Krittanawong, C.; Zhang, H.; Wang, Z.; Aydar, M.; Kitai, T. Artificial Intelligence in Precision Cardiovascular Medicine. *J. Am. Coll. Cardiol.* 2017, 69, 2657–2664. [CrossRef]
29. Ahuja, A.S. The impact of artificial intelligence in medicine on the future role of the physician. *PeerJ* 2019, 7, e7702. [CrossRef]
30. Turhan, B. On the dataset shift problem in software engineering prediction models. *Empir. Softw. Eng.* 2012, 17, 62–75. [CrossRef]
31. Campbell, N.R.; Chockalingam, A.; Fodor, J.G.; McKay, D.W. Accurate, reproducible measurement of blood pressure. *CMAJ* 1990, 143, 19–24.
32. Quan, X.; Liu, J.; Roxlo, T.; Siddharth, S.; Leong, W.; Muir, A.; Cheong, S.M.; Rao, A. Advances in Non-Invasive Blood Pressure Monitoring. *Sensors* 2021, 21, 4273. [CrossRef]
33. Gesche, H.; Grosskurth, D.; Kuchler, G.; Patzak, A. Continuous blood pressure measurement by using the pulse transit time: Comparison to a cuff-based method. *Eur. J. Appl. Physiol.* 2012, 112, 309–315. [CrossRef]
34. Huang, K.H.; Tan, F.; Wang, T.D.; Yang, Y.J. A Highly Sensitive Pressure-Sensing Array for Blood Pressure Estimation Assisted by Machine-Learning Techniques. *Sensors* 2019, 19, 848. [CrossRef]
35. Chowdhury, M.H.; Shuzan, M.N.I.; Chowdhury, M.E.H.; Mahbub, Z.B.; Uddin, M.M.; Khandakar, A.; Reaz, M.B.I. Estimating Blood Pressure from the Photoplethysmogram Signal and Demographic Features Using Machine Learning Techniques. *Sensors* 2020, 20, 3127. [CrossRef]
36. Khalid, S.; Liu, H.; Zia, T.; Zhang, J.; Chen, F.; Zheng, D. Cuffless Blood Pressure Estimation Using Single Channel Photoplethysmography: A Two-Step Method. *IEEE Access* 2020, 8, 58146–58154. [CrossRef]
37. Elgendi, M.; Fletcher, R.; Liang, Y.; Howard, N.; Lovell, N.H.; Abbott, D.; Lim, K.; Ward, R. The use of photoplethysmography for assessing hypertension. *NPJ Digit. Med.* 2019, 2, 60. [CrossRef]
38. Zheng, Y.; Poon, C.C.; Yan, B.P.; Lau, J.Y. Pulse Arrival Time Based Cuff-Less and 24-H Wearable Blood Pressure Monitoring and its Diagnostic Value in Hypertension. *J. Med. Syst.* 2016, 40, 195. [CrossRef]
39. Pandian, P.S.; Mohanavelu, K.; Safeer, K.P.; Kotresh, T.M.; Shakunthala, D.T.; Gopal, P.; Padaki, V.C. Smart Vest: Wearable multi-parameter remote physiological monitoring system. *Med. Eng. Phys.* 2008, 30, 466–477. [CrossRef]
40. Plante, T.B.; Urrea, B.; MacFarlane, Z.T.; Blumenthal, R.S.; Miller, E.R., 3rd; Appel, L.J.; Martin, S.S. Validation of the Instant Blood Pressure Smartphone App. *JAMA Intern. Med.* 2016, 176, 700–702. [CrossRef]
41. Zhang, Q.; Zhou, D.; Zeng, X. Highly wearable cuff-less blood pressure and heart rate monitoring with single-arm electrocardiogram and photoplethysmogram signals. *Biomed. Eng. Online* 2017, 16, 23. [CrossRef]
42. Radha, M.; de Groot, K.; Rajani, N.; Wong, C.C.P.; Kobold, N.; Vos, V.; Fonseca, P.; Mastellos, N.; Wark, P.A.; Velthoven, N.; et al. Estimating blood pressure trends and the nocturnal dip from photoplethysmography. *Physiol. Meas.* 2019, 40, 025006. [CrossRef]
43. Hare, A.J.; Chokshi, N.; Adusumalli, S. Novel Digital Technologies for Blood Pressure Monitoring and Hypertension Management. *Curr. Cardiovasc. Risk Rep.* 2021, 15, 11. [CrossRef]
44. Nour, M.; Kandaz, D.; Ucar, M.K.; Polat, K.; Alhudhaif, A. Machine Learning and Electrocardiography Signal-Based Minimum Calculation Time Detection for Blood Pressure Detection. *Comput. Math. Methods Med.* 2022, 2022, 5714454. [CrossRef]
45. Kumar, P.S.; Rai, P.; Ramasamy, M.; Varadan, V.K.; Varadan, V.K. Multiparametric cloth-based wearable, SimpleSense, estimates blood pressure. *Sci. Rep.* 2022, 12, 13059. [CrossRef]
46. Mase, M.; Mattei, W.; Cucino, R.; Faes, L.; Nollo, G. Feasibility of cuff-free measurement of systolic and diastolic arterial blood pressure. *J. Electrocardiol.* 2011, 44, 201–207. [CrossRef]
47. Park, M.; Kang, H.; Huh, Y.; Kim, K.C. Cuffless and noninvasive measurement of systolic blood pressure, diastolic blood pressure, mean arterial pressure and pulse pressure using radial artery tonometry pressure sensor with concept of Korean traditional medicine. *Annu. Int. Conf. IEEE Eng. Med. Biol. Soc.* 2007, 2007, 3597–3600. [CrossRef]
48. Kachuee, M.; Kiani, M.M.; Mohammadzade, H.; Shabany, M. Cuffless Blood Pressure Estimation Algorithms for Continuous Health-Care Monitoring. *IEEE Trans. Biomed. Eng.* 2017, 64, 859–869. [CrossRef]
49. Monte-Moreno, E. Non-invasive estimate of blood glucose and blood pressure from a photoplethysmograph by means of machine learning techniques. *Artif. Intell. Med.* 2011, 53, 127–138. [CrossRef]

50. Peng, R.C.; Yan, W.R.; Zhang, N.L.; Lin, W.H.; Zhou, X.L.; Zhang, Y.T. Cuffless and Continuous Blood Pressure Estimation from the Heart Sound Signals. *Sensors* **2015**, *15*, 23653–23666. [CrossRef]
51. Khalid, S.G.; Zhang, J.; Chen, F.; Zheng, D. Blood Pressure Estimation Using Photoplethysmography Only: Comparison between Different Machine Learning Approaches. *J. Healthc. Eng.* **2018**, *2018*, 1548647. [CrossRef]
52. Yan, C.; Li, Z.; Zhao, W.; Hu, J.; Jia, D.; Wang, H.; You, T. Novel Deep Convolutional Neural Network for Cuff-less Blood Pressure Measurement Using ECG and PPG Signals. *Annu. Int. Conf. IEEE Eng. Med. Biol. Soc.* **2019**, *2019*, 1917–1920. [CrossRef]
53. Rastegar, S.; Gholamhosseini, H.; Lowe, A.; Mehdipour, F.; Linden, M. Estimating Systolic Blood Pressure Using Convolutional Neural Networks. *Stud. Health Technol. Inform.* **2019**, *261*, 143–149.
54. Tison, G.H.; Singh, A.C.; Ohashi, D.A.; Hsieh, J.T.; Ballinger, B.M.; Olgin, J.E.; Marcus, G.M.; Pletcher, M.J. Abstract 21042: Cardiovascular Risk Stratification Using Off-the-Shelf Wearables and a Multi-Task Deep Learning Algorithm. *Circulation* **2017**, *136*, A21042. [CrossRef]
55. Banerjee, R.; Choudhury, A.D.; Sinha, A.; Visvanathan, A. HeartSense: Smart phones to estimate blood pressure from photoplethysmography. In Proceedings of the 12th ACM Conference on Embedded Network Sensor Systems, Memphis, TN, USA, 3–6 November 2014.
56. Ye, C.; Fu, T.; Hao, S.; Zhang, Y.; Wang, O.; Jin, B.; Xia, M.; Liu, M.; Zhou, X.; Wu, Q.; et al. Prediction of Incident Hypertension Within the Next Year: Prospective Study Using Statewide Electronic Health Records and Machine Learning. *J. Med. Internet Res.* **2018**, *20*, e22. [CrossRef]
57. Kanegae, H.; Suzuki, K.; Fukatani, K.; Ito, T.; Harada, N.; Kario, K. Highly precise risk prediction model for new-onset hypertension using artificial intelligence techniques. *J. Clin. Hypertens.* **2020**, *22*, 445–450. [CrossRef]
58. Golino, H.F.; Amaral, L.S.; Duarte, S.F.; Gomes, C.M.; Soares Tde, J.; Dos Reis, L.A.; Santos, J. Predicting increased blood pressure using machine learning. *J. Obes.* **2014**, *2014*, 637635. [CrossRef]
59. Huang, S.; Xu, Y.; Yue, L.; Wei, S.; Liu, L.; Gan, X.; Zhou, S.; Nie, S. Evaluating the risk of hypertension using an artificial neural network method in rural residents over the age of 35 years in a Chinese area. *Hypertens. Res.* **2010**, *33*, 722–726. [CrossRef]
60. Held, E.; Cape, J.; Tintle, N. Comparing machine learning and logistic regression methods for predicting hypertension using a combination of gene expression and next-generation sequencing data. *BMC Proc.* **2016**, *10*, 141–145. [CrossRef]
61. Li, Y.H.; Zhang, G.G.; Wang, N. Systematic Characterization and Prediction of Human Hypertension Genes. *Hypertension* **2017**, *69*, 349–355. [CrossRef]
62. Pei, Z.; Liu, J.; Liu, M.; Zhou, W.; Yan, P.; Wen, S.; Chen, Y. Risk-Predicting Model for Incident of Essential Hypertension Based on Environmental and Genetic Factors with Support Vector Machine. *Interdiscip. Sci.* **2018**, *10*, 126–130. [CrossRef]
63. Maxwell, A.; Li, R.; Yang, B.; Weng, H.; Ou, A.; Hong, H.; Zhou, Z.; Gong, P.; Zhang, C. Deep learning architectures for multi-label classification of intelligent health risk prediction. *BMC Bioinform.* **2017**, *18*, 523. [CrossRef]
64. Sakr, S.; Elshawi, R.; Ahmed, A.; Qureshi, W.T.; Brawner, C.; Keteyian, S.; Blaha, M.J.; Al-Mallah, M.H. Using machine learning on cardiorespiratory fitness data for predicting hypertension: The Henry Ford ExercIse Testing (FIT) Project. *PLoS ONE* **2018**, *13*, e0195344. [CrossRef]
65. Fernandes, M.; Olde Rikkert, M.G.M. The new US and European guidelines in hypertension: A multi-dimensional analysis. *Contemp. Clin. Trials* **2019**, *81*, 44–54. [CrossRef]
66. McCormack, T.; Boffa, R.J.; Jones, N.R.; Carville, S.; McManus, R.J. The 2018 ESC/ESH hypertension guideline and the 2019 NICE hypertension guideline, how and why they differ. *Eur. Heart J.* **2019**, *40*, 3456–3458. [CrossRef]
67. Diciolla, M.; Binetti, G.; Di Noia, T.; Pesce, F.; Schena, F.P.; Vagane, A.M.; Bjorneklett, R.; Suzuki, H.; Tomino, Y.; Naso, D. Patient classification and outcome prediction in IgA nephropathy. *Comput. Biol. Med.* **2015**, *66*, 278–286. [CrossRef]
68. Lafrenière, D.; Zulkernine, F.H.; Barber, D.; Martin, K. Using machine learning to predict hypertension from a clinical dataset. In Proceedings of the IEEE Symposium Series on Computational Intelligence (SSCI), Athens, Greece, 6–9 December 2016; pp. 1–7.
69. Hermida, R.C.; Smolensky, M.H.; Ayala, D.E.; Portaluppi, F. Ambulatory Blood Pressure Monitoring (ABPM) as the reference standard for diagnosis of hypertension and assessment of vascular risk in adults. *Chronobiol. Int.* **2015**, *32*, 1329–1342. [CrossRef]
70. Pierdomenico, S.D.; Cuccurullo, F. Prognostic value of white-coat and masked hypertension diagnosed by ambulatory monitoring in initially untreated subjects: An updated meta analysis. *Am. J. Hypertens.* **2011**, *24*, 52–58. [CrossRef]
71. Asayama, K.; Thijs, L.; Li, Y.; Gu, Y.M.; Hara, A.; Liu, Y.P.; Zhang, Z.; Wei, F.F.; Lujambio, I.; Mena, L.J.; et al. Setting thresholds to varying blood pressure monitoring intervals differentially affects risk estimates associated with white-coat and masked hypertension in the population. *Hypertension* **2014**, *64*, 935–942. [CrossRef]
72. Poplin, R.; Varadarajan, A.V.; Blumer, K.; Liu, Y.; McConnell, M.V.; Corrado, G.S.; Peng, L.; Webster, D.R. Prediction of cardiovascular risk factors from retinal fundus photographs via deep learning. *Nat. Biomed. Eng.* **2018**, *2*, 158–164. [CrossRef]
73. Persell, S.D.; Peprah, Y.A.; Lipiszko, D.; Lee, J.Y.; Li, J.J.; Ciolino, J.D.; Karmali, K.N.; Sato, H. Effect of Home Blood Pressure Monitoring via a Smartphone Hypertension Coaching Application or Tracking Application on Adults With Uncontrolled Hypertension: A Randomized Clinical Trial. *JAMA Netw. Open* **2020**, *3*, e200255. [CrossRef]
74. Williams, B.; Mancia, G.; Spiering, W.; Agabiti Rosei, E.; Azizi, M.; Burnier, M.; Clement, D.L.; Coca, A.; de Simone, G.; Dominiczak, A.; et al. 2018 ESC/ESH Guidelines for the management of arterial hypertension. *Eur. Heart J.* **2018**, *39*, 3021–3104. [CrossRef]
75. Koren, G.; Nordon, G.; Radinsky, K.; Shalev, V. Machine learning of big data in gaining insight into successful treatment of hypertension. *Pharmacol. Res. Perspect.* **2018**, *6*, e00396. [CrossRef]

76. Duan, T.; Rajpurkar, P.; Laird, D.; Ng, A.Y.; Basu, S. Clinical Value of Predicting Individual Treatment Effects for Intensive Blood Pressure Therapy. *Circ. Cardiovasc. Qual. Outcomes* **2019**, *12*, e005010. [CrossRef]
77. Ye, X.; Zeng, Q.T.; Facelli, J.C.; Brixner, D.I.; Conway, M.; Bray, B.E. Predicting Optimal Hypertension Treatment Pathways Using Recurrent Neural Networks. *Int. J. Med. Inform.* **2020**, *139*, 104122. [CrossRef]
78. da Silva, V.J.; da Silva Souza, V.; Guimaraes da Cruz, R.; Mesquita Vidal Martinez de Lucena, J.; Jazdi, N.; Ferreira de Lucena Junior, V. Commercial Devices-Based System Designed to Improve the Treatment Adherence of Hypertensive Patients. *Sensors* **2019**, *19*, 4539. [CrossRef]
79. Matthews, H.; Hanison, J.; Nirmalan, N. "Omics"-Informed Drug and Biomarker Discovery: Opportunities, Challenges and Future Perspectives. *Proteomes* **2016**, *4*, 28. [CrossRef]
80. Monte, A.A.; Vasiliou, V.; Heard, K.J. Omics Screening for Pharmaceutical Efficacy and Safety in Clinical Practice. *J. Pharm. Pharm.* **2012**, *S5*, 001. [CrossRef]
81. Unger, T.; Borghi, C.; Charchar, F.; Khan, N.A.; Poulter, N.R.; Prabhakaran, D.; Ramirez, A.; Schlaich, M.; Stergiou, G.S.; Tomaszewski, M.; et al. 2020 International Society of Hypertension global hypertension practice guidelines. *J. Hypertens.* **2020**, *38*, 982–1004. [CrossRef]
82. Chang, W.; Liu, Y.; Xiao, Y.; Yuan, X.; Xu, X.; Zhang, S.; Zhou, S. A Machine-Learning-Based Prediction Method for Hypertension Outcomes Based on Medical Data. *Diagnostics* **2019**, *9*, 178. [CrossRef]
83. SCORE2-OP Working Group; ESC Cardiovascular Risk Collaboration. SCORE2-OP risk prediction algorithms: Estimating incident cardiovascular event risk in older persons in four geographical risk regions. *Eur. Heart J.* **2021**, *42*, 2455–2467. [CrossRef]
84. Crea, F. The new SCORE2 risk prediction algorithms and the growing challenge of risk factors not captured by traditional risk scores. *Eur. Heart J.* **2021**, *42*, 2403–2407. [CrossRef]
85. Conroy, R.M.; Pyorala, K.; Fitzgerald, A.P.; Sans, S.; Menotti, A.; De Backer, G.; De Bacquer, D.; Ducimetiere, P.; Jousilahti, P.; Keil, U.; et al. Estimation of ten-year risk of fatal cardiovascular disease in Europe: The SCORE project. *Eur. Heart J.* **2003**, *24*, 987–1003. [CrossRef]
86. Sabovcik, F.; Ntalianis, E.; Cauwenberghs, N.; Kuznetsova, T. Improving predictive performance in incident heart failure using machine learning and multi-center data. *Front. Cardiovasc. Med.* **2022**, *9*, 1011071. [CrossRef]
87. Diller, G.P.; Kempny, A.; Babu-Narayan, S.V.; Henrichs, M.; Brida, M.; Uebing, A.; Lammers, A.E.; Baumgartner, H.; Li, W.; Wort, S.J.; et al. Machine learning algorithms estimating prognosis and guiding therapy in adult congenital heart disease: Data from a single tertiary centre including 10 019 patients. *Eur. Heart J.* **2019**, *40*, 1069–1077. [CrossRef]
88. Santhanam, P.; Ahima, R.S. Machine learning and blood pressure. *J. Clin. Hypertens.* **2019**, *21*, 1735–1737. [CrossRef]
89. Wu, X.; Yuan, X.; Wang, W.; Liu, K.; Qin, Y.; Sun, X.; Ma, W.; Zou, Y.; Zhang, H.; Zhou, X.; et al. Value of a Machine Learning Approach for Predicting Clinical Outcomes in Young Patients With Hypertension. *Hypertension* **2020**, *75*, 1271–1278. [CrossRef]
90. Huan, T.; Meng, Q.; Saleh, M.A.; Norlander, A.E.; Joehanes, R.; Zhu, J.; Chen, B.H.; Zhang, B.; Johnson, A.D.; Ying, S.; et al. Integrative network analysis reveals molecular mechanisms of blood pressure regulation. *Mol. Syst. Biol.* **2015**, *11*, 799. [CrossRef]
91. Srivastava, P.; Srivastava, A.; Burande, A.; Khandelwal, A. A Note on Hypertension Classification Scheme and Soft Computing Decision Making System. *ISRN Biomath.* **2013**, *2013*, 342970. [CrossRef]
92. Rimoldi, S.F.; Scherrer, U.; Messerli, F.H. Secondary arterial hypertension: When, who, and how to screen? *Eur. Heart J.* **2014**, *35*, 1245–1254. [CrossRef]
93. Arar, M.Y.; Hogg, R.J.; Arant, B.S., Jr.; Seikaly, M.G. Etiology of sustained hypertension in children in the southwestern United States. *Pediatr. Nephrol.* **1994**, *8*, 186–189. [CrossRef]
94. Pedrosa, R.P.; Drager, L.F.; Gonzaga, C.C.; Sousa, M.G.; de Paula, L.K.; Amaro, A.C.; Amodeo, C.; Bortolotto, L.A.; Krieger, E.M.; Bradley, T.D.; et al. Obstructive sleep apnea: The most common secondary cause of hypertension associated with resistant hypertension. *Hypertension* **2011**, *58*, 811–817. [CrossRef]
95. Reel, P.S.; Reel, S.; van Kralingen, J.C.; Langton, K.; Lang, K.; Erlic, Z.; Larsen, C.K.; Amar, L.; Pamporaki, C.; Mulatero, P.; et al. Machine learning for classification of hypertension subtypes using multi-omics: A multi-centre, retrospective, data-driven study. *EBioMedicine* **2022**, *84*, 104276. [CrossRef]
96. Miller, D.D. Machine Intelligence in Cardiovascular Medicine. *Cardiol. Rev.* **2020**, *28*, 53–64. [CrossRef]
97. Chen, J.; Qian, L.; Urakov, T.; Gu, W.; Liang, L. Adversarial Robustness Study of Convolutional Neural Network for Lumbar Disk Shape Reconstruction from MR images. *SPIE Med. Imaging Image Process.* **2021**, *11596*, 1159615.
98. D'Angelo, G.; Della-Morte, D.; Pastore, D.; Donadel, G.; De Stefano, A.; Palmieri, F. Identifying patterns in multiple biomarkers to diagnose diabetic foot using an explainable genetic programming-based approach. *Future Gener. Comput. Syst.* **2023**, *140*, 138–150. [CrossRef]
99. Goldstein, A.; Kapelner, A.; Bleich, J.; Pitkin, E. Peeking inside the black box: Visualizing statistical learning with plots of individual conditional expectation. *J. Comput. Graph. Stat.* **2015**, *24*, 44–65. [CrossRef]
100. Petch, J.; Di, S.; Nelson, W. Opening the Black Box: The Promise and Limitations of Explainable Machine Learning in Cardiology. *Can. J. Cardiol.* **2022**, *38*, 204–213. [CrossRef]

101. Tat, E.; Bhatt, D.L.; Rabbat, M.G. Addressing bias: Artificial intelligence in cardiovascular medicine. *Lancet Digit. Health* **2020**, *2*, e635–e636. [CrossRef]
102. Krittanawong, C.; Bomback, A.S.; Baber, U.; Bangalore, S.; Messerli, F.H.; Wilson Tang, W.H. Future Direction for Using Artificial Intelligence to Predict and Manage Hypertension. *Curr. Hypertens. Rep.* **2018**, *20*, 75. [CrossRef]
103. Chen, S.; Ji, Z.; Wu, H.; Xu, Y. A Non-Invasive Continuous Blood Pressure Estimation Approach Based on Machine Learning. *Sensors* **2019**, *19*, 2585. [CrossRef]

Disclaimer/Publisher's Note: The statements, opinions and data contained in all publications are solely those of the individual author(s) and contributor(s) and not of MDPI and/or the editor(s). MDPI and/or the editor(s) disclaim responsibility for any injury to people or property resulting from any ideas, methods, instructions or products referred to in the content.

MDPI
St. Alban-Anlage 66
4052 Basel
Switzerland
www.mdpi.com

Journal of Cardiovascular Development and Disease Editorial Office
E-mail: jcdd@mdpi.com
www.mdpi.com/journal/jcdd

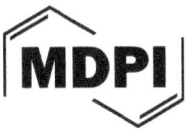

Disclaimer/Publisher's Note: The statements, opinions and data contained in all publications are solely those of the individual author(s) and contributor(s) and not of MDPI and/or the editor(s). MDPI and/or the editor(s) disclaim responsibility for any injury to people or property resulting from any ideas, methods, instructions or products referred to in the content.

www.ingramcontent.com/pod-product-compliance
Lightning Source LLC
LaVergne TN
LVHW070633100526
838202LV00012B/796